The Quality Improvement Challenge

The Quality Improvement Challenge

A Practical Guide for Physicians

Richard J. Banchs, MD

Associate Professor of Anesthesiology
Associate Head, Department of Anesthesiology
Director, Quality and Safety
University of Illinois Hospital and Health Sciences System
USA

Michael R. Pop, SSMBB, MBA

Director of Business Process Improvement
Omron Automation Americas
USA

WILEY Blackwell

Registered Office(s)
John Wiley & Sons, Inc., 111 River Street, Hoboken, NJ 07030, USA
John Wiley & Sons Ltd, The Atrium, Southern Gate, Chichester, West Sussex, PO19 8SQ, UK

Editorial Office
9600 Garsington Road, Oxford, OX4 2DQ, UK

For details of our global editorial offices, customer services, and more information about Wiley products visit us at www.wiley.com.

Wiley also publishes its books in a variety of electronic formats and by print-on-demand. Some content that appears in standard print versions of this book may not be available in other formats.

Library of Congress Cataloging-in-Publication Data

Names: Banchs, Richard J., author. | Pop, Michael R., author.
Title: The quality improvement challenge : a practical guide for physicians
 / Richard J. Banchs, Michael R. Pop.
Description: First edition. | Hoboken, NJ : Wiley-Blackwell, 2021. |
 Includes bibliographical references and index.
Identifiers: LCCN 2020039053 (print) | LCCN 2020039054 (ebook) | ISBN
 9781119698982 (paperback) | ISBN 9781119699002 (adobe PDF) | ISBN
 9781119699019 (epub)
Subjects: MESH: Quality Improvement | Physician's Role | Quality of Health
 Care–organization & administration
Classification: LCC R690 (print) | LCC R690 (ebook) | NLM WX 153 | DDC
 610.69/5–dc23
LC record available at https://lccn.loc.gov/2020039053
LC ebook record available at https://lccn.loc.gov/2020039054

Cover Design: Wiley
Cover Image: © Artur Debat/Getty Images

Set in 10.5/13pt STIXTwoText by SPi Global, Pondicherry, India

C9781119698982_290321

To Dr. David E. Schwartz, my Chair, who believed in me and supported me in my endeavors; to Alexander, Brandon, Kristian, and Luca, my kids, who patiently read my drafts and asked many thought-provoking questions; and to Sharon, my wife, who stands by me with every new adventure.

Richard J. Banchs, MD

To my beautiful wife, Lorelle, who continues to support me on my continuous improvement journey through life. She makes me a better man.

Michael R. Pop, SSMBB, MBA

Contents

Why This Book?

Efforts to improve the quality of healthcare have focused on increasing accountability, measurements, and new payment models. These and other efforts have failed to achieve a meaningful and sustainable improvement. Patients continue to experience fragmented, impersonal, inconvenient, and unsafe care while providers are increasingly becoming burned out by a system overburdened with administrative tasks. The current approach seems at odds with the mission of providing high-quality care. A fundamental change is needed in how we deliver care, and how we go about improving it.

It is widely accepted that physician leadership is an essential requirement for successful quality improvement efforts. Yet physicians have been reluctant to engage, either because of the constraints of their overbooked clinical schedules, their perception of QI, or because quality priorities are often set by outsiders rather than chosen by physicians based on their insights, experience, and expertise. As a result, physicians have been marginally involved in operational improvement, and for the most part, have relinquished that responsibility to managers and hospital administrators. A strategy for improving healthcare delivery that continues to ignore the engagement of physicians is doomed to fail. Physicians should lead improvement efforts: they are well positioned to accept the improvement challenge. They have valuable insights into processes, have been trained as problem-solvers, and making things better speaks to their intrinsic motivation. Their engagement is critical, will serve their patients well, and may be the new role physicians need to gain a sense of purpose, restore their identity, and decrease burnout.

This new role is going to require knowledge and skills that graduate and postgraduate education has not provided. To date, medical education has focused almost exclusively on the acquisition of scientific knowledge and clinical facts. This book has been written to fill this knowledge gap. Principles and practices of improvement methodology, team dynamics, and organizational change management are presented in a straightforward and clear way for any physician, young or seasoned, seeking a template for an improvement initiative. The material in this book synthesizes current knowledge on the subject from multiple authoritative sources and combines disciplines as diverse as Lean, Six Sigma, Human-Centered Design, and Neurosciences for organizational change. The goal is to provide the reader with an integrated and systematic approach to quality improvement projects and a roadmap to address the unique, change-resistant features associated with the healthcare environment. It is our hope that physicians everywhere will embark on an improvement journey, for the benefit of their patients, organizations, and themselves.

Richard J. Banchs, MD
Michael R. Pop, SSMBB, MBA

About the Authors

Richard J. Banchs, MD is a board-certified pediatric anesthesiologist. He is a Lean Six Sigma Black Belt and Change Management Experienced Practitioner. Since 2007 he has been combining his clinical responsibilities with improvement work. He has successfully used the improvement framework described in this book in the deployment of a broad variety of large- and small-scale projects in the US and abroad. These improvement initiatives have included QI projects in operating rooms, emergency departments, outpatient clinics, and inpatient units both in small hospitals and large academic centers with the goals of improving quality, performance, and patient and provider's satisfaction.

Dr. Banchs compiles his improvement knowledge and years of clinical experience in the front lines into a road map for healthcare practitioners to achieve success in their quality improvement projects. By being on both sides of the equation, he can offer a global perspective on the nature of improvement work and the best strategies to overcome the barriers to improvement in healthcare. In this book, he shares his knowledge and expertise with any physician wishing to successfully improve the practice of medicine.

Since 2013, Dr. Banchs has been teaching improvement methodology to staff, residents, and faculty at the University of Illinois Hospital in Chicago. He has served as the senior director of the Organizational Process Improvement (OPI) office, and is currently the Associate Head for Quality and Safety for the Department of Anesthesiology.

Michael R. Pop, SSMBB, MBA is a Lean Six Sigma Master Black Belt. He is an accomplished Quality Professional with 30 years of experience enhancing operations and leading teams through the implementation of effective solutions to permanently resolve quality issues. He is currently the director of Business Process Improvement for the Omron Automation Americas group. Prior to his current role, he was a senior consultant with Illinois Business Innovation Services spending the majority of his career providing Quality Systems Management, Lean, Six-Sigma, Quality Management, and Quality Engineering support to various industries, including diversified manufacturers, education, healthcare, government and not-for-profits.

He has assisted multiple hospitals and clinics in implementing Lean Six Sigma Operations and has coached and mentored numerous healthcare leaders in the use of Statistical Process Control techniques to improve both process and healthcare services. As a quality consultant, Mr. Pop has assisted numerous organizations with becoming registered to ISO 9001, a set of international standards on quality management and quality assurance. He has trained over 200 Lean Six Sigma Black Belts and 500+ Green Belt students, helping them implement effective, efficient, and cost-effective processes resulting in more than $20 million in savings for their organizations.

Michael R. Pop has a Master of Business Administration and a bachelor's degree in Mechanical Engineering Technology, both from Purdue University, and is a Certified Six Sigma Master Black Belt, Certified Quality Engineer, and a Certified Quality Auditor. He is currently a senior member of the American Society for Quality (ASQ).

List of Stories, Examples, Exercises and Case Studies

Stories from the Front Lines of Healthcare
- Martha Sanchez, the Head of Housekeeping (Chapter 4)
- Turn-Around Time for X-rays in the ED (Chapter 5)
- Andrea, the QI Project Manager (Chapter 10)
- Wait Time in the Orthopedic Outpatient Clinic (Chapter 18)
- The Early Discharge QI Project at Memorial Hospital (Chapter 23)
- The NICU Team at St. Agnes Hospital (Chapter 25)
- Brandon, the Ambulatory Clinic manager (Chapter 26)
- "Make It Happen" (Chapter 29)

Examples
- First-Case On-Time-Start Accuracy at Fond-du-Lac Medical Center (Chapter 4)
- Patient Arrival-to-Departure Time at the PCP Clinic (Chapter 4)
- A SIPOC diagram for St. Barnabas Preoperative Evaluation Clinic (Chapter 7)
- The "Customer" of a STAT Arterial Blood Gas (ABG) (Chapter 8)
- Supply Chain Management for Patient Care Units (Chapter 8)
- Patient Satisfaction with UI Health Outpatient Care Center (Chapter 8)
- Improving the Organization of Medical Supplies in the EDRR (Chapter 8)
- Improving MRI Patient Throughput (Chapter 9)
- Improving STAT Chest X-Rays in the ICU (Chapter 12)
- Temperature Management on Arrival to the ED (Chapter 13)
- Stratification Factors for "Time from Order to Arrival of TPN Bag" (Chapter 13)
- Order-to-Result Time at Mercy Hospital (Chapter 15)
- Narcotic Discrepancies at Chicago Med (Chapter 15)
- C-section Rate at London Memorial (Chapter 15)
- The Individuals and Moving Range (I-mR) Chart of a Patient's SBP (Chapter 16)
- Door-to-Infusion Time at Huron Medical Center (Chapter 16)
- Improving DVT Prophylaxis (Chapter 17)
- Medication Error before Initiating CPB (Chapter 18)
- Patient Satisfaction with the ED Visit (Chapter 18)

Exercises

- A Problem Statement and Project Charter for Your QI project (Chapter 4)
- The QI team at Heart Medical Center (Chapter 6)
- CTQs for the New Women's Center (Chapter 8)
- Mapping "Ordering Blood from the Blood Bank" (Chapter 10)
- Identifying "Waste" in the Pediatric Unit (Chapter 11)
- In-training Examination at Mass General Hospital (Chapter 18)

Case Studies

- Improving RTA Time at St. Michaels Hospital (Chapter 14)
- Door-to-Infusion Time at Huron Medical Center (Chapter 16)
- The New Balloon Angioplasty Catheter at UIC (Chapter 17)
- Decreasing Unplanned Readmissions after Tonsillectomy (Chapter 20)

About the Companion Website

This book is accompanied by a companion website:

www.wiley.com/go/banchs/quality

The website includes:

Powerpoints of supplementary material of project templates and forms.

Scan this QR code to visit the companion website.

PART I

THE BASICS

CHAPTER 1

The Problem with Healthcare

SO, WHAT'S THE PROBLEM?

In the last 20 years, science has made a number of transformational changes that have impacted the way we think about healthcare. Targeted cancer therapy, drug-eluting cardiac stents, 3D printing, and the human genome project are but a few of the advances that have revolutionized medicine. Yet how we deliver care and the healthcare experience have not improved at the same rate. Despite significant efforts, regulatory mandates, and the sacrifice of many in the front line we have not achieved our goals of providing safe, efficient, and cost-effective care for all. Standards and benchmarks often lag or fail to be followed, best-practices have been slow to spread, and quality differences have persisted among providers and geographic areas. These accounts, coupled with highly publicized medical malpractice litigation, have eroded patients' trust in the healthcare system.

The current crisis isn't new. It has evolved over the last 30 years to the current level of intensity that we now face and can no longer ignore. Reports including the Institute of Medicine's "To Err Is Human" (Kohn 2000), "Crossing the Quality Chasm" (IOM 2001), and "Transforming Healthcare: A Safety Imperative" (Leape 2009) have highlighted the inability of the healthcare system to reliably provide safe, high quality, cost-effective patient care. The crisis has deepened by rising expectations of patients who are accustomed to a retail setting, where services are customer-driven, efficient, and accessible 24/7 through mobile connectivity, and are demanding the same from healthcare. A true "patient-to-consumer revolution" (Wyman 2014) is demanding

The Quality Improvement Challenge: A Practical Guide for Physicians, First Edition.
Richard J. Banchs and Michael R. Pop.
© 2021 John Wiley & Sons Ltd. Published 2021 by John Wiley & Sons Ltd.
Companion website: www.wiley.com/go/banchs/quality

increased access, service, personalization, and speed from a healthcare system that is slow, inconvenient, confusing and difficult to navigate. Competition among healthcare organizations is no longer based solely on reputation, but on service, value, and price.

In this environment, healthcare organizations face a significant pressure to provide high-quality, state-of-the-art patient care while lowering costs and improving patients' care experiences. These demands exist in the context of heightened accreditation requirements, uncertain governmental mandates, decreasing reimbursement, and overwhelmed clinicians and administrators. The negative results are experienced by both patients and healthcare professionals.

HOW DID WE GET HERE?

Many factors have contributed to the current state of affairs and the inability of healthcare to reliably deliver safe, high-quality, cost-effective patient care. Worth mentioning is an out-of-date business model, healthcare's organizations' inefficient organizational structure, the traditional quality paradigm, and an ineffective physician compensation model.

- **The business model.** Healthcare organizations have been anchored in a business model that may have been successful in the past but has outlasted the circumstances that created the need for it. Despite the needs of the current marketplace, healthcare organizations have continued to focus on providing a full spectrum of healthcare services, that is, all services to all patients. Clayton Christensen in his book *The Innovator's Prescription* (Christensen 2009) describes two types of business models that any organization can follow: a **solution shop,** where a healthcare organization focuses on diagnostic activities, and a **value-adding process** where the focus is on the efficient delivery of care and specific treatments. Christensen argues that these two models are different, and they require different resources, processes, organizational structures, and profit models. With the current technological and scientific progress, healthcare challenges, and diversity of needs, trying to provide all services to all patients is the wrong value proposition. The combination of these two models under one roof creates a system that requires an enormous amount of resources, and results in inefficiencies, waste, and duplication of efforts. It creates a system that functions, as Michael Porter describes, as a "confederation of stand-alone units that replicate services" (Porter 2016). For every dollar spent, a reported 30 cents are wasted in steps that do not add value, the result of excessive bureaucracy, defensive medicine, and duplication of services.
- **Organizational structure.** Healthcare organizations have customarily been organized according to clinical specialties. While this originally arose from the need to maintain the competency of clinicians to deliver high-quality care, this structure has created **clinical silos** that have resulted in fragmented care and dysfuntional workflow across the healthcare organization. Rather

than organizing care around specialty departments and special services, care should be organized around medical conditions with multiple subspecialties and teams converging on the specific patient condition. In the current system, effective synchronization, collaboration, and communication are often not present and are more often than not the cause of rework, mistakes, complications, and wasteful spending.

- **The quality paradigm.** In the **traditional quality paradigm**, quality was defined by the provider and by the effectiveness of care. In this view, quality is achieved when the right treatment is administered in response to a specific recognizable pattern, and results in the elimination of the disease condition. This long-held view of quality ignored additional dimensions of quality care, such as the need for efficiency, timeliness, and patient-centeredness (IOM 2001). Focusing only on effective care resulted in a healthcare experience that fell short of patients' expectations. The traditional quality paradigm, a lack of oversight, and the inability of physicians to regulate their own profession has had a significant impact on the quality of care. As a result, we have seen unethical practices, high rates of patient injuries, and injustices in the ability to access care (Berwick 2016).

- **The physician compensation model.** Incentives for payment have been completely misaligned with the goals of improving the quality of care. Providers and healthcare organizations have been paid for number of procedures performed (volume-driven payment) rather than for the outcome and quality of care (value-driven payment). This has resulted in excessive and unnecessary procedures, overly used diagnostic services, increased insurance premiums, and procedure-related complications.

THE CHALLENGES TO IMPROVE HEALTHCARE

Efforts to improve the quality of care have focused on performance metrics, complex incentive formulas, and increased scrutiny from regulatory agencies. These and other measures have not addressed the real problem and, for the most part, have not significantly improved the quality of care. Patients continue to be disappointed with the healthcare experience, and staff and providers are getting increasingly burned out from the overwhelming day-to-day administrative burden. There is a generalized frustration among providers working in a system that is inefficient, overcomplicated, and seemingly at odds with the mission of providing high-quality care. Despite significant efforts to improve, we have not achieved our goals. Accountability based on metrics developed by outsiders has failed to engage physicians, and too much of the efforts of healthcare organizations is spent on submitting reports, preparing for accreditation surveys, and ensuring adherence to regulatory mandates. Meeting the objectives of specific organizational metrics has become an all-consuming activity, rather than developing a strategic and comprehensive improvement agenda. There is no question that the work involved to ensure survey readiness and regulation compliance is important, but too much effort is directed at achieving core measure targets and not enough on system redesign. By prioritizing improvement initiatives that address the underlying processes related to the regulatory compliance and core measure targets, we could address both regulatory mandates and improve the health-care experience.

> **Quotable quote: *"We are faced with a series of great opportunities bril-liantly disguised as insoluble problems." John W Gardner***

Healthcare organizations continue to invest resources to improve the delivery of care but face unique challenges that impact the effectiveness of the improvement efforts they pursue. Process improvement is not easy, and it requires a clear understanding of the barriers:

- **The culture.** The primary role of a healthcare organization is to provide care to patients, a high-stakes undertaking that may exacerbate patients' clinical con-ditions if errors occur. As a result, healthcare professionals are risk averse, con-servative, and hesitant to try new things compared to other industries. When quality improvement (QI) teams and organizations try to implement changes, they often encounter a resistant culture that labors to maintain the status quo. Incongruously, providers and staff often resist the adoption of standards and other evidence-based guidelines that support improved patient outcomes in favor of time-honored, and sometimes outdated, traditional approaches to patient care.

- **Silos.** Improvement initiatives are difficult in healthcare organizations unac-customed to leveraging teamwork across silos to accomplish their goals. Silos not only exist within the clinical specialties but also exist between the clinical and the operational areas in healthcare organizations. These silos often cut from the top of the organization down to the front line staff members. They impact the effectiveness of any improvement initiative, ultimately leading to a fragmented operational approach that focuses only on individual tasks and departments without considering the entire patient experience. Coordination and collaboration give way to "suboptimization," where every unit pursues its own "targets" independent of the needs and aims of the organization as a whole.

- **A lack of IT support.** Improvement initiatives depend on and should be guided by data. But QI teams often find it difficult to get their basic needs ful-filled, having to allocate additional team resources, or rely on manual data col-lection to obtain the data they need. It is difficult to understand why staff and providers have to struggle to get a report of the same data they just entered into the hospital's electronic medical record.

- **A lack of active participation of senior hospital leaders.** The role of the leader is to legitimize improvement projects and facilitate the work of the improvement team. The leader establishes priorities for competing initiatives;

provides resources for the team; resolves cross-functional issues, and removes roadblocks that impede the success of the project. Senior leaders in healthcare are often not visible, active, or engaged in QI projects. When leaders are not present, projects flounder, have difficulty reaching their objectives, and often fail. Leaders are vital in building a coalition of key sponsors to achieve project success and facilitating change.

- **A lack of improvement experience.** Healthcare professionals often lack the experience and formal training needed to address the complex performance problems of the healthcare delivery system. Postgraduate healthcare education continues to be almost exclusively focused on the acquisition of scientific and clinical facts, and has not included the knowledge and skills that define competency in improvement work. QI competency needs to be developed with rigor, heightened focus, and consistency like any other discipline. Because they lack experience, often staff and providers rely on their subject-matter expertise to complete a QI project. They fail to follow the required structured systematic approach and cannot achieve the goals of the improvement initiative. Improvement knowledge does not come as a natural evolution of clinical expertise. Improvement capability is not a natural ability!

- **The team dynamics.** QI teams in healthcare are often multidisciplinary in nature and are convened in an ad-hoc manner, from different areas or departments. There is usually very little time to ensure cohesive functioning of the team members to avoid "silo" mentality. Physicians, nurses, staff, and administrators are brought together and expected to work as a team, even if they have never done so in the clinical arena.

- **A top-down approach to improvement.** With multiple competing clinical priorities, improvement projects are often left in the hands of leaders and small teams of specialized subject-matter experts (SMEs). This traditional model is no longer effective and cannot achieve the operational improvements in the large scale that are needed in today's healthcare organizations. Engagement of the front line is critical to succeed and, yet, is not always present. This traditional approach to QI perpetuates the belief that *process improvement is the responsibility of a small number of individuals in the organization and it does not have the same critical nature as the "clinical side" of care.* Even when the front line is engaged, organizations don't provide sufficient time, resources, or support. It becomes challenging to convene regular meetings with key stakeholders who must juggle their clinical and nonclinical responsibilities with project activities.

- **Lack of a robust change management strategy.** There is often more focus on the technical or clinical aspects of the problem than on how the solution will be received by the front line. It is important to remember that *all improvement is a change, and change is going to have a significant effect on the professionals in the front line.* Change management is often an afterthought, with the main focus being on designing, testing, and deploying the solution that addresses the needs of the project. Managing the effects of change is often reactive, and implemented without a clear plan. Communication and engagement with the front lines is not given sufficient emphasis leaving the project team unable to implement the much-needed solution.

- **Too many competing initiatives.** In healthcare, there are too many competing initiatives that result in **improvement fatigue.** Healthcare providers face a constant barrage of mandates to change practice from external stakeholders, including accrediting organizations, regulatory bodies, third-party payers, and professional associations. Front lines often become overwhelmed by the number of changes that occur in their work routines. There is a lack of leadership with proper selection, stratification, and improvement focus at the front line.

- **Excessive focus on the methodology rather than the improvement opportunity.** In the late 1980s, healthcare organizations began incorporating industrial quality-management methodologies including Lean, Six Sigma, and Lean Six Sigma in their strategies to improve delivery of care. The Lean Six Sigma approach attempts to address the non-value-added activities, inefficient workflows, and disorganized work environments that interfere with clinicians' ability to provide safe, high-quality patient care. It merges the customer-orientation and waste-reduction techniques of Lean (time-driven focus) with the more statistical and data-driven systematic error reduction strategies of Six Sigma (quality-driven focus). When implemented as an overarching management system and organizational philosophy, Lean Six Sigma process improvement methodology has been shown to improve patients' experience, staff and providers' work environment, and the quality of patient care (Nicolay 2012). Not all QI projects have been successful using Lean Six Sigma. Some teams have had disappointing results. For these teams, Lean Six Sigma lacked some of the critical elements they needed for success. When applied to medicine, industrial quality management methodologies have several problems:

  o Heavy use of technical and business terminology. These improvement methodologies are derived from the manufacturing sector and often carry with them an overemphasis on improvement jargon that seems complex, counterintuitive, and far removed from the clinician's front line.

  o Improvement is often carried out by small teams of certified Lean Six Sigma practitioners who make up their own distinct department. These SMEs lead improvement efforts in a "top-down" approach but often fail to create the conditions for the front line stakeholders to engage. Changes are pushed through without the front line professionals' involvement in developing, revising, or monitoring the performance of key processes.

Physicians have a limited understanding of these improvement methodologies and in general regard them as something outside of the scope of medicine, showing little interest in learning them. Most industries make great products with average employees working with brilliant processes. *Healthcare does great work with brilliant employees working with mediocre processes.*

WHAT IS THE PHYSICIAN'S ROLE IN PROCESS IMPROVEMENT?

It is widely accepted that physician engagement is an essential requirement for any successful quality improvement project, and yet we have not seen the full engagement of clinicians. Physicians have a pivotal role within the organization. However, they are often not involved in healthcare organization improvement efforts, either because of the constraints of their overbooked clinical schedules or because of the perception that they are not directly responsible for the improvement of the operational aspects of delivering care.

Physicians express a strong support for QI projects, but often have a different view of what this entails. Although this is probably not you (the reader!), physicians in general

- View improvement projects as taking time away from patient care, interfering with their schedule, and adding complexity to their workflow, even when that very workflow is the cause of the problem. This unfavorable view of QI projects is further perpetuated when their improvement efforts are not recognized with professional advancement or other incentives.
- Are often reluctant to participate in QI projects because they believe the improvement initiative will be ineffective.
- View quality assessment as an integral element of the practice of medicine and resist any improvement initiative that challenges this view.
- View clinical guidelines and pathways as hampering individual provider's freedom.
- Have a lack of expertise in project management, team dynamics, and communication.

Physicians have historically been responsible for the quality of clinical care by virtue of their credentials. This has resulted in their implicit expectation that the burden of operational improvement should be left to staff and hospital administration, a tenet described by Kornacki as "The Physician Compact" (Kornacki 2012): *"The Physician Compact is an implicit psychological contract that defines the actions physicians believe are expected of them and the response they expect in return from their employers."*

According to this compact, physicians believe their role is to treat patients, provide quality care (as defined by the physician), advance research, and support medical education. In return, they expect to be given clinical autonomy, protection from market forces, and the resources needed to resolve operational problems. In contrast, hospitals and healthcare organization need standardization, improved efficiencies, lower costs, and physician engagement in operational challenges. There is an internal incongruence between physicians' expectations and hospital needs that results in resentment, misunderstandings, and a lack of physician engagement in operational improvement (Kornacki 2015). Efficiency and standardization are often perceived by physicians as a restriction to their ability to integrate their knowledge, experience, and assessment skills in their clinical practice. Ironically, it is often the physicians who initially identify processes that are dysfunctional and are open to becoming engaged in "their project" when there is adequate facilitation and coordination by another staff member.

REFERENCES

1. Berwick D. (2016). Era 3 for medicine and health care. *JAMA* 315: 13.
2. Christensen Cl. (2009). *The Innovator's Prescription*. McGraw Hill.
3. Institute of Medicine. (2001). *Crossing the Quality Chasm: A New Health System for the 21st Century*. National Academy Press, March.
4. Kohn LT. (2000). *To Err Is Human: Building a Safer Health System. Institute of Medicine Committee on Quality of Health Care in America*. National Academies Press.
5. Kornacki MJ. (2015). *A New Compact: Aligning Physicians and Organization Expectations to Transform Patient Care*. Health Administration Press.
6. Kornacki MJ. (2012). *Leading Physicians through Change*. ACPE.
7. Leape L. (2009). Transforming healthcare: a safety imperative. *Qual Saf Health Care* 18: 424–428.
8. Nicolay CR. (2012). Systematic Review of the application of quality improvement methodologies from the manufacturing industry to surgical healthcare. *British Journal of Surgery* 99: 324–335.
9. Porter M. (2016). *The Future Perioperative Physician: Leaders in Value Based Health Care Delivery*. Keynote Speaker. ASA Annual Meeting. Chicago.
10. Wyman O. (2014). *The Patient to Consumer Revolution. How High Tech, Transparent Marketplaces, and Consumer Power Are Transforming US Healthcare*. Health and Life Sciences.

CHAPTER 2

We Need to Improve the Way We Improve

WHAT'S THE GOAL OF A QI PROJECT?

First, Define Quality

The goal of healthcare is to provide quality care. The traditional quality paradigm was centered on the provider's point of view and the notion that quality care was **effective care**. But expectations have changed, and the paradigm has evolved to one centered on the patient's perspective, which includes not only the treatment but the healthcare experience. Quality is no longer just "effective" care. Quality is now defined as much by the therapeutic intervention as by how we meet patients' expectations. In 2001, the Institute of Medicine defined quality along six dimensions: **effective, efficient, timely, safe, patient-centered,** and **equitable** (IOM 2001). In this new paradigm, assessing quality requires us to evaluate "what" was provided i.e. effective and safe care, as well as "how" it was provided, i.e. efficient, timely, culturally sensitive, and equitable care (see Figure 2-1).

Patients remain at the center of our delivery system because they are the reason healthcare organizations exist. Clinicians provide care to patients and expert services to other providers. Leaders and ancillary staff support the providers' clinical practice within a complex, multidimensional system. Together, their efforts yield the patient's outcomes and experiences. Our aim is to provide care that is effective in addressing the disease process, and is delivered in an efficient, timely, safe, patient-centered, and equitable manner. This paradigm shift has redefined not only quality but the role of the healthcare provider. It is no longer sufficient to provide treatment for a patient's

The Quality Improvement Challenge: A Practical Guide for Physicians, First Edition.
Richard J. Banchs and Michael R. Pop.
© 2021 John Wiley & Sons Ltd. Published 2021 by John Wiley & Sons Ltd.
Companion website: www.wiley.com/go/banchs/quality

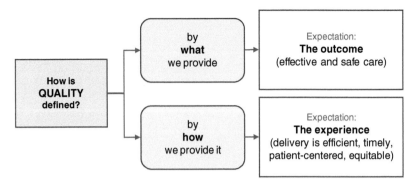

FIGURE 2-1　The new quality paradigm.

clinical condition; we must also improve the quality of the healthcare delivery system to address patients' expectations of the holistic care experience.

Then, Define Improvement

Improving the quality care for our patients cannot be achieved just by increasing resources and cost in a wasteful manner. Improvement is centered on **value**. There are numerous definitions of value. For now, let's consider value as the **outcomes achieved (therapeutic intervention + patient experience), divided by resources used in achieving the outcomes**. To improve, we need to focus on achieving quality care while optimizing the quantity of resources such as time, personnel, and money consumed in working to achieve it (see Figure 2-2).

Quotable quote: "The biggest room is the room for improvement."
Chinese proverb

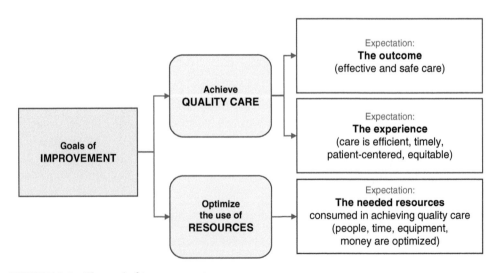

FIGURE 2-2　The goal of improvement.

A BETTER IMPROVEMENT STRATEGY

The identified barriers and characteristics of currently used improvement practices have contributed in part to failed improvement projects and frustrated healthcare leaders and clinicians. Healthcare is a complex and dynamic system, and the pressure of the current healthcare marketplace requires "organic and continuous improvement initiated and sustained at all levels and areas of the organization" (Pennington 2017). We need to move beyond the small, dedicated teams of subject-matter experts that lead and support specific priority initiatives. Healthcare professionals throughout the organization need to acquire the knowledge, behaviors, and skills that define competency in quality improvement work, and become the drivers of the healthcare transformation. Improvement needs to be embedded in the DNA of healthcare organizations. Rather than imposed from the "top-down," improvement must come from the "bottom-up," inspired by a vision that enlists professionals in a common cause. "Top-down" and "bottom-up" approaches have to converge.

> **Improvement needs a problem-solving approach that engages frontline professionals in creating solutions through a focus on the needs and values of the patients the solutions will serve, and the staff and providers who will deliver them.**

Frontline professionals will need to be involved in all aspects of QI. Their engagement is critical to develop, revise, and monitor the performance of core care processes. Engagement of the frontline professionals depends on three enablers:

1. **Engaged leadership.** Leaders need to be actively engaged in creating an improvement agenda and providing the needed resources. Leaders are key in assuring the success of a QI project. They provide guidance, resources, and can be instrumental in creating a network of middle-level leaders to support the changes. Successful improvement initiatives must rely on the collective efforts of all leaders, both clinical and operational.
2. **Shared knowledge.** Improvement competency needs to be supported and shared throughout the organization. For a healthcare organization to be successful with its improvement agenda, a large portion of the front line must be trained in the knowledge and skills that define improvement competency. Improvement knowledge needs to be **democratized.** Improvement capability cannot just be in the hands of a small team of experts while the front line lacks the skillset to successfully complete a QI project. Outsourcing process improvement expertise (i.e., hiring a consultant) cannot be the only solution. Relying solely on expert consultants often results in short-lived success and considerable expense. *Investing in human capital and broadening the base of improvement experts within an organization is a more cost-effective and permanent*

strategy. To that end, educating healthcare providers and staff to become the future leaders of improvement initiatives keeps the path moving toward an improved healthcare delivery system.

3. **Physician driven.** Physicians need to look at the practice of medicine through a new paradigm: knowledge of **patient processes** – how diseases affect physiology – is as important as the knowledge of **system processes** – how the system and its components affect the delivery of care. While therapeutic interventions improve the health of our patients, redesigning processes improves the health of the system in which care is delivered. Physicians need to be engaged and drive the improvement and change management initiatives. They have a pivotal role and are the linchpin that drives the success of improvement efforts. Today's physicians have two roles: *deliver outstanding clinical care and improve the quality of the healthcare delivery system.*

GUIDING PRINCIPLES

These five guiding principles are the values that establish our framework for all improvement efforts in the healthcare environment:

1. **Problems need to be approached using the lens of the customer.** To understand a problem, we need to see the problem from the lens of the people who experience them; we need to "walk" in their shoes, understand their issues, and be willing to address their needs. Improvement is only realized when we place the end user's needs and experiences at the heart of the process. Value is created by focusing the efforts of staff and providers on the needs and expectations of the patient or the end user. End users are the experts of their own experience, and are central to the process of creating a solution that delivers on their expectations.

2. **Consider the people who deliver care as the key to the solution.** The people who deliver care and experience the problems of the system are the key; we need to bring them along in the improvement process because they are the ones who understand the system and hold the key to the solution. Healthcare professionals see and understand the challenges our patients face. Their understanding of the process and proximity to the patients makes them uniquely suited to identify and deliver potential solutions that can improve the healthcare experience. To improve, we must engage providers and staff. They have a pivotal role and are the linchpin that makes possible the success of the improvement efforts. Front line stakeholders have valuable insights into their processes and the barriers they face in delivering high-quality patient care, but they often have minimal opportunity to share that proficiency in modifying their workflows. In most organizations, there is an enormous reservoir of "energy, ideas, and engagement that is never tapped into because of

management practices that reduce intrinsic motivation and hinder joy and creativity in work" (Rena Awdish 2018).

3. **Be willing to try, fail, and try again.** Improvement in healthcare is complicated. Improvement is an imperfect process that requires our willingness to design and test solutions, and when they fail, to learn from our mistakes. In a risk-averse culture such as healthcare, improvement is difficult. We just need to make sure that our failures do not harm our patients. Engaging in the right kind of testing produces the right kind of failures from which we can learn.

Quotable quote: "Fall seven times. Stand up eight." Japanese proverb

4. **To improve, sometimes we must think "out of the box."** The traditional formula of continuous incremental improvements sometimes delivers disappointing results when it comes to the operational side of healthcare. We may not achieve the dramatic results we expected, largely because we may have been trying to improve the "old way" of doing things. Sometimes we have to stop focusing on improving what appears to be outdated models that were successful in the past but have outlasted the circumstances that created the need for them. For these processes, improvements cannot address what is fundamentally wrong with them. They have underlying deficiencies in their conceptualization, structure, job design, workflows, and control mechanisms because they were designed to address the needs of a different time. Improvement cannot succeed when it relies on an obsolete paradigm. When this is the case, we must redesign our processes using our knowledge, and a clear understanding of the needs of our patients.

5. **Consider all improvement a change.** All improvement is a change, and change is always met with varying degrees of resistance. For change to occur, QI teams must create a space where growth can develop, giving the frontline professionals the opportunity to understand the problem, discuss barriers to success, and engage in the co-creation and implementation of solutions. The effectiveness of our improvement effort results not only from the quality of the solution but also from the engagement and buy-in of the frontline professionals. If staff and providers do not accept the change, it is very unlikely that improvement will succeed. We must understand what drives change at the front line, and then design strategies to overcome the natural resistance that so often derails our improvements efforts. Change cannot succeed without the commitment of the people that it will affect.

THE FIVE "RS" OF EVERY QI PROJECT

All projects need a structured approach that moves through several distinctive phases. To achieve the goals of any QI project, an improvement team needs to successfully transition through five phases (see Figure 2-3). These phases define a logical flow to problem solving that starts with understanding the problem and continue through dissecting the process to identify root causes of defects and breakdowns, and creating solutions that address the needs of the people that experience the problem.

Each phase follows the **Project Roadmap,** drawing from a set of steps and tools to help reach the final destination (see Figure 2-4).

The first "R": The Right Project. First, identify project opportunities. Once you have selected your project, ask yourself: Is this the right project? Is this project feasible? Can the project goals be achieved? Confirm feasibility, jot down some ideas, and write the first draft of your Problem Statement. Then create your Project Charter. The Problem Statement and Project Charter will help you and your team focus on the right project.

The second "R": The Right People. All projects must have the "right people on the bus" (Bossidy 2002). Projects need a senior leader (primary sponsor) to legitimize the project, provide resources, and resolve cross-functional issues. The primary sponsor must be present and active throughout the lifecycle of the project. Project teams need a competent leader and team members from the front line with subject-matter expertise and the appropriate mix of skills.

The third "R": The Right Problem. We must "walk in the shoes" of the customers or end users to understand the problem; learn about their experiences and understand their expectations. Collect the voice of the people that "do the work." Understand their needs. What are their challenges? What barriers prevent them from meeting the customers' expectations? Summarize the resulting insights into a clear explanation of the problem you are trying to address. This phase will help your team focus on the right issues.

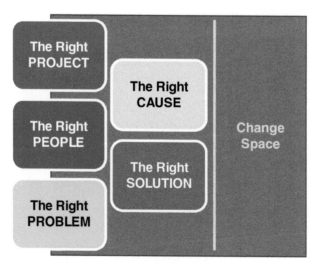

FIGURE 2-3   The five "Rs" of all successful QI projects.

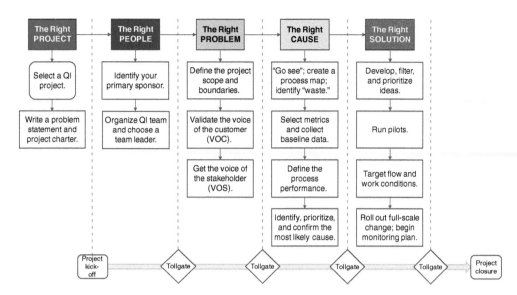

FIGURE 2-4   The Project Roadmap.

The fourth "R": The Right Cause. The first step in finding the cause is to "go see." Understand how work is really done. "Walk the process" to identify areas of improvement. Eliminate waste where you can see it. Once you understand the process, select the measurements that matter. Define your metrics and collect baseline data. What is our baseline performance? Can we meet our customers' needs? Are we meeting our customers' needs? How often are we meeting these needs? Organize and stratify your data and use your process knowledge to discover the most likely cause of the problem. Then test your assumptions and confirm the cause-and-effect relationship.

The fifth "R": The Right Solution. Use tools to energize your creative thinking. Generate a list of improvement ideas. Evaluate your options and prioritize the best solution. Create low-fidelity mock-ups and work with the end users and frontline stakeholders to test your ideas. Make this process iterative. Modify and refine the original idea as needed by uncovering performance gaps that need to be addressed. Learn from your testing. Once you have a winner, roll it out with the support of the key stakeholder who will be implementing it over the long term.

These five phases may be iterative and overlapping, require the completion of several steps, and end with project deliverables as shown on the **Project Checklist** (See Table 2-1). Starting after the second phase and continuing throughout the project, the QI team should meet with the Primary Sponsor for a **tollgate review** (see Chapter 24). A tollgate review is a go/no-go decision point where project activities and deliverables are reviewed to assure that the project is on track. Likewise, after each step, the QI team should plan for **communication** with the frontline stakeholders. Effective communication is a critical aspect of any quality improvement project and is recognized as a key component of behavior change in any change management effort (see Chapter 25).

TABLE 2-1 THE QI PROJECT STEPS CHECKLIST

Project Steps	
Phase	**Steps**
The Right Project	• Identify **project opportunities** (Chapter 3)
	• Assess & confirm **project feasibility** (Chapter 3)
	• Write a **Problem Statement** (Chapter 4)
	• Create a draft of your **Project Charter** (Chapter 4)
The Right People	• Identify your **Primary Sponsor** (Chapter 5)
	• Organize a **QI team** and choose a **team leader** (Chapter 6)
Complete first tollgate review (chapter 24); Communicate with front line (Chapter 25)	
The Right Problem	• Set a "kickⴙoff" date and launch the project
	• Define the **scope and boundaries** of the project (Chapter 7)
	• Validate the **Voice of the Customer** (Chapter 8)
	• Get the **Voice of the Stakeholder** (Chapter 9)
	• Complete the final draft of your **project charter**
Complete second tollgate review (Chapter 24); communicate with front line (Chapter 25)	
The Right Cause	• Go see at the **"gemba"** and create a **Process Map** (Chapter 10)
	• Quick wins: identify and eliminate **"waste"** (Chapter 11)
	• Measure what matters: select key **project metrics** (Chapter 12)
	• Plan data collection and collect **baseline data** (Chapter 13)
	• Define **baseline process performance** (Chapters 14–17)
	• Identify and prioritize the most likely **cause** (Chapter 18)
	• Confirm the **cause & effect** relationship (Chapter 19)
Complete third tollgate review (Chapter 24); Communicate with front line (Chapter 25)	

(Continued)

TABLE 2-1 (CONTINUED)

Project Steps	
Phase	**Steps**
The Right Solution	• Develop, filter, and prioritize **improvement ideas** (Chapter 20)
	• Test the effectiveness of your ideas with a **pilot** (Chapter 21)
	• Target and improve **flow** and **work conditions** (Chapter 22)
	• Create an **implementation plan** (Chapter 23)
	• Roll out the **full-scale** change(s) (Chapter 23)
	• Create and begin **monitoring plan** (Chapter 23)
Complete fourth tollgate review (Chapter 24); Project Closure (Chapter 23)	

THE CHANGE SPACE

A QI project is always a change project. Change rolled out "top down" often fails because it is rarely embraced, and results in doubt, pushback, and even open resistance. To be embraced, change must be **socially constructed** (Hamel 2016). Successful change requires an engaged front line. Engagement

- happens when the front line is given the opportunity to be involved in the improvement process, and;
- requires participation in the search for causes and the creation of possible solutions.

Quotable quote: "In times of change the learners will inherit the earth, while the knowers will find themselves beautifully equipped to deal with a world that no longer exists." Eric Hoffer

Frontline professionals must share responsibility for change needs. All successful projects need a change space, or framework, that engages frontline professionals in a shared vision of the problem and the co-creation of solutions. The role of the improvement team is not to find solutions and implement changes but to create the conditions and provide the tools that enable the front line to find solutions.

REFERENCES

1. Awdish R. (2018). *Keynote Speaker.* Institute for Healthcare Improvement National Forum.

2. Bossidy L. (2002). *Execution: the discipline of getting things done.* Random House.

3. Hamel G. (2016). *Build a change platform, not a change program.* McKinsey & Company.

4. Pennington R. (2017). The Pennington Group. www.penningtongroup.com.

PART II

THE FIRST "R": THE RIGHT PROJECT

CHAPTER 3

The Project Selection Process

WHERE DO I START?

Ask the Right Questions

Improvement projects are launched to address patients' expectations for quality and service; frontline staff and providers' workflow issues; a department's strategic initiatives; or disappointing performance and undesirable outcomes. If you clearly know what problem you are going to address, then you are ready to move to the next steps. But if you are not sure where to focus your efforts, start with the right questions.

Scan the environment, listen to people, and observe the work environment around you. Start by asking yourself these four questions:

1. **What is important to my patients**? What are their needs and expectations? What do they want from the care we provide? Where does our performance fall short?
2. **What are the needs of providers and staff?** What do they need to succeed? What are their challenges? What are their "pain points"?
3. **What is my area struggling with?** What are the issues affecting us (unit or department)? What are the strategic initiatives planned for this year? Where do we fall short in our performance?

The Quality Improvement Challenge: A Practical Guide for Physicians, First Edition.
Richard J. Banchs and Michael R. Pop.
© 2021 John Wiley & Sons Ltd. Published 2021 by John Wiley & Sons Ltd.
Companion website: www.wiley.com/go/banchs/quality

4. **What is my hospital struggling with?** What are some of the hospital's strategic initiatives, and how do these translate to my daily work? What issues affect our hospital (healthcare organization)?

The answer to these and other questions may give you an insight into what improvements are most urgently needed. Sometimes a quality improvement (QI) project idea may come from your **own daily experience**. What are you struggling with? What are the challenges and barriers that prevent you from doing your work? What can be improved in your work environment?

Your personal experience, the needs of your patients, and challenges of the frontline staff and providers are all sources of project ideas. If you are a healthcare leader, all ideas should be considered: top-down from supervisors and leaders and bottom-up from providers and frontline staff. Anyone should be able to suggest an improvement idea. Timely, constructive feedback should be provided by leaders to those who forward an improvement idea, regardless of the final decision to move ahead with a QI project.

Consider the Three "Voices" for Project Ideas

In general, project ideas come from three sources. We call them the **voices**. They are the "Voice of the Customer," the "Voice of the Stakeholder," and the "Voice of the Process" (see Figure 3-1).

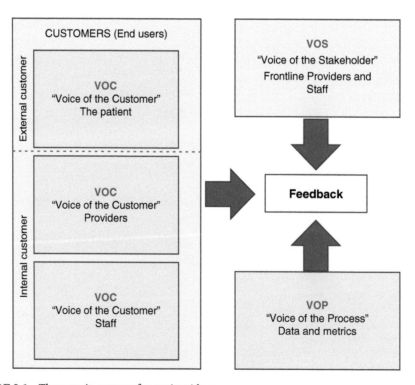

FIGURE 3-1   Three main sources for project ideas.

The Voice of the Customer (VOC)

The VOC is the expression of the *needs and expectations of the customers*. In health-care, patients are our "customers," and their needs and expectations should drive our QI efforts. However, as in healthcare, most organizations have two types of customers:

1. **External customers**. These are our **patients**. We launch improvement pro-jects to address their needs, concerns, and expectations. When we listen to our patients at the point-of-care, review patient surveys, or speak to their fam-ilies we may find patients' expectations are not met. We may then ask our-selves, how can we improve the care we provide and make their experience a better one?

2. **Internal customers**. The internal customers are the **staff** and **providers** at the front line. Sometimes the customer is not the patient. Frontline staff and providers depend on others for the work they do. They are the **end users**. Clinical practice involves caring for patients. But to care for patients, providers and staff need consultations, diagnostic imaging, lab work, demographic and insurance information, nutritional services, and so on. Providers and staff provide services to patients, but in turn depend on other providers and staff for their work. When these providers and staff receive the work product of other providers and staff, we call them **customers**. The providers and staff that perform services for other providers and staff are called **stakeholders**. Stakeholders are the professionals "doing the work." Improvement initiatives sometimes are needed to improve the work products our internal customers receive. *Example: When you, as a provider, order a chest X-ray, you are the "cus-tomer," not the patient. The patient will benefit from the treatment approach you prescribe and is the ultimate and last customer. But for the chest X-ray, you are the customer. What will happen if the radiology technician routinely takes an hour to show up? What if the official reading of a STAT chest X-ray takes a day? What if a large number of chest X-rays are overpenetrated, underpenetrated, or miss the costo-phrenic angle? You, the customer, will not be happy (and rightfully so!). Based on the VOC (internal customer), the radiology department may decide to initiate a QI project.*

The Voice of the Stakeholder (VOS)

The VOS is the expression of the *needs and requirements of the frontline professionals*. Stakeholders are the frontline staff and providers; they are the people "doing the work"; they are the professionals with the subject-matter expertise and knowledge of the process. *Stakeholders understand the system and are the experts needed for the process to deliver what the customer needs and expects.* Stakeholders may be staff, phy-sicians, nurses, or technicians involved in providing care. Stakeholders work on the process to provide a **work product**. When serving patients, the work product is "care and the healthcare experience"; when serving other providers and staff, the work product may be "information, supplies, results, etc."

Stakeholders want to do a good job. To perform optimally, they need equipment, supplies, information, and resources, on time, every time. They also need standards, updated policies, and proper procedures. If there is a problem with their performance, we need to ask ourselves: Do they have what they need? What are their challenges? Stakeholders' inability to deliver the service the customer needs and expects may be related to problems with the system: Do needed supplies arrive on time? Is the equipment in working condition? Is the work process standardized? Perhaps frontline stakeholders don't have the equipment and supplies they need, or the people responsible for supplying them with what they need are not doing so in a timely fashion. In any case, a QI project may need to be launched to find the causes of poor performance and address stakeholders' needs.

The Voice of the Process (VOP)

The VOP is *how the process communicates performance against customer needs and expectations.* This communication is done through process measures and in the form of data. Sometimes a QI project is launched to address process performance on a specific metric. This is the case when financial reports, clinical audits, and other types of data show a gap in performance. There may be an increased number of complications or readmission rates. Even if we don't have a VOC or VOS, the VOP (increased costs, slow response times, miscoded charts, increased narcotic discrepancies in the MICU, etc.) may be reasons why you and your team decide to launch a QI project.

Quotable quote: "If opportunity doesn't knock, build a door." Milton Berle

THE PROJECT SELECTION PROCESS

The Goal

The goal of the Project Selection Process is to select a QI project that is important to you and your organization in addressing critical issues of patient care, healthcare experience, costs, and resource utilization. A weak, undefined Project Selection Process makes improvement efforts more difficult and time consuming. A strong, defined, communicated and ingrained Project Selection Process can really make a significant difference in a healthcare organization's improvement efforts. A strong project selection process has the following characteristics:

- Projects are selected from both leadership and the front line (top down and bottom up); anyone can initiate a project idea.
- Criteria for prioritizing potential projects has been operationally defined and accepted by key leaders.
- Projects are selected based on their relationship to the hospital's (area, unit, department) strategic initiatives and goals.

- Leadership actively supports selected projects and is willing to provide the necessary resources.

Successful projects are those that are important to you and at the same time have the support of the leaders. Spend time during the project selection process to make sure you screen project ideas, focus your approach, and select the project that best delivers on the needs of your organization. If your project is not addressing the most pressing issues, you may not generate the support and get the resources you need. When that is the case, leadership buy-in may be difficult, mid-level manager's resistance may be high, and your team will struggle. The eventual outcome of your QI efforts may be less than ideal.

Project Selection Criteria

For each problem you have identified, define the current state of performance and compare it to the ideal state of performance. Do you have data you can use? What is the gap between the current state and ideal state of performance? How will we know we need to improve if we don't have data? What issues are critical? Narrow down the list of projects to those that address critical issues or are directly related to them. For each project, write a summary statement that details the current state versus ideal state and the gap between them. Define your project's desired outcomes.

Consider the scope and complexity of the improvement effort. What resources are available? Choose wisely! Consider your availability as well as the availability of project leaders, team leaders, and team members, especially if their involvement in the project is not part of their primary role. Remember, you still have a full-time job!

Several criteria are important to consider when selecting your project:

- **The Aim/ Purpose.** Every QI project must be related back to the overall strategic initiatives and goals of the organization (department, unit) via the metrics of the project. Project metrics such as **safety, quality, productivity, or costs** must be traceable both up and down throughout the organization. What is the gap between the ideal state and current state of the process performance? How do you know? Is the project targeting the internal or the external customer?
- **Scope.** What work process will be the focus of your QI project? What will be the start point and what will be the end point? What performance gap are you trying to close? Is your project overly ambitious for the time allowed? Make sure the scope of your project is realistic and you are not trying to take on too much, often referred to as "trying to boil the ocean."
- **Leadership.** Make sure senior and local leadership can actively engage in supporting the project and are willing and able to provide the necessary resources (time, personnel, administrative assistance, money). Remember, one of the most important resources is time! Time away from clinical duty is needed to actually be able to successfully complete and implement the QI project.
- **Timeline.** Can the project realistically be completed within a one- to six-month

period? A good rule of thumb is for the first couple of projects to set the target to one to three months. If the project duration extends longer than six months, other issues may arise that will make it difficult to complete your project.

- **Competing priorities.** Will any other initiatives be affecting the process targeted for improvement?

What Does a Good Project Idea Look Like?

There are several characteristics of a good project, including the following:

- The project is connected to the hospital's (area, unit, department) strategic objectives and addresses the current priorities of leadership.
- The problem addressed by the project is recognized to be of major importance and addresses issues of quality, safety, productivity, or cost.
- There is a clear primary metric that the project is trying to improve.
- The project scope and boundaries are not too ambitious, and the project timeline is acceptable.
- The project will have support from senior and local leadership.

Project Selection Steps

Project selection follows these four steps (see Figure 3-2):

1. **Scan.** Generate a list of project ideas. Review the VOC, VOS, and VOP if available. Review your clinical and operational metrics. Discuss ideas with leadership.
2. **Select.** Select 3 to 5 important issues. Identify your frontline staff's "pain points" and areas of poor performance based on available information and data. Using the above information, develop a list of potential projects; add any other ideas you may have. Focus on problems of quality, safety, productivity, or cost.

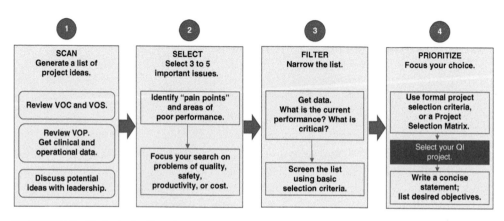

FIGURE 3-2   Project selection steps.

3. **Filter.** Narrow the list. Get data (if available). What is the current performance? What is critical? What needs to be addressed? Screen your list with basic criteria outlined in the previous section. Sort any of those that do not meet the necessary criteria. Write a concise statement listing desired objectives.

4. **Prioritize.** Focus your choice. Evaluate and prioritize the remaining potential projects. Use the Project Selection Criteria or a Project Selection Matrix; Once you have selected a project, plan how you are going to get the necessary support and resources. Write a brief summary of the problem to validate the potential project.

Be careful not to "bite off more than you can chew." It is generally better to do two or three projects really well rather than to focus on the total number of projects completed. The goal of a QI initiative is not to do projects but to improve processes. Be patient – worthwhile QI projects take time to properly complete.

Once you have selected your QI project, you should have the following:

- A defined and agreed on aim/purpose that is related up and down the organization via metrics;
- A focused problem statement that is clear and easy to understand, and that accurately describes the gap in performance;
- A competent team leader and team members who want and have the motivation to improve; and
- An engaged leader with the authority and willingness to support the QI initiative.

See these requirements in the next chapters.

THE PROJECT SELECTION MATRIX: A TOOL TO PRIORITIZE QI PROJECTS

> **The Project Selection Matrix is a tool that combines project selection criteria with weighted scores used to prioritize the most relevant projects.**

In this example we use a Project Selection Matrix to compare two projects. The Project Selection Matrix uses four columns to assess each project:

1. **Column A: Project Criteria.** List general project selection criteria that are important for your projects and organization.

2. **Column B: Priority Score.** List the numeric values assigned to each criterion. These values are assigned by senior leadership, mid-level leaders, or the QI team to highlight the most relevant requirements for the projects. Use a scale

from 1 to 10, with 1 being assigned to the criterion you have decided is least importance and 10 to the criterion with the highest relevance.

3. **Column C: Correlation Score**. Evaluate the correlation of each project against each of the criterion. Use a scale of 1 to 10, where 1 has the weakest match with the proposed criterion and 10 is assigned to the criterion that best matches the project characteristics. Starting out, it may be easier to use a simpler and cleaner approach, using a scale of 0, 3, 5, and 9 so that it is easier to discern between projects with 0 = no relationship, 3 = weak relationship, 5 = moderate relationship, 9 = strong relationship.

4. **Column D: Product Score**. This is the calculated numerical value or weighted score derived from multiplying column B (Priority Score) by column C (Correlation Score).

Complete the process for each criterion. Add all the weighted scores to calculate the total score. Repeat for each project. Select the project with the highest total score. Be careful to not get caught up in making sure we have the "perfect" score! See an example of a Project Selection Matrix template in Table 3-1.

TABLE 3-1 Template for a Project Selection Matrix

	Project Selection Matrix					
	Project A			Project B		
Column A Project Criteria	Column B Priority Score	Column C Correlation Score	Column D Product Score	Column B Priority Score	Column C Correlation Score	Column D Product Score
The project relates via metrics to goals of the organization.						
The project is supported by senior and local leadership.						
The project has defined goals and a narrow scope.						
The project will improve patient safety.						
The project will improve efficiency and patient flow.						

(Continued)

TABLE 3-1 (Continued)

	Project A			Project B		
	Project Selection Matrix					
	Column B	Column C	Column D	Column B	Column C	Column D
Column A Project Criteria	Priority Score	Correlation Score	Product Score	Priority Score	Correlation Score	Product Score
The project aims to decrease operational costs.						
The project will improve patient experience.						
Frontline stakeholders will support the project.						
The project can be completed in less than six months.						
The project will not interfere with ongoing QI initiatives.						
TOTAL SCORE						

A PROJECT TYPE FOR EVERY PROBLEM

Project strategy and resource requirements vary according to the specific type of project that is undertaken. While all projects follow the principles of improvement described in previous pages, not all projects require the same amount of effort, resources, tools, data, or statistical analysis. In the clinical arena, there are several project types and approaches to improvement. We have chosen to call them type I, type II, and type III.

Type I. These are the **quick wins** and "**just do it**" projects. These are rapid-improvement projects usually initiated by an individual or a small team to address a simple problem that affects a limited area. People are just trying to make their workflow or work environment better. This type of project usually seeks a practical and inexpensive solution, which is typically already known or requires little investigation. The project needs a loose framework and can be done in a couple of days. Examples of a project type I are: Improve the organization and prioritization of incoming faxes; make sure patient demographic information is documented in the chart accurately and in a timely fashion; organize a supply room.

Type II. The project addresses a simple performance problem that affects a small area or department. The root causes of the problem may be known or unknown, but the solution in general is not known. The project requires some data, the use of some improvement tools, and basic statistics. There is a low to moderate risk if the solution fails. These projects are done using different frameworks and tools. For example

- **Kaizen events.** A *Kaizen* event (the word comes from the Japanese) is a focused, short-term project event attended by leaders, mid-level managers, and frontline staff and providers to make improvements to an existing process for which they are responsible for. A Kaizen event is traditionally scheduled as a week-long event.
- **A3 projects.** A3 is a structured problem-solving and continuous improvement approach that is simple, visual, and provides a structure to guide individuals or teams in problem solving. The approach typically uses a single sheet of ISO-A3-size paper to document all the information that relates to the project. The A3 sheet includes seven common sections: background, current conditions, goals, analysis, solutions, plan for improvement, and follow-up.
- **Rapid Cycle Improvement.** A team leader takes mid-level managers and frontline staff and providers through a four-step improvement cycle called the PDSA cycle: Plan-Do-Study-Act (see chapter 21). The PDSA cycle helps the team understand the problem, formulate a hypothesis, develop a solution, create a plan of action, test the solution, and learn from the experience. Solutions are developed quickly and implementation can be done rapidly.

Type III. These projects require the engagement of a formal QI team in order to address a complex performance problem that affects a core process. These are big projects. The root causes of the problem and the solution/s are unknown. These projects usually require the QI team to come up with a multifaceted solution. The change will affect multiple departments and/or locations, and may impact a large number of people. Type III improvement projects require an in-depth analysis of the problem, a stepwise structured approach, and a large amount of data used for statistical analysis. There is high organizational risk if the solution fails. Adequate resources and leadership are critical. Examples: Improve throughput in the Emergency Department; improve turnover time in the operating rooms; decrease complication rates on the patient care units.

PROJECT TYPES FROM THE LENS OF CHANGE

All improvement is a change, and change is always met with varying degrees of resistance. You can also sort projects according to the amount of effort required to find a solution and the engagement or push-back you can expect (see Figure 3-3).

- **Type A.** These projects require a small investment of time to find the right solution. Once the solution has been appropriately trialed, the proposed changes will be well received and rapidly adopted by staff and providers. These types of projects require a small team and limited resources.
- **Type B.** These projects require significant efforts to find the best solution. However, the proposed changes will be generally well accepted and rapidly adopted by the front line. These projects require leaders and teams to focus on finding the best solution.
- **Type C.** These projects require a formal investigation of the causes, and a structured approach to finding the solution. Changes will be met with pushback and resistance from the front line. These projects are common in the clinical setting, where best-practice and clinical pathways are being implemented.
- **Type D.** These are complex projects. They require significant resources to find the most likely cause of the problem and the best solution. Once the solution is rolled out full-scale, the QI team is going to encounter significant pushback and resistance from key stakeholders. These projects are resource intensive for leaders, teams, and healthcare organizations, and require experience in both project and change management.

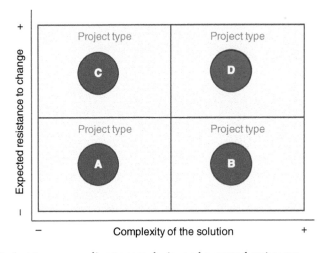

FIGURE 3-3   Project types according to complexity and expected resistance.

HOW TO ESTABLISH YOUR PROJECT'S TIMELINES

Administrators, sponsors, and clinical leaders may require an estimated project duration to monitor the project and ascertain when they can expect project deliverables. Other project stakeholders and frontline employees may need to know the estimated project timeline to evaluate the feasibility of their participation in the project. All face multiple competing priorities every day. They may hesitate to become involved in your project if they fear the project is going to interfere with their other responsibilities. You should develop a project schedule based on realistic estimates of activity duration prior to engaging team members. The two most common scheduling practices are schedule set and PERT:

- **Schedule set.** The QI team may receive the expected timeline for implementation of process improvements by senior leadership or the primary sponsor. Based on the expected date of project completion, you may have to work backward to determine the amount of time you can allocate for each activity to develop the project schedule. Schedule activity estimates can be a one-point, best-guess estimate based on your quality improvement experience in conducting similar process improvement projects, or historical information from the organization's subject-matter experts. These estimates can provide a general guide to a projected project timeline, initially with progressive specificity as the project activities unfold.
- **Program Evaluation and Review Technique (PERT).** Another way to develop a schedule is to use the Program Evaluation and Review Technique, which relies on historical information or expert opinions to approximate optimistic, pessimistic, and most likely estimates of the duration of each activity, which are then combined to yield the project schedule. The formula for determining the activity duration using **PERT is: $(O + P + 4ML) / 6$**, where O is the optimistic estimate, P is the pessimistic estimate, and ML is the most likely estimate.

Regardless of the method of estimating that is used, the schedule will need to be updated when new information becomes available. You may need to align your project activities with the schedule, as the project team members, leaders, local sponsors, and frontline stakeholders usually have multiple conflicting priorities with restricted availability for project work. When the schedule gets off track, two schedule-compression techniques may be employed in an attempt to restore the timeline:

- **Parallel processing** involves performing two activities that are usually completed in a sequential manner in a parallel manner instead. This technique increases the risk of rework due to the change in the process.
- **Crashing** involves using additional human resources to complete the activity faster. This technique impacts the cost of the project according to the type and

number of resources used. It may also be performed to conduct a pilot to evaluate the effectiveness of the new process and justify additional resources.

By developing a tentative project schedule and updating it as new information becomes available, you will be able to estimate and manage project resources more efficiently and effectively.

CHAPTER 4

Frame Your Challenge: The Problem Statement and Charter

STORIES FROM THE FRONT LINES OF HEALTHCARE: MARTHA SANCHEZ, THE HEAD OF HOUSEKEEPING

> *"I think the problem is that we don't have enough people in the morning shift to clean the rooms so we can keep patients moving," said Martha Sanchez, the head of housekeeping. "If we are to decrease the time patients have to wait to be seen, we need to clean the rooms faster after the doctor sees the patient. I am going to speak to the director of the clinic; I said it many times: we need more staff!"*

> **Describe the situation. How is the problem defined? Why is the way Martha Sanchez "sees the problem" a problem?**

THE PROBLEM STATEMENT

What Is a Problem Statement?

You should start every improvement effort by creating a clear and concise statement of: what problem you are trying to address, why you are launching a project, and what your overall objectives are.

The Quality Improvement Challenge: A Practical Guide for Physicians, First Edition.
Richard J. Banchs and Michael R. Pop.
© 2021 John Wiley & Sons Ltd. Published 2021 by John Wiley & Sons Ltd.
Companion website: www.wiley.com/go/banchs/quality

> **The *problem statement* is a clear, concise, and specific explanation of the problem that does not include any causes of the problem.**

What's not working? What is wrong? How is performance falling short of customers' expectations? What is the magnitude of the problem, and who does it affect? What's the challenge? **The problem statement frames the issues and is critical to the success of your improvement efforts.** The time spent defining the problem is not a waste: it's time well spent!

The primary purpose of a problem statement is to focus the efforts and attention of the QI team. A good problem statement should

- Be clear.
- Use precise language without unnecessary medical or technical jargon.
- Describe the problem to the level where the root cause is not yet known.
- Incorporate data, if any is available.
- Include the undesirable results and outcomes from the patient, providers, or staff's perspective.
- Be agreed upon and fully supported by all core team members.

Why Do We Need a Problem Statement?

When people describe a problem, they often describe it in vague terms and use what they think is the cause to define it. Defining the problem by the cause creates a narrow-minded focus that, at best, restricts creativity and, at worst, sets in motion a process that culminates in rolling-out solutions that do not address the true nature of the problem. By simply and properly defining the problem, you will create a better solution. The most apparent problem is often the tip of the iceberg, which upon further investigation reveals a multitude of underlying problems that leads to what at first glance seems obvious.

To describe a problem, put yourself "in the shoes" of the customer and try and describe it from the perspective of the people affected by the problem. Properly defining a problem is the most commonly overlooked step for many QI teams, and yet it is the step that provides the greatest return on investment. Healthcare providers and QI teams often jump to searching for solutions without having clearly defined and agreed on the actual problem. Teams spend a great deal of time debating the "best" solution but seldomly ask themselves: do we clearly and fully understand the problem?

Quotable quote: "Without changing our patterns of thought, we will not be able to solve the problems that we created with our current patterns of thought." Albert Einstein

How to Write a Focused Problem Statement

Problem statement investigation efforts should include

- The reasons why we should address the problem,
- The consequences of not addressing the problem,
- The "why now?" are we addressing the problem, and
- How the project is linked to the organizational priorities.

Remember, the problem statement should not include any potential causes of the problem or possible solutions to resolve it. One way to create a problem statement is to divided it in three parts: define what we consider the "ideal state" (or standard); define the current state; and identify the gap between the current state and the ideal state. Write a short paragraph addressing each one while answering the relevant questions:

- **Ideal state.** What would be the ideal performance? What would success look like? What is the standard?
- **Current state.** What's the failure? What is the rate of failure (how often is it happening)? How long has it been going on? What's the background? Who does it affect? What is the patient or customer's perspective? What is the stakeholder's perspective? What metrics are currently used to measure the problem? Where is the data coming from? What is the current performance? What is the key output metric that needs to be improved?
- **Gap.** What is the gap between our current state and the ideal state? What needs to happen?

A problem statement is often supported by a **goal statement**. The goal statement should be brief and specific, use the same metrics as the problem statement, and include a specific date by which the project should be completed successfully. A goal statement often accompanies the problem statement and defines the targets of the QI project.

THE PROBLEM STATEMENT IS YOUR "ELEVATOR SPEECH"

Imagine you walk into an elevator and the CEO of the hospital comes in right after you. He politely greets you and then asks you about your project. He has heard from your chair that you want to launch a QI project to improve the current situation in the cath lab. What are you going to say? Well, here are some of the questions you may want to address: What's the problem? How is the problem affecting your patients? Why is it important? Why address the problem now? What are your goals? You may have a clear idea of what you want to improve, but you should be able to articulate it in a succinct and clear fashion.

Quotable Quotes: "A problem that is poorly defined has an infinite number of solutions but a problem well defined is a problem half solved."
Wally Davis

A Problem Statement May Include a "Burning Platform"

The problem statement may include a "burning platform" or statement that provides a brief explanation of the reasons why we should address the problem now. The burning platform establishes what makes this project a priority now, versus, let's say, something else. The burning platform or business case should answer the following questions:

- Why are we addressing the problem now?
- What benefits can we expect for our patients, staff, physicians, and healthcare organization?
- How does this project support /relate to the overall strategic goals of your department?
- How is it aligned with the strategies of the hospital?

The burning platform may also include a statement about the consequences of not addressing the issues now, and a statement that establishes a clear link between the project and the strategic business / clinical priorities of the hospital (or area, unit, department).

Example: First-case on-time-start accuracy at Fond-du-Lac Medical Center

The Problem Statement

Ideal state: First-case on-time start accuracy should be above the 50th percentile of cohort performance. One hundred percent of the causes of delay should be appropriately documented in our EMR.

Current state: Data from Surgical Compass® Cohort Benchmark analysis shows a first-case on-time-start accuracy rate of 16 percent (160/1000) (< 25th percentile of cohort performance) in our operating room. Delayed on-time-start is the cause of decreased quality, loss of productivity, and ongoing dissatisfaction among our patients, surgeons, and OR staff. Preliminary data reveal that in up to 65 percent (546) of the delays, the appropriate cause is not well documented, which is preventing our efforts to address the situation.

Gap: 25 percent difference between ideal state and current state, with 546 causes not being fully documented.

THE PROJECT CHARTER

What Is a Project Charter?

After the problem has been clearly defined with a Problem Statement, it is time to agree on the nature and specifics of the project. The Project Charter is the most important document of your project.

The Project Charter is a document that serves to gain agreement between the Primary Sponsor and the QI team as to the nature, scope, goals, and timeline of the project. The Project Charter concisely delineates the who, what, when, where, how, and why of the project.

The Project Charter is key to helping the QI team achieve the goal of the project because

- It helps everyone understand the aim, scope, and goals of the project.
- It serves to gain agreement between all parties.
- It authorizes the project's initiation and use of resources by the QI team.

The **Project Charter** serves as an *informal contract between the* **Primary Sponsor** *and the project team* as to the scope, roles, responsibilities, and nature of the project. An initial draft of the Project Charter must be complete at the beginning of the project. It must also specify who the Project Sponsor, physician sponsors and project manager / leader are. Once the team is formed, the Project Charter can include the project team members, team leader, and key stakeholders when they become known.

The Project Charter can be referred to throughout the project's life cycle when questions arise regarding expected project performance, deliverables, and timelines. It is a *living document* that should be updated throughout the project as new information becomes available.

A Project Charter is not a project management plan. It is not a comprehensive document detailing all the steps and actions necessary to complete the project. Instead, the Project Charter is the *compass that sets the direction* for the QI team, clearly outlining the participants, scope, metrics, and goals of the project.

> *Quotable quotes: "To solve a problem or to reach a goal, you don't need to know all the answers in advance. But you must have a clear idea of the problem and the goal you want to reach." W. Clement Stone*

The Project Charter "Must-Haves"

The Project Charter must have the following six important components:

1. A **Problem Statement.** A Project Charter must have a problem statement to clearly define the focus of the project; What's the problem? Reasons for action? What's the background? A burning platform may be a part of the problem statement. The problem statement provides the reasons for prioritizing the project at this time, the anticipated consequences if the project is not undertaken, and the project's financial or clinical implications if known.

2. **The scope and boundaries.** What are we going to improve?, and very importantly, what is not going to be addressed now? What is in-scope and out-of-scope? The scope and boundaries of the project help the team focus on the work that needs to be done, the areas or issues that will not be addressed at this time, and the expected deliverables.

3. **Key metrics.** What are we going to measure? How will we know we have improved? This section describes what will be measured and how the project success will be defined and evaluated.

4. **Goals and objectives.** What do we want to achieve? What will success look like? This section defines the proposed project goals. Remember, goals should be **SMART**: Specific, Measurable, Attainable, Realistic, and Time-Bound. If the current baseline performance is not known, specific project goals can be set at a later date after the current process performance is defined (see Chapters 14–17). Project goals should be agreed upon with the Primary Sponsor and Key Stakeholders.

5. **Milestones and timeline.** By when do we want to achieve it? Estimate the dates when specific deliverables will be produced. There are numerous tools to estimate timelines. A great way to visualize a project's timeline is by creating a **Gantt chart**, a type of horizontal bar chart that outlines all the tasks involved in a project shown against a timescale that serves to give the reader an instant overview of the entire project, together with information on the order of the tasks and when each task needs to be completed.

6. **Signatures.** Who are the parties involved? A Project Charter should bear the signature of the key parties:
    1. as a sign the project has been approved by the Primary Sponsor;
    2. as a sign of commitment by the team leader and the members of the QI team; and
    3. to establish a clear agreement on the nature, scope, goals, and timeline of the project.

The Project Charter is a valuable tool to provide direction to a QI team as well as to establish performance expectations of both the Project Sponsor and the QI team that senior leadership can use to track performance of all parties.

Example: The patient arrival-to-departure time at the PCP clinic

Figure 4-1 is an example of a Project Charter for you. The charter includes the Primary Sponsor, project team members, reason for action, project scope and boundaries, key

PROJECT CHARTER

	Start date	Complete
	May2, 2016	March 2017

Title: Decreasing patient arrival-to-departure time (lead time) in the PCP Clinic

PRIMARY SPONSOR

Rachel Miller

PROJECT TEAM

Jonathan Tomasso MD (Team Leader)	Paul Brown (Administrative Aid)
Amy Casper (Clinic Director)	Christine Dash (Pharm D)
Meggan Peebe (Administrative Nurse)	Veronica Martinez (Customer Service)

REASON FOR ACTION Problem Statement: Ideal State, Current State, Gap

The Institute for Healthcare Improvement (IHI) suggests a typical office visit should take 1.5 times the actual time spent with a provider. For an average 20-minute visit, a patient should spend no more than 30 minutes in the clinic. The total time spent in the clinic (patient arrival-to-departure time) is called lead time. Preliminary data obtained from our PCP (Primary Care Plus) clinic shows an average lead time of 70 minutes, for an average 20 minutes provider visit. This shows a gap of 40 minutes for the average patient visit. Long lead times are a source of concern because they negatively affect patient satisfaction and the overall care experience, medical compliance, and patient return show rates.

PROJECT SCOPE & BOUNDARIES

In-scope	The Organizational Process Improvement (OPI) Office partnered with the Chief Ambulatory Officer and a seven-member clinic team lead by Dr. Rachel Miller to work on improving patient arrival-to-departure time. The project scope includes all clinic visits in a 12 h period (7:00 a.m. to 7:00 p.m.) Monday to Friday.
Out-of-scope	The QI project will not address patient arrival-to-departure time during Saturday schedule.

KEY METRICS

Primary metric: : Patient arrival-to-departure time

Secondary metric: The team decided to include patient satisfaction. Satisfaction will be measured with a "satisfaction bundle" that includes four service attributes linked to satisfaction with the clinic experience: "greeted with a smile," "treated with respect," "kept informed of changes and delays," and "receiving the appropriate information to understand what to do once I leave the clinic."

PROJECT GOALS

Primary metric:
< 40 minutes arrival to departure time for MD and PhamD visits
< 30 minutes arrival to departure time for RN visits
Secondary metric:
50% success rate with the satisfaction bundle (% of patients that respond "yes" to all four service attributes)

TIMELINES

Current State Analysis completed by September 1, 2016
Pilots and full-scale implementation by January 2017
Project completed by March 2017

ELECTRONIC SIGNATURES

Primary Sponsor	Rachel Miller
Team Leader	Jonathan Tomasso
OPI Office	Richard Banchs

The Organizational Process Improvement (OPI) Office

FIGURE 4-1   The patient arrival-to-departure time at the PCP clinic.

metrics, goals of the project, timelines, and electronic signatures. We have created our own template, but, of course, you can build your own.

EXERCISE: A PROBLEM STATEMENT AND PROJECT CHARTER FOR YOUR QI PROJECT

Think of a problem you would like to address and the project you would launch. Using what you have learned so far

- Write a short paragraph describing the problem you aim to address, reasons why you should address the problem, the consequences of not addressing the problem, and the "why now?" you are addressing the problem. Be careful not to include the causes of the problem or possible solutions in your problem statement.
- Write your first draft of a Project Charter; make sure it has the six "must-haves." You will probably have to estimate the goals and timelines.

SUMMARY QUIZ

1. What are three common steps used when writing a problem statement?
   A. The ideal state, current state, and gap
   B. The current state, ideal state, solutions
   C. The pain points, current state, solutions
   D. The root causes, solutions, current state
   E. Type A, type B, and type C
2. What is a Project Charter?
   A. An important document for every project
   B. A definition of the scope and objectives of the project
   C. A cooperative effort between the Primary Sponsor, the team leader, and the QI team
   D. A living document that can be modified as more information becomes available
   E. All of the above
3. What are some of the critical elements for all Project Charters?
   A. Suppliers, inputs, processes, and outputs
   B. The Voice of the Customer and the Voice of the Stakeholder
   C. The Problem Statement, scope, metrics, targets, and timelines
   D. The problem and the data to support the problem
   E. The primary and supplemental sponsors
4. Once you create a Project Charter, it is "set in stone."
   A. True
   B. False

5. What is a statement that defines the problem and the undesirable outcomes from the customer's perspective?
   A. A need statement
   B. A Project Charter
   C. A SIPOC diagram
   D. A Problem Statement
   E. An aim statement

6. Which of the following statements defines a well-written Problem Statement?
   A. Is clear, precise, without unnecessary medical or technical jargon
   B. Explains the extent of the problem
   C. Describes the problem at the level where the root cause is not yet known
   D. Provides available supporting data
   E. All of the above

7. A "business case" includes all the following EXCEPT
   A. a brief explanation of the reasons to address the problem;
   B. the consequences of not addressing the problem;
   C. the causes of the problem;
   D. the link between the problem, the project, and the clinical priorities; or
   E. the goals we want to achieve.

Key: 1a, 2e, 3c, 4b, 5d, 6e, 7c

PART III

THE SECOND "R": THE RIGHT PEOPLE

CHAPTER 5

Don't Go at It Alone: Find a Primary Sponsor

STORIES FROM THE FRONT LINES OF HEALTHCARE: TURN-AROUND TIME FOR X-RAYS IN THE ED

Dr. Ashley Nixon was an Emergency Department (ED) physician at Mercy Hospital. She and her colleagues staffed the surgical care track of the ED. She took pride in her work and her ability to provide high-quality, efficient care to her patients but was becoming increasingly concerned about the long turn-around time for X-rays. The time to get an X-ray result once the order was in had more than doubled in the last six months. This was affecting patient flow and her ability to provide timely care for her patients. Dr. Nixon decided to launch a QI project to improve the situation. After evaluating the current process, she decided to make some changes she thought would improve turn-around time for X-rays. She discussed these changes with Dr. Edward Mosley, a colleague. He agreed that she had a good plan and that the changes would help expedite the turn-around time for results. Dr. Nixon emailed the revised process to the ED nurse managers and the radiology manager, indicating they would start the revised process the following week. On Monday morning, Dr. Nixon met significant resistance. Nurses and radiology techs said they didn't know anything about the revised process and would need their managers' approval before proceeding with "doing anything differently." When asked for advice, Dr. Mosley suggested to Dr. Nixon that she talk directly to the nurse and radiology manager. Over the

The Quality Improvement Challenge: A Practical Guide for Physicians, First Edition.
Richard J. Banchs and Michael R. Pop.
© 2021 John Wiley & Sons Ltd. Published 2021 by John Wiley & Sons Ltd.
Companion website: www.wiley.com/go/banchs/quality

ensuing months, several meetings were scheduled, but without the active involvement of a senior leader, no progress was made. Delays continued with X-rays in the ED.

What was the problem? How did Dr. Nixon approach it? What was the result? Why did this happen?

THE PRIMARY SPONSOR

What Is a Primary Sponsor?

All projects need a sponsor. A Primary Sponsor can be a physician leader, departmental chair, division chief, executive leader, director, or high-level unit manager.

> **A Primary Sponsor is the senior leader who has access to the necessary resources and the authority to ensure the success of the improvement project or change initiative.**

As a senior leader in the organization, the Primary Sponsor can **"open doors"** for the improvement team. The Primary Sponsor uses connections, influence, and a power base to increase buy-in, resolve cross-functional issues, and mitigate resistance from the frontline stakeholders.

The Critical Role of a Primary Sponsor

The role of the Primary Sponsor in the QI project is critical. The Primary Sponsor serves an essential function for the project team in helping move the project forward and achieve objectives. These are the most important functions of the Primary Sponsor:

- Establish priorities for competing initiatives.
- Resolve cross-functional issues.
- Remove roadblocks; the Primary Sponsor serves as the point person to address barriers that interfere with the project's progression.
- Help manage change by building a coalition of key stakeholders to support the change.

One of the most common causes of QI project failure is the *absence or lack of meaningful involvement of the Primary Sponsor to provide the necessary leadership and support for the change initiative.* The Primary Sponsor needs to be visible, engaged, and active throughout the lifecycle of the project.

The role of the Primary Sponsor is crucial in the team's ability to manage change. Improvement teams often start a project without involving a senior leader and then struggle unnecessarily throughout the project. The Primary Sponsor is the project facilitator and the **change leader**. Ronald Heifetz, professor of leadership at the John F. Kennedy School of Government at Harvard University, defines the change leader as "the person that provides the technical solution while preparing people for the adaptive change by understanding their loss, providing hope, and explaining the process" (Heifetz 2002).

To appropriately fulfill the role, the Primary Sponsor must spend time communicating directly with the front lines to help the QI Team gain buy-in for the project. One of the greatest contributors to success in change initiatives is an active and visible Primary Sponsor. The greatest obstacle to success is ineffective change management sponsorship to support the QI project (Prosci 2016).

WHO SHOULD BE YOUR PRIMARY SPONSOR?

You may be approached by a senior leader with a request for an improvement project. Most likely this leader will become your Primary Sponsor. If you have the opportunity to choose your Primary Sponsor, there are a number of requirements you should keep in mind. While all Primary Sponsors are senior leaders, not all senior leaders should be the Primary Sponsor. Ideally, the leader you have chosen to be your project's Primary Sponsor has the following characteristics:

- is well respected by both the team and key stakeholders,
- is considered a credible leader,
- has the authority and appropriate leadership level to be able to resolve cross-functional issues when they arise,
- has experience in leading projects and change management initiatives, and
- has the willingness and ability to actively participate in the crucial phases of the project.

Many healthcare organizations have a matrix reporting structure that complicates the selection of the Primary Sponsor. You may need to select a Primary Sponsor and ask for the assistance of a second senior leader. In these situations, clear communication with all leaders involved is necessary. While not ideal, you may need to choose two sponsors for your project.

REFERENCES

1. Heifetz R. (2002). *Leadership on the Line*. Harvard Business Review Press.
2. Prosci®. (2016). Best-Practices in Change Management. Best-Practices Report. Edition.

REVIEW QUIZ

1. What is a Primary Sponsor?
   A. A person that will support your QI project
   B. A high-level leader that can ensure the success of your project
   C. A leader that establishes the priorities of the QI project
   D. A leader that is actively engaged in the change initiative
   E. All of the above

2. One of the greatest contributors to project success is the active and visible participation of a Primary Sponsor.
   A. True
   B. False

3. A Primary Sponsor is generally a senior leader (executive, high level manager, physician leader) in the organization who can "open doors" for the QI team.
   A. True
   B. False

4. An effective Primary Sponsor must have the appropriate leadership level to be able to resolve cross-functional issues.
   A. True
   B. False

5. One of the greatest obstacles to the success of change initiatives is ineffective change management support by the Primary Sponsor.
   A. True
   B. False

6. To be an effective Primary Sponsor of a QI project, you need to be visible, engaged, and active throughout the life-cycle of the project.
   A. True
   B. False

7. Which of the following is NOT a typical role of the Primary Sponsor?
   A. Provide resources for the improvement team
   B. Establish priorities for competing initiatives
   C. Resolve cross-functional issues
   D. Analyze baseline data and create a graphic summary of the findings
   E. Engage key stakeholders to support the change and manage any resistance

8. To effectively support an improvement team, a Primary Sponsor must
   A. be a leader with authority,
   B. have the appropriate leadership level in the organization,
   C. be respected,
   D. be able to be actively engaged in the QI project, or
   E. all of the above

   Key: 1e, 2a, 3a, 4a, 5a, 6a, 7d, 8e

CHAPTER 6

Organize Your QI Team and Select the Team Leader

THE QI TEAM

Improvement Is a Team Sport

There are projects that are simple, straightforward, and quick that an individual can do without a team. These are the "quick-win" projects. In general, however, QI projects are better done as a team. Teams are integral parts of healthcare organizations, both operationally and clinically. Typically, teams are built in order to solve problems or complete work that exceeds an individual's capacity or requires the expertise of a diverse group of individuals. In general improvement is a "team sport." *Teams outperform individuals acting alone* especially when performance requires multiple skills, judgments, and experiences.

There are two significant benefits to working as a team:

1. **Higher quality of solutions.** Diversity of opinions creates better solutions. People in teams share their competencies and experiences, and combine their unique talents to fuel creative and innovative problem solving and optimal solution generation.
2. **Increased productivity and motivation.** Alignment of team members toward a common purpose focuses their efforts and accountability toward an agreed-on target; timelines facilitate successful project completion.

The Quality Improvement Challenge: A Practical Guide for Physicians, First Edition.
Richard J. Banchs and Michael R. Pop.
© 2021 John Wiley & Sons Ltd. Published 2021 by John Wiley & Sons Ltd.
Companion website: www.wiley.com/go/banchs/quality

The Challenge for QI Teams in Healthcare

The formation of a high-functioning team dedicated to improvement tasks is difficult in healthcare. QI teams face three main challenges:

- **Time.** Teams in healthcare often struggle with getting off quickly to a productive start and finding the time to carry on their project activities. Patient care is always the priority for clinicians; QI activities are often seen as less important. Resource constraints related to staffing and scheduling requirements limit the availability of key stakeholders to participate regularly on QI project teams. As a result, teams are composed in an indiscriminate way with an underrepresentation of front line clinicians because they cannot be relieved from their patient care responsibilities.
- **Silos.** The culture of the healthcare environment also makes improvement work difficult. Healthcare silos (doing what is best for me or my department/unit/function instead of what is best for the patient, team, or organization) foster group mentality and functionality rather than team performance. Competing priorities create confusion and adherence to dysfunctional loyalties, making the task of improving difficult.
- **Pushback.** QI teams in healthcare often struggle with the lack of buy-in from the front lines; under these conditions, it is difficult to have a successful hand-off of their recommendations to the people who "do the work."

The Key to Addressing These Challenges

These three challenges require separate, specific approaches:

- **The challenge of time.** A team needs to focus their team on productive activities. A QI team needs
  - A leader willing to get the right people on the team, provide the needed resources, and "open doors" when problems arise.
  - A leader that is willing to deal with the cross-functional issues and political barriers as they arise.
  - A leader that provides clarity regarding the team's purpose and goals, so that QI teams get off to a quick, productive start. Clarity on the team's purpose is always made easier with a clear, well written, and agreed-upon Project Charter.
- **The challenge of silos.** A QI team needs to work together to develop clarity in the team's purpose, goals, and work strategy. This will enable team members to develop common commitment and trust; commitment and trust can overcome silo mentality and the disconnect between the members of the team. Open and effective communication among team members must be present to achieve this critical affective component (see Chapter 27).

- **Pushback and lack of buy-in.** Support for the project depends on
  - the leaders and their active participation throughout the life cycle of the project;
  - the QI team supporting, training, and coaching frontlines professionals;
  - effective communication; and
  - an early engagement of the front line in the co-creation of the solutions (see Chapter 29).

Quotable quote: "There are two types of people – ones who do the work and ones who take the credit. Try to be in the first group. There is less competition there." Indira Gandhi

WHO SHOULD BE ON YOUR QI TEAM?

Selection Criteria

"Who should be sitting at the table"? Make sure your QI team has the right professionals from the front lines. It is important to include the people that "do the work" from all levels of the value stream. Improvement teams often have too many supervisors, managers, and directors, but not enough front line stakeholders who have the "know-how" of the process that needs to be improved. Without first-hand knowledge of the process, improvement ideas are usually inadequate, too broad, or too restrictive. These ideas are seen as out-of-touch with the reality of the daily work because they have been developed by a QI team lacking the technical expertise or process knowledge of the intimate details of how work is actually done. Without first-hand knowledge of the process, improvement suggestions are usually not supported by the people who actually "do the work." How do *you* feel when regulatory agencies and administrators tell you how to "improve" your clinical practice?

In general, a QI team should have a mixture of stakeholders, supervisors, and leaders with stakeholders > supervisors > leaders, in that order.

- Stakeholders are the people who **do the work.** They are the front line. Make sure the stakeholders who will have to implement the changes are part of the team.
- Supervisors are the people **responsible for the work.** They are the nurse managers, division chiefs, directors, and other responsible parties.
- Leaders are hospital or departmental level leaders who **support the project.** A leadership position in the organization is not by itself a good selection criterion to become a member of a QI team.
- Some teams may need additional members, such as subject-matter experts, project facilitators, and consultants.

Selecting the people that you get along with is not the best strategy to create a high-functioning team. Because we usually get along with like-minded people, filling a team with the people we get along with will probably result in **group thinking.** To create an effective team, choose front line professionals who bring the appropriate **mix of skills.** Choose a good mix of "experts, "doers," and "schmoozers." These people have the following attributes:

- **Process knowledge.** Teams must have at least one person who knows the process.
- **Organization.** Every team needs members who have the ability to organize and get things done.
- **Creativity.** Creatives know how to work though problems and find solutions.
- **Good interpersonal skills.** Effective communicators can explain the team's message and reach the front line professionals.

"Thanks, But No Thanks"

One of the reasons most people hesitate to become part of a QI project is the perception that project activities will increase the workload of an already resource-stretched front line. In some organizations, QI projects have historically resulted in nothing more than additional work requirements for the front line to negotiate. Be careful when pulling together a group of stakeholders who are already struggling with challenging workloads in order to form your project team. Frontline professionals need to have the appropriate resources and see the value in participating in a QI project. Here are some suggestions to encourage participation in QI projects:

- Critically evaluate the time demands you are placing on those involved. Create as close of a timeline as you can.
- Make sure participating members get the appropriate support from their supervisors. People need time away from clinical responsibilities for project activities. **"Improving after five o'clock"** is not the best strategy.
- Share realistic estimates of the time required to participate in the project with team members and their supervisors.
- Adhere to strict professional behavior during project-related interactions, such as adequately preparing for activities, scheduling meetings for the minimum time necessary to complete activities, and clearly communicating accountabilities and deadlines, etc.
- Adopt a flexible approach to the completion of project requirements to accommodate project team members' needs and conflicts with clinical work.
- Avoid wasting project team members' time by first acknowledging that there is a cost associated with every project-related activity. Eliminate non-value-added project work; make sure team meetings are efficient and achieve their intended goals (see Chapter 26).

How Many Team Members Do You Need?

In general, a QI project team should have *four to eight members*. A team of this size is better able to work through their "individual, functional, and hierarchical differences toward a common plan and hold themselves jointly accountable for the results" (Katzenbach 1993). When teams are either too small or too big, three things tend to happen:

1. **Group thinking.** A team that is too small may run into "group thinking" with lack of diversity in the team's analytical and creative thinking.
2. **Difficulty managing the team.** A team that is too big may run into a number of problems, including scheduling, managing, and decision-making.
3. **The Ringelmann's effect.** Ringelmann's famous study — often called the Ringelmann effect — analyzed people alone and in groups as they pulled on a rope. Ringelmann then measured the pull force and found that as he added more and more people to the rope, the total force generated by the group rose, but the average force exerted by each decreased. When teams are very large, team members tend to decrease the intensity of their work because they expect or assume other members will "pull their weight."

THE TEAM LEADER

Who Should Lead Your Improvement Team?

If you are the person who initiated the project, you will most likely be the team leader. However, be aware that the leader of the QI team can be any one in the improvement team. Also, the team leader may or may not be the project leader responsible for the QI project, depending on the healthcare organization, composition of the team, the requirements of the project, and the strengths/ limitations of the project leader. What is important to know is that the effectiveness of a QI team is, in general, a reflection of the team leader's skill in coaching and supporting the team's work. The person chosen to be the team leader should meet certain requirements:

- Have a good process knowledge or subject-matter expertise (a must!).
- Be respected by the front line professionals (staff, nurses, doctors, key stakeholders).
- Have excellent interpersonal, facilitation, and communication skills.
- Have the ability to give helpful and effective feedback, as well as to create and lead an environment of constructive conflict.
- Have good problem-solving and decision-making ability.
- Be able to recognize others and celebrate the team's achievements.

What Is the Role of the Team Leader

In general, the team leader sets the project's strategy and facilitates the team's progress in meeting milestones and achieving the project objectives. Specifically, the team leader's role is to

- Provide a framework for the team's purpose that builds commitment and drives the project.
- Collaborate and help team members clearly delineate their roles and responsibilities.
- Help coordinate the completion of the project work according to the specified time frames.
- Coach the team to accomplish both effective communication and constructive conflict resolution.

The responsibility of the leader is to *establish clarity on the activities and goals that the team must achieve and then give them the tools they need to achieve them.* The role of the leader is not to do everything but to facilitate the work of the QI team members. Many leaders feel a great deal of pressure to operate like surgeons (you have a problem, *I* can take it off of you) rather than a psychiatrist (you have a problem, let me help you figure out a way *you* can solve the problem) (Heifetz 2002). Having said that, as Larry Bossidy and Ram Charan state in their book *Execution. The Discipline of Getting Things Done*, a successful leader needs to be "engaged personally and deeply in the substance and sometimes the detail of the execution" (Bossidy 2002).

THE TRUE ROLE OF THE QI TEAM

All improvement is a change, and acceptance of the need to change comes naturally when the front line is engaged in discovering the reason for poor performance and participating in the co-creation of innovative solutions. **"People support what they help create."** Given the importance of front line engagement in the improvement efforts, the role of the QI team is not to work independently to find solutions and implement them top down. *A QI team is most effective when its members help create the conditions that allow key stakeholders to solve the problem that directly affects them.*

A QI project is a *partnership* between four key actors: The Primary Sponsor, the Local Sponsor, the frontline professionals, and the QI team. The Primary Sponsors are the senior leaders who provide resources and legitimize the project; the Local Sponsors are the mid-level leaders, managers, division heads, and departmental leaders who support the project, engage the front line in project activities, and support the change; the front line professionals are the people responsible for operationalizing the improvement and change; and finally, the QI team. The fundamental role of the QI team is to be the facilitator (see Figure 6-1):

- **Facilitate the role of the Primary Sponsor.** The Senior leaders and Primary Sponsor are the **project authority.** The role of the Primary Sponsor is general oversight and legitimization of the process improvement efforts; allocation of resources; communication and influencing opinion; and opening doors for the QI team. The QI team can help the Primary Sponsor by providing continuous updates on the progress of the project, coordinating the calendar of activities for meetings with the front line, and providing message content for written communication, meetings, and presentations.

- **Facilitate the role of the Local Sponsor.** The Local Sponsors (managers, division heads, departmental leaders) are responsible for the success of the project at the front line; they are the QI team's **project partners.** When the Local Sponsors support the project, they are important **ambassadors** for the change; they have a key role in project activities and acceptance of the change. Local Sponsors are responsible for making the improvement possible. They keep the front line informed and engaged, provide resources, coach performance, and arrange for training. The QI team can facilitate their role by providing continuous updates on the progress of the project, helping them coordinate calendar of activities for meetings with the front line, providing message content for written communication, meetings and presentations; and sharing tools, processes, and techniques to help sponsors with project activities and change management.

- **Help the front line be engaged and succeed.** The front line has a crucial role. They are the **project owners** and should be engaged in understanding the problem, finding possible causes of poor performance, co-creating solutions, and working through the technical aspects of the change. The QI team can facilitate their engagement by frequent sharing of information, creating

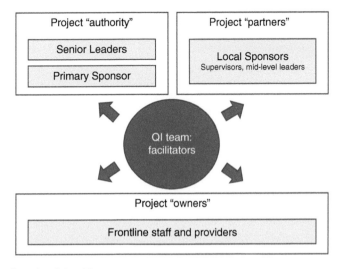

FIGURE 6-1   The role of the QI team.

the conditions for change (the Change Space), and providing coaching and training on the new process.

THE FIRST TOLLGATE REVIEW

Periodically, the improvement team needs to confirm that they are on the right track to achieve their project objectives. This is best done through a tollgate review with the Primary Sponsor. A tollgate review is a go/no-go checkpoint where the team leader, team members and the Primary Sponsor meet to discuss ongoing project activities, review results and deliverables, and assure that the project is on track. The first toll-gate review should be scheduled with the Primary Sponsor soon after organizing your team, at the end of the first "R": the "Right People" (see Chapter 25).

EXERCISE: THE QI TEAM AT HEART MEDICAL CENTER

The Leadership at Heart Medical Center would like to reduce the long patient wait times in the emergency room (ER). Preliminary work has identified turnaround times (TAT) on routine blood and urine analysis in the main chemistry lab as the major causes of delay. You have been asked to assemble a team to address the issue. Using the hospital's list of available personnel (see Table 6-1), select six team members for your QI project.

TABLE 6-1   Heart Medical Center Hospital Roster

Hospital Roster: ER & Labs		
Name	Department	Position
Alens, F	Laboratory	Shift supervisor
Andrews	Laboratory	Lab tech
Anselmo, L	Administration	Hospital CMO
Bronch, G	Laboratory	Lab tech
Constatnts, D	Laboratory	Lab clerk
Deli, M	ER	ER physician
Dormund, M	Laboratory	Senior lab tech a.m. shift
Efram, N	ER	ER clerk
Gild, R	ER	ER nurse
Goldsmith, H	ER	ER nurse

(Continued)

TABLE 6-1 (Continued)

Hospital Roster: ER & Labs

Name	Department	Position
Goldstein, S	ER	ER physician
Hussain, H	ER	ER clerk
Kundenman, B	Laboratory	Lab tech
Libra, F	ER	ER physician
Manheim, N	ER	ER nurse
Monroe, J	ER	ER medical director
Opostini, C	Laboratory	Senior lab tech p.m. shift
Smith, A	Pathology	Director of Pathology
Vitorini, K	ER	ER physician
Woldenbaum, B	Laboratory	Shift supervisor

REFERENCES

1. Bossidy R. (2002). *Execution: The Discipline of Getting Things Done*. Random House.
2. Heifetz R. (2002). *Leadership on the Line: Staying Alive through the Dangers of Leading*. Harvard Business Review Press.
3. Katzenbach R. (1993). *The Discipline of Teams*. Harvard Business Review Press.

REVIEW QUIZ

1. A team leader should be chosen on the basis of all the following characteristics EXCEPT
   A. good process knowledge,
   B. respected by the front line professionals,
   C. excellent interpersonal and communication skills,
   D. leadership position in the organization, or
   E. good facilitator.
2. All of the following characterize a group of people performing as a team EXCEPT
   A. complementary skills,
   B. common purpose,
   C. focus on individual goal achievement,
   D. mutual accountability, or
   E. common approach.

3. Regarding the composition of a QI team
   A. front-line professionals need to have the largest representation.
   B. the ideal team size is 4–8 members.
   C. it is important to have team members that bring subject-matter expertise.
   D. it is important for the team to have a mix of skills.
   E. all of the above.

4. Team members should be preferentially selected on the basis of all the following characteristics EXCEPT
   A. bring process knowledge,
   B. have a high-ranking leadership position in the organization,
   C. have technical expertise,
   D. have problem-solving skills, or
   E. have great interpersonal skills.

5. A team leader's role is to facilitate the team's success in achieving the project's goals.
   A. True
   B. False

6. The formation of high-performing QI teams in healthcare is made more difficult by
   A. clinical silos,
   B. prioritization of patient care,
   C. resource constraints,
   D. conservative culture, or
   E. all of the above

7. What is the role of the QI team during an improvement project?
   A. share findings and communicate through all project phases.
   B. provide message content for written communication to senior leaders.
   C. provide material and audiovisual support for meetings and presentations.
   D. provide or facilitate coaching and training of the front line.
   E. all of the above

Key: 1d, 2c, 3e, 4d, 5a, 6e, 7e.

Exercise key: While the problem affects the ER and the professionals working in the ER, the root of the problem for a long turnover time of routine samples is in the lab. In this example, team members should be chosen preferentially for their subject-matter expertise: processing samples. ER staff and providers are the customers of the process; lab personnel are the stakeholders. Given these roles, your QI team should include a majority of lab personnel, who are the stakeholders with the best process knowledge. The stakeholders do the work and therefore have the expertise. Chose a majority of front line workers and some supervisors. A customer (ER staff or provider) can also be a member of the QI team helping team members have a better perspective of "what the customer needs."

PART IV

THE THIRD "R": THE RIGHT PROBLEM

CHAPTER 7

What Is the Scope of the Project? The SIPOC Diagram

YOU NEED TO KNOW YOUR PROJECT'S SCOPE AND BOUNDARIES

What process does the problem relate to? What is the target of the improvement? Where does work begin and end? The process boundaries clearly define the extent of the project scope and serve as an effective way for making decisions about the project activities. The project scope *establishes the limits of the project work, defines the inclusions and exclusions, and helps define the expected outcomes of the QI project.*

The easiest way for all key stakeholders to agree with the scope and boundaries of your project is to show the beginning and the end of the process that is going to be targeted for improvement. This can be done well with a **high-level process diagram**, such as the SIPOC diagram.

THE TOOL: A SIPOC DIAGRAM

What Is a SIPOC Diagram?

SIPOC is an acronym for Suppliers, Inputs, Process, Outputs, and Customers. Although the name originated in the manufacturing industry, the SIPOC diagram has achieved widespread acceptance in healthcare.

The Quality Improvement Challenge: A Practical Guide for Physicians, First Edition.
Richard J. Banchs and Michael R. Pop.
© 2021 John Wiley & Sons Ltd. Published 2021 by John Wiley & Sons Ltd.
Companion website: www.wiley.com/go/banchs/quality

> **The SIPOC diagram shows a process snapshot and captures all the key activities and relevant elements in a process in order to help define the scope and boundaries of a project.**

The SIPOC diagram

- provides an easy way to visualize the process in its entirety;
- presents the process in 4–6 high-level steps;
- visually documents the relationship between suppliers, inputs, outputs, and customers; and
- clearly identifies the start and end of the process.

It is critical to understand the **start** and **end** of a process because they impact the stakeholders, the criteria used to select who should be involved in the improvement team, and the scope of the project.

Advantages of the SIPOC Diagram

Despite a lack of familiarity with its terminology, most QI teams in healthcare find the SIPOC diagram to be a great tool to define the scope and boundaries of their project. The SIPOC diagram offers numerous benefits:

- It provides an easy way to visualize the process in its entirety and to quickly understand the limits of the project. The diagram facilitates an understanding of the flow of the process for all team members.
- The team and the Primary Sponsor are better aligned with the scope and boundaries of the project.
- Relevant elements that are needed when considering the project scope are quickly captured.
- It presents a graphical depiction of the relationship between process inputs and outputs, and between suppliers and customers.
- The key stakeholders are delineated. The SIPOC diagram makes clear who needs to be included in project communications.
- Discussion is better focused on the key elements of the project.

The SIPOC diagram helps get the **Primary Sponsor,** QI team members, and key stakeholders on the same page. It also helps prevent **scope creep**, which is the tendency for ill-defined project scopes to expand over time, resulting in projects that cannot accomplish the objectives or produce the expected deliverables in the agreed upon time frame.

HOW TO DRAW A SIPOC DIAGRAM

A SIPOC diagram has five distinguishable elements (see Figure 7-1):

1. **A list of suppliers.** A supplier is a person, team, or department that provides inputs into the process. Suppliers can be technicians, physicians, nurses, materials management crews, blood bank personnel, or an entire clinical department. Suppliers, in general, do not perform the work. They provide what the "people that do the work" need to perform their duties.

2. **A list of inputs.** An input is what flows into the process. This can be people, materials, supplies, equipment, information, or data.

3. **A list of outputs:** An output is the finished product(s) or service(s) from the process or, if more detail is needed, each process step.

4. **A list of customers or end users.** As we explained in Chapter 3, a customer is the end user who receives the work product or output of the process. The ultimate customer is the patient, but in healthcare, customers can also be other end users such as physicians, nurses, technicians, or other front-line staff.

5. **A high-level view of the process.** These are the 4–6 high-level steps that are required to achieve the output.

Figure 7-2 presents a completed SIPOC diagram, for the "prescription to medication delivery" process, highlighting the suppliers, inputs, outputs, customers, and the high-level view map or steps of the process.

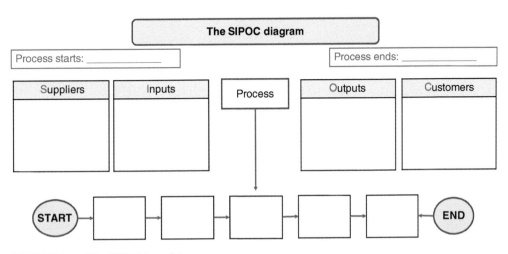

FIGURE 7-1   The SIPOC template.

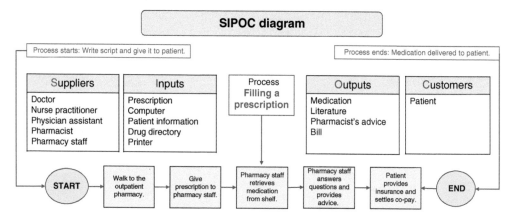

FIGURE 7-2   SIPOC diagram for "prescription to medication delivery."

Steps to Creating a SIPOC Diagram

- Identify the process's beginning and ending steps.
- Add the main process steps, selecting a maximum of 4–6 high-level steps.
- Identify the key outputs.
- Identify customers in the downstream steps, while focusing on the critical few.
- Identify the key inputs and suppliers in the upstream steps.
- Identify the critical to quality requirements for each input, process steps, and outputs.

Example: SIPOC Diagram for St. Barnabas' Preoperative Evaluation Clinic

The Preoperative Evaluation Clinic (PEC) at St. Barnabas Medical Center is staffed with three physician assistants (PAs) and one full-time anesthesiologist. At a recent meeting of the Surgical Services, a number of surgeons complained about the performance of the clinic, specifically, about delays in getting patients scheduled and a high cancellation rate on the day of surgery (DOS). Cancellations negatively affect the OR throughput, surgeon's satisfaction, and the "bottom line" for the organization. The chair of Anesthesiology decided to launch a QI project. The goal of the project was to improve efficiency by reducing the number of cancellations on the day of surgery that are due to incomplete preoperative workup. After writing a Problem Statement, and drafting their first Project Charter, the QI team decided to set the project scope and boundaries creating a SIPOC diagram (see Figure 7-3).

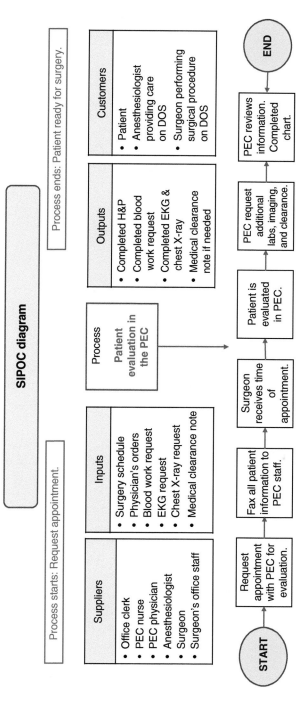

FIGURE 7-3   A SIPOC diagram for "patient evaluation in the PEC clinic."

CHAPTER 8

Who Are the "Customers," and What Do They Need?

IN HEALTHCARE, WE ALSO HAVE "CUSTOMERS"

Who Is the "Customer"?

Improving the quality of care requires a meaningful and actionable strategy and a well-organized approach. The appropriateness of the strategy, and the effectiveness of the approach, depend on a clear understanding of the problem from the customer's perspective. To clearly understand the problem we should "walk a mile in the customer's shoes." So, who is the customer?

> **The customer is the person who requires and benefits from our work product; the customer is the end user, the person who receives the output of the process we are considering.**

Before we can address a problem and understand the nature of the problem, we must identify the customer. Problems in QI can only be understood from the **customer's perspective**. If we ignore the customer, it will be difficult to truly understand the issue, focus our improvement efforts, and move the project in the right direction. *Problems should be defined using the lens of the people who experience them.*

In manufacturing, the customer is well known, and the customer's needs are well defined. Improvement efforts are focused on delivering **value** to the

The Quality Improvement Challenge: A Practical Guide for Physicians, First Edition.
Richard J. Banchs and Michael R. Pop.
© 2021 John Wiley & Sons Ltd. Published 2021 by John Wiley & Sons Ltd.
Companion website: www.wiley.com/go/banchs/quality

customer. The same happens in healthcare. Staff and providers in healthcare organizations create value for their customers. Their efforts are focused on delivering quality care and an outstanding healthcare experience. So, who are the customers in healthcare?

Three Types of Customers

In healthcare, the patient is always the ultimate and final customer. But there may be additional customers, as we described in Chapter 3. The word *customer* applies to any person who receives the work product or output of a process. **The customer is the end user of the process outcome**. Generally, there are three main customers for a QI project team to consider (see Figure 8-1):

- **Patients.** The patient is the customer. The patients' needs must drive our improvement projects. Many of our QI efforts are launched to address our patients' needs and expectations. Patients expect care that is safe, timely, effective, efficient, equitative, and patient-centered (the six dimensions of the Institute of Medicine). The patient is called the **external customer**.
- **Providers.** Sometimes the customer is not the patient. Sometimes the customer is a provider. A QI project may be initiated to address the concern of a provider or group of providers. Providers need the work product of others to do their job. Providers need: reliable information, diagnostic services, lab services, imaging services, on-time deliveries of supplies, and so on. Providers need the work product of others so they can provide effective and efficient care to their patients. Providers are called **internal customers.**
- **Staff.** The customers of a QI project can be the staff. Staff enable the delivery of care. These professionals also depend on others for information, equipment, and supplies to perform their duties and support patient care. Other people in the care value chain may be responsible for providing them with what they need to do their job. A QI project may be initiated to address their needs. Staff are also **internal customers.**

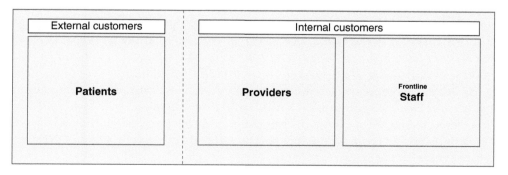

FIGURE 8-1   The three types of customers in QI projects.

Example: The Customer of a STAT Arterial Blood Gas (ABG)

The customer of a STAT ABG is the provider. The provider is the person who needs to interpret the results to make critical decisions about patient care. If the results take too long, it may affect a timely treatment. During a crisis, the timely report of the results in the EMR may be critical. What if it takes too long? A QI project may be initiated at the request of these customers to address the issue of STAT ABGs taking too long. Staff, providers, and the organization are the internal customers. Ultimately, the patient will benefit from the provider's therapeutic decisions and, of course, will always be the final customer.

THE "CUSTOMER CONTINUUM"

Within the care process, the professionals who receive the end product of a process (customers) can become, in turn, the professionals who do the work and supply services for customers of the next process. Depending on your perspective and the process you are trying to improve, a person can be the customer of a process, or the frontline professional delivering a service to another customer: a stakeholder. The customer who receives a service (the output of a process) may become the person who supplies services for the next process. The problem you are trying to address and the process you are trying to fix will determine which customer you should consider. *That is why clarity about the process's start and end is so important.* The process limits determine who you consider the customer and who are the stakeholders (the people that do the work).

Example: Supply Chain Management for Patient Care Units

Materials management receives the supplies that have been ordered from a vendor. If we consider the target the process "supply delivery to the hospital," the vendor is the stakeholder, and materials management staff are the customers. Subsequently, patient care units' supply rooms are restocked by materials management. Nurses use these supplies to restock carts in the hallways that are used by physicians on rounds. If the QI project aims to improve "the supply chain management for patient care units," the customer is the nurse, and the suppliers are materials management staff. The carts are used by the physicians on rounds to provide wound care and re-dress patient's wounds. If the QI project aims to improve the "availability of supplies during rounds," nurses become the suppliers, and physicians, the customers. This example illustrates the customer continuum, a chain with three "suppliers of service" and three customers receiving the output of the process. Depending on which portion of the process continuum (value stream) we focus on, the QI team changes and so do the boundaries and scope of the project.

The supplier (professional providing a work product)	The customer (end user that receives a work product)
Vendor: Delivers ordered supplies to the hospital	*Materials management: Receives ordered supplies*
Materials management: Stocks patient care units' supply room	*Nurse: Finds the supplies needed in the supply room*
Nurse: Restocks supply carts with wound dressing supplies	*Physician: Finds needed supplies. Uses wound dressing supplies from supply cart to change patients' dressings*

THE VOICE OF THE CUSTOMER (VOC)

What Is the "Voice of the Customer"?

A successful improvement project cannot be launched on the basis of our opinions, beliefs, or assumptions about the problem. It must be substantiated by a true assessment of the situation that includes a clear understanding of the nature of the problem from the perspective of the internal or external customer.

> **The Voice of the Customer (VOC) is the expression of the collective needs, wants, preferences, and expectations of the customers.**

The first step in finding the "Right Problem" is to understand and define the problem from the perspective of the customer. The VOC uses the customer's input to define the needs and requirements of the service or care that is being provided. As discussed previously, customers can be patients, providers, or staff. The VOC is critical to the project team because

- It helps us understand the main drivers of quality and customer satisfaction.
- It allow us to focus our improvement efforts.
- It sets the priorities, scope, and goals for the project.

Quotable quote: "The first step in exceeding your patients' expectations is to know those expectations." Roy H. Williams

The "What" and "How" of the Voice of the Customer

Patients, providers, and staff are the customers of our healthcare processes. They expect an outcome (VOC). The outcome must have certain **attributes** and must be delivered within certain **requirements**. The VOC therefore has two distinct components (see Figure 8-2):

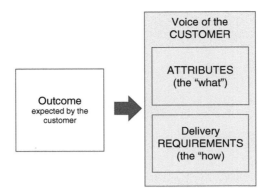

FIGURE 8-2   The outcome expected by the customer (VOC) is defined by attributes and requirements.

1. **The "what" (attributes).** This is the needed outcome, and the attributes of the outcome the customer (patient, provider, or staff) expects. A patient expects an "effective treatment," "clear instructions," and "clean facilities." Alternatively, when a physician is the customer of a process, he or she might expect an "accurate diagnosis," a "centered chest X-ray," or the "correct demographic information."
2. **The "how" (requirements).** These are the requirements that characterize the outcome (output). Patients expect care delivered "on-time" or in a "culturally sensitive" manner. Physicians would expect a chest X-ray (needed outcome) to show up in the EMR "in a timely fashion," and the radiologist's official reading to be "easily found in the EMR."

The customer (patient, staff, or provider) defines quality by identifying

- the needed (expected) outcome.
- the attributes of the outcome, and
- the requirements that characterize the outcome.

Fulfilling the attributes (the "what") and requirements (the "how") of the VOC results in customer satisfaction. Achieving customers' satisfaction is the ultimate goal of the QI project.

HOW DO WE COLLECT THE VOC?

Interviews

Interviews allow QI teams to get qualitative information about the needs and preferences of customers. Speaking to people that are the end users of the process and experience the problem can help us gain valuable information about the nature of the problem. It allows us to learn what the customer deems important and helps create a clear image about the customer's needs and expectations. Interviews with the customers should be conducted at the beginning of the project to understand the issues. Interviews can also be conducted in the middle of a project to clarify important points, better understand the problem, or test potential ideas with the customers. Before conducting an interview, be clear about the what you are trying to achieve and the goal of the interview. Here are some steps you should take to maximize the return on investment of your interview.

Before the interview:
- Select your customer's segment carefully.
- Decide on the criteria you are going to use for selecting interviewees.
- Prepare a list of questions.
- Decide on the interview method (face-to-face, phone, other).
- Set an appropriate time and place.

During the interview:
- Introduce yourself.
- Clearly define the purpose of the interview.
- Get consent if needed.
- Listen carefully and take good notes.
- Practice active listening.
- Collect additional information about the customer if needed.
- Thank all participants when done.

It's best to get the VOC in person; talking to patients, staff, or providers at the time and location where they receive the end product of the process, whether that be receiving care (patients), or what they need to perform their work (staff and providers). If this is not possible, try to fund other alternatives that get you as close as possible.

One type of interview is a **focus group**. A focus group is a gathering of a selected number of people from the population of interest who participate in a facilitated discussion intended to elicit their opinions and perceptions about a particular issue or service. A focus group allows guests to interact. The format is flexible and follows a loose structure. It allows different groups to be invited around a single area of interest.

Surveys

A survey provides quantitative and qualitative information about a large population of customers. A survey can also be used as preliminary tool to gather information and identify a target population, and subsequently conduct an interview. When preparing a survey, we recommend these steps:

1. Develop the objectives.

2. Calculate the sample size. Use standard formulas as needed (you can easily find them online).

3. Draft each question and determine the measurement scale. Numeric scales are often easier to work with but qualitative scales are sometimes needed. If necessary, include a "not applicable" category.

4. Determine how you are going to code the survey to maintain anonymity.

5. Make sure you conduct a pilot to assure the questions probe the correct issues and the answers are appropriate to the questions. Nothing is more disappointing than to find the survey you worked hard to design and administer is not fulfilling its purpose.

6. Decide how you will send the survey (email, mail, fax, download from web page, etc.).

7. Decide on the timeline and how you are going to get the surveys back.

Questionnaires designed in the United States may not be valid when applied to patients from other countries, as there may be disparities in patient expectations and cultural biases.

When direct methods for soliciting feedback are not available, indirect ways such as emails, phone interviews, or letters can be used to ensure that the needs and expectations of the customers are known.

CRITICAL-TO-QUALITY (CTQ)

What are the CTQs?

Patients, providers, and staff are customers in our healthcare processes. They expect an outcome:

- The outcome must have certain **attributes** and must be delivered within certain **requirements** (VOC).
- The customer also defines the **specifications** for both the attributes and requirements of the final outcome.

> **The customer (patient, staff, or provider) defines quality by identifying the outcome, the attributes of the outcome, and the requirements that characterize the outcome. The customer also defines the specifications for both the attributes and the requirements.**

Patients know what they mean when they say that something is "good." Our job is to help translate their statement into specific attributes and requirement that can be measured, tracked, and improved.

Patients' needs and expectations are at times vague and nondescriptive. Specificity is needed to address the identified gaps between our current performance and the needs of our customers. A method designed to focus on the critical issues needed to achieve customers' satisfaction with the outcome involves developing Critical-to-Quality (CTQ) requirements, or CTQs.

The CTQs are key measurable characteristics of service or care whose performance standards or **specifications** must be met in order to satisfy the customer (see Figure 8-3).

Patient or customer needs and expectations come in all forms, shapes, and length of detail. Before we can move forward, these expectations need to be identified, organized, and understood. The CTQs help with this important task. The CTQs translate

> **The CTQs translate general and difficult-to-measure customer needs or desires into very *specific* and *measurable* attributes and requirements of customer satisfaction. The CTQs are the quantifiable expectations of the customer.**

the broad needs and requirements of the customer (patients, staff, and providers), the VOC, into specific, actionable, and measurable performance attributes and requirements that provide direction for the project's goals and activities.

Remember, improving a process and achieving patient or customer satisfaction are the underlying targets of the QI project. Developing CTQ requirements allows us to define the expectations of the customer (i.e. quality from the customer's perspective), and set the goal and aims of the project. Once we understand what is critical for the customer, we can

- Define our current performance.
- Define the gap in performance and understand the magnitude of the problem.
- Set the scope for the project.

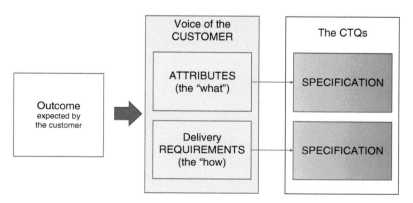

FIGURE 8-3   The CTQs are the specifications of the Voice of the Customer

- Define the goals of the improvement initiative.
- Set the targets we need to achieve.

Because patients, providers, and staff are the customers of our healthcare processes, CTQs are the **critical patients' requirements**, **critical physicians' requirements**, or the **critical staff's requirements** whose performance standards or specifications must be met in order to meet their expectations.

THE CRITICAL-TO-QUALITY TREE

From the Voice of the Customer, the CTQs can be developed using a tree diagram. **The CTQ tree** is a diagram-based tool used to organize identified specifications of an outcome's attributes and requirements that the customer expects.

A tree diagram provides the clarity and structure needed to develop CTQs and focus our improvement efforts. To create a CTQ tree, follow these six steps:

1. **Define the customer.** First, find the customer of your process.
2. **Get the Voice of the Customer**. Use interviews, surveys, or any other means to get the customer's needs and expectations. Record the VOC statements. Make sure you write down the attributes and requirements of each outcome they expect.
3. **Aggregate the VOC statements into families with similar meaning.** Combine the statements from the VOC according to categories or topics. Group ideas or statements with similar meaning. Topic categories could be: "expectations of the clinic environment"; "quality of clinical care"; "staff and physician interaction"; "the registration process" and so on. You may want to repeat these steps for each customer segment.
4. **For each family, create the drivers.** For each family or group of statements, create the "drivers" or single word or short sentence that defines the group. Ask yourself, "What do all these statements have in common? What attributes or requirements of the outcome are customers referring to?" Use the word or sentence that best describes the idea.
5. **Develop the specifications or CTQs.** For each driver or group of statements, drill down to the specifics. What does the driver mean to the customer (patient, staff, provider)? What are the technical characteristics? How can it be measured? What are the specifics? How can you operationalize it in the clinical setting? Identify one or more specific and measurable characteristics for each driver, that the process must satisfy to provide the high-quality care or level of service the customer expects. You may need to go back to the patients or customer groups and clarify the exact meaning and specifics for each driver.
6. **Validate the CTQ tree.** Validate the CTQs (attributes and requirements) with the customer. Ask the customers if this is what they mean and ask them if they agree with your characterization of their needs and expectations.

Once you and your team create the CTQ requirements, you will have a better chance to define metrics and focus the QI project on specifics. Project metrics are key to evaluating the success of the project in meeting the patient or customer's expectations.

Example: Patient Satisfaction with UI Health Outpatient Care Center

If our QI project aimed to improve patient satisfaction with UI Health Outpatient Care Center, we would first need to define what are the attributes and requirements of a visit to the Center that deliver the experience the patient expects. The first step would be to get the Voice of the Customer. Remember, these statements are usually too broad and lack specificity to be used as guidance in our improvement efforts. Once we got the VOC, we would develop the CTQs, or specifications that are going to make our patients' statements meaningful, specific, and more importantly, measurable. To do this, we would group the VOC statements with similar meaning into families and then ask ourselves, "What do these statements have in common?" We would then summarize each group or family of statements into single-word descriptors or "drivers" of patient satisfaction. We may need to dig deeper within the VOC statements to find specifics, or go back to patients to ask questions about the drivers. This would allow us to create one or more CTQ for each driver. The CTQs are the specifications for the attributes and requirements of the outcome the patient expects. In the UIH clinic example, CTQs would be: "greeted with a smile"; "registered within 5 minutes"; "accurate information"; "seen by provider within 30 minutes of my arrival"; and "availability of guest features." The great thing about a CTQ is that it can be measured to establish our current performance, and audited to assess the degree to which we are continuing to achieve patient satisfaction (see Figure 8-4).

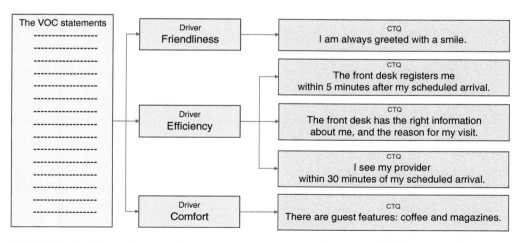

FIGURE 8-4   The attributes and requirements for patient satisfaction (CTQs) at UI Health Outpatient Care Center.

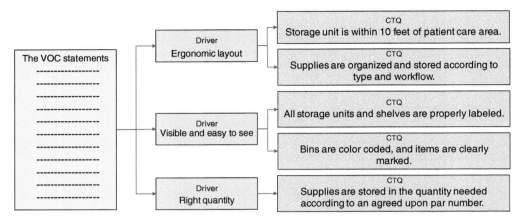

FIGURE 8-5   The attributes and requirements for staff and provider satisfaction (CTQs) with the organization of clinical supplies in the ED's resuscitation room.

Example: Improving the Organization of Medical Supplies in the EDRR

Assume you wanted to improve the organization of medical supplies in the emergency department's resuscitation room (EDRR). First, you would need to define what attributes and requirements characterize a well-organized EDRR. What does "well-organized" really mean for providers and staff (the customer!)? How do they define it? What are the specific characteristics of the layout, organization of cabinets, and shelving that make it so? Following the steps outlined before, we would collect the Voice of the Customer, find the "drivers," and, with a bit more work, develop one or more CTQs for each driver. It is always a good idea to validate the CTQs with front line providers and staff (see Figure 8-5).

EXERCISE: CTQS FOR THE NEW WOMEN'S CENTER

The new Women's Center at Lake Hospital had been up and running for the last three months. Dr. Sonia Watson decided it was time to launch a couple of improvement projects to improve patient care. She was eager to provide the community with the kind of service they had long waited for and deserved. For her first QI project, she decided to focus her efforts on mammographies, specifically to improve the appointment, registration, and follow-up processes. Dr. Watson and her staff held several focus groups within the community to better understand their patients' needs and expectations, get feedback from previous experiences, and identify critical requirements of patient satisfaction. The team recorded the following statements from their interviews:

- "When I go to a clinic, it's really important for me to have staff that is kind and understanding."
- "Mammograms are no fun! A smile at the other end is always welcomed."

- "I really appreciate it when I receive a timely phone call from the doctor with my test results; ideally I should get it within a day or two after my scheduled appointment."
- "My technician took good care of me during the procedure; she let me know what she was doing so I knew what to expect."
- "It's frustrating when I call to make an appointment and I cannot be seen for a month; I should be able to be seen in a week."
- "The technologist that did my mammogram listen to my concerns and explained the procedure well."
- "A text message is helpful to keep my appointments on track."
- "I find it stressful to wait for test results for days on end and not hear back from my doctor; I think we should be called with results within a day or two."
- "The staff at the clinic were really helpful; they gave me clear instructions as to when I would be getting my results back."
- "I want to be able to get the results of a mammogram within a day or two in case it's cancer! I don't want to wait."
- "I prefer to be seen sooner than later; the procedure is not pleasant and it makes me nervous having to wait to come in."
- "I like when follow-up appointments are scheduled during my appointment so I don't have to call back once I leave."
- "The clinic should provide us with some kind of written material so we can understand what is going to happen, as well next steps in case there is something wrong with my mammogram."
- "Written instructions at the time of discharge are really helpful for me."
- "Having a lump in your breast and not knowing if it is cancer is horrible, and the wait is agonizing."
- "A text or an email reminder is a great thing to remind me when I am due for my next appointment; it really helps me not to forget my annual visits."
- "My technologist was really helpful during the procedure; she smiled and made me feel comfortable."

From the VOC, develop the CTQs. Follow these steps:

- Group customer feedback (VOC) into families of statements with similar meaning. If needed, use an affinity diagram.
- For each family of statements, create the drivers, single words or short sentences, that summarize the idea, need, or expectation expressed by the VOC statements.
- For each driver, develop one or more CTQs; drill down to the specifics. Ask yourself: What does the driver or key word really mean to the patient? How can we measure it? Can you assign a specific descriptor? Make sure your CTQs are specific and measurable.

REVIEW QUIZ

1. What does VOC stand for?
   A. Vick's Organic Cough-drops
   B. Victory over crisis
   C. Voice of the Customer
   D. Very old canary
   E. Voice of the Consumer

2. In the healthcare environment, we call a "customer"
   A. the supplier of a product or service,
   B. the person who does the work,
   C. the person who provides a product or service,
   D. the person who receives a product or service: the end user, or
   E. the goal of the improvement project.

3. Which of the following statements is TRUE?
   A. The customer is the person who requires and benefits from our work product.
   B. In healthcare, the customer is always the patient.
   C. Providers and hospital staff are always the stakeholders, never the customers.
   D. Patients are the internal customers.
   E. Providers and staff are the external customers.

4. All the following statements regarding the VOC are true EXCEPT
   A. the VOC defines needs and requirements of the customer,
   B. the VOC is how the customer defines quality,
   C. the VOC is always clear and needs no further clarification,
   D. the VOC sets the priorities of the QI project, or
   E. the VOC helps focus improvement efforts.

5. Critical Customer Requirements
   A. facilitate prioritizing the most important issues to address,
   B. translate very general and difficult to measure customer needs and desires,
   C. need to be specific and measurable,
   D. allow us to organize and categorize customer needs and expectations, or
   E. all of the above

Key: 1c, 2d, 3a, 4c, 5e

CHAPTER 9

Who Are the "Stakeholders," and What Challenges Do They Have?

THE FRONTLINE STAKEHOLDERS

The frontline professionals are called stakeholders. Stakeholders are the people doing the work. Stakeholders include staff, providers, clinical leaders, and hospital administrators.

> **Stakeholders are the professionals with the subject-matter expertise and knowledge of the process who understand the system and do the work.**

The stakeholders have a vested interest in the functioning of the process. They are sometimes referred to as the **Process Owners**. They are the people who experience either the "pain or the gain" of the process' performance. If the process is not performing well, stakeholders are directly impacted and suffer the consequences. Therefore, they are an interested party in the improvement project and an important component of the improvement efforts. Stakeholders have the expertise we need to improve.

THE VOICE OF THE STAKEHOLDERS

> **The Voice of the Stakeholder (VOS) is the expression of the requirements of the frontline professionals.**

The Quality Improvement Challenge: A Practical Guide for Physicians, First Edition.
Richard J. Banchs and Michael R. Pop.
© 2021 John Wiley & Sons Ltd. Published 2021 by John Wiley & Sons Ltd.
Companion website: www.wiley.com/go/banchs/quality

The perspectives of the frontline stakeholders must be considered if we are to get a clear understanding of the problem and develop optimal solutions. We cannot fully address the needs and requirements of our customers (patients, providers, and staff) without understanding and addressing the challenges experienced by the stakeholders. *Customer requirements, and the ability of the stakeholder to fulfill their needs and expectations, are intimately interrelated.*

Critical-to-Quality (CTQs) requirements help us understand the specific and measurable requirements for customer satisfaction. This information is critical to guide our improvement effort, but it is not enough if we want sustainable improvements. We also need to understand the issues that prevent frontline stakeholders from delivering the services that customers expect. The perspective of the front line is critical to understanding the *nature of the problem, the drivers of stakeholder's performance and motivation, and ultimately to gain stakeholder's project buy-in.*

The VOS adds an additional dimension to understanding the nature of the problem from the perspective of the people who actually "do the work." This "work" can be caring for patients, delivering supplies, educating residents, collecting insurance information, communicating with patients, or providing diagnostic services. The VOS is a critical element of every project. Without it, we may not be able to understand the true nature of the problem.

The VOS

- lends credibility to our efforts to improve the process,
- creates motivation for improvemen,
- helps obtain the front line's buy-in for the QI project, and
- helps sustain the improvements once they have been implemented.

Let's say we want to improve patient flow in the pediatric clinic. You decide to assemble a QI team. Baseline performance shows long **lead times** for patients (patient-in to patient-out time). What's the problem? You decide to document the VOS, stakeholders being the frontline professionals (physicians, nurses, physician assistants, and administrative staff) who provide services and care for patients coming to the clinic. How is their ability to deliver quality care impacted? Are the scheduled visit times appropriate for the type of patients that come to the clinic? Do administrative personnel at the front desk have all the information they need to register patients? Are there enough examining rooms to make the flow of work efficient? When physicians perform a physical exam, do they have what they need? These and other factors affect the flow of work and may be responsible for the long lead time that patients experience. Without understanding the problem from the stakeholders' perspective, any attempts to improve workflow will fail.

As with the Voice of the Customer (VOC), we can get the Voice of the Stakeholder (VOS) using interviews, surveys, and, of course, face-to-face at staff meetings and other informal gatherings.

THE CRITICAL NEEDS OF THE STAKEHOLDERS

What Are the Critical Needs?

Stakeholders know what they need to do their jobs. But often the expression of what they need lacks the specificity required to be used as one of the goals of our QI project. Developing the Critical Needs (CN) help translate general statements into more specific requirements for performance that can be measured, tracked, and improved.

> **The Critical Needs (CNs) translate very general and difficult-to-measure requirements of stakeholders (VOS) into very specific and measurable needs and requirements of the front line's ability to deliver quality care.**

The CNs need to be specific, actionable, and measurable to optimize stakeholders' *performance.* The CNs of the stakeholder can be developed using a diagram–based tool such as the **Critical Needs tree.** The CN tree follows the same format used to develop CTQ attributes and requirements of customer satisfaction. A tree diagram provides the clarity and structure needed for focusing the improvement efforts. The CNs tree allows us to drill down to the specific needs that stakeholders must have to do their "job" properly and successfully. *Critical needs can be measured, tracked, and improved.*

Example: Improving MRI Patient Throughput

You are a leader of a QI team tasked with improving patient throughput in the *MRI suite. After collecting the VOC and developing your CTQs, you proceed to* *collect the VOS. Stakeholders are the MRI technician and supervisors for the two* *MRI shifts. Using the VOS, you proceed to develop a CNs tree. The critical needs* *and requirements of these stakeholders drive MRI performance. In this example,* *"patients arrive on-time," "MRI orders are appropriate, complete and accurate,"* *and "patients are ready to be scanned" would be the main drivers of stakeholder* *performance* (see Figure 9-1).

THE SECOND TOLLGATE REVIEW

Periodically, the improvement team needs to confirm that they are on the right track to achieve their project objectives. This is best done through a tollgate review with the primary sponsor. A tollgate review is a go/no-go checkpoint where the team leader,

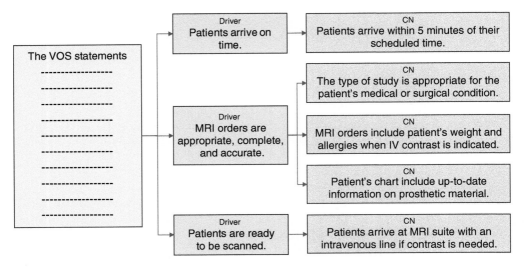

FIGURE 9-1   Critical Needs tree defining the requirements for optimal performance of the MRI staff.

team members, and the primary sponsor meet to discuss ongoing project activities; review results and deliverables; and assure the project is on track. The second tollgate review should be scheduled with the primary sponsor soon after completing the CNs tree, at the end of the second "R": the "right problem" (see Chapter 25).

REVIEW QUIZ

1. What is another name for a stakeholder?
    A. Supplier
    B. Frontline professional or process owner
    C. Team leader
    D. Customer
    E. Patient

2. Stakeholders
    A. are the frontline healthcare professionals,
    B. are professionals directly affected by the QI project,
    C. have the subject-matter expertise,
    D. experience the "pain or gain" of the process, or
    E. all of the above

3. Which of these methods can be used to obtain the Voice of the Stakeholder (VOS)?
    A. Surveys
    B. Face-to-face discussions
    C. Emails
    D. Staff meetings
    E. All of the above

4. Regarding the VOS, all of the following are true EXCEPT
   A. collecting the VOS lends credibility to our QI efforts,
   B. the VOS helps us deliver services and care that meet the needs of the patients,
   C. the VOS is not important for the success of the QI project,
   D. collecting the VOS helps get buy-in for the QI project from the front lines, or
   E. the VOS is needed to understand the determinants of stakeholders' performance.

5. The Critical Needs (CNs) of the stakeholder
   A. can be developed using a tree diagram,
   B. translate the broad needs of the stakeholder into actionable and measurable requirements,
   C. are specific,
   D. are measurable, or
   E. all of the above

Key: 1b; 2e, 3e, 4c, 5e

PART V

THE FOURTH "R": THE RIGHT CAUSE

CHAPTER 10

To Understand a Process, You Need to "Go See" and Create a Map

STORIES FROM THE FRONT LINES OF HEALTHCARE: ANDREA, THE QI PROJECT MANAGER

Andrea agreed with the hospital's senior leadership team to work to improve the emergency department's (ED) core measure results. It was decided the focus would be on the "door-to-provider (DtP) time," or the time it took for a patient to see a provider after entering the ED. After reviewing the available data, Andrea interviewed the ED's medical director, nursing director, and nursing manager. Andrea then decided it was time to walk the process for her first direct contact and observation. She sat at the greeter's desk with the ED clerk, who was the first point of contact for every walk-in patient. The clerk's job was to ask the patients why they had come to the ED, and perform a quick registration before sending them to a side room to wait for the triage nurse to call them. At one point during the observation, Andrea noticed several people lined up and waiting at the greeter's desk. The ED clerk asked patients politely to fill a short form, and then methodically entered the information in the computer while the patient stood at the front desk. One after the other, patients waited their turn to give the information to the clerk. When all was done, Andrea inquired about the reason to have patients wait while the information was entered in the computer. The ED clerk responded that this was the "way we have always done registration."

The Quality Improvement Challenge: A Practical Guide for Physicians, First Edition.
Richard J. Banchs and Michael R. Pop.
© 2021 John Wiley & Sons Ltd. Published 2021 by John Wiley & Sons Ltd.
Companion website: www.wiley.com/go/banchs/quality

What was affecting workflow efficiency? How did Andrea uncover the problem?

THE FIRST STEP IS TO "GO SEE"

Every improvement project must start with a visit to the place where staff and providers interact with the customers. Remember, customers can be internal (staff and providers) or external (patients). To truly understand the nature of the problem you must first "go see." Without a clear understanding of how work is being performed, you may miss valuable clues and may be unable to find the true causes of the problem you are trying to address.

The "gemba"

To see, you must go to the gemba. The word *gemba,* meaning "the actual place," comes from Japan, the birthplace of Lean methodology.

> **The gemba is the place where work is done and value is created. We go to the gemba to see the process in motion.**

The gemba can be the operating room, the emergency room, central supply, the main laboratory, or the neonatal intensive care unit. Important information about how work is performed is often not shared with the QI team verbally because it is so ingrained in the culture and status quo of the work place that it becomes second nature to the frontline stakeholders. By going to the gemba, we can truly see how work is performed. Our goal in going to the gemba is to accomplish the following:

- Directly observe the work being done.
- Understand the sequence and order of the steps of the processes.
- Elicit the input and perspective of the people who do the work; these are the stakeholders or subject-matter experts.
- Verify whether the information shared by the frontline stakeholder matches what is actually done.
- Confirm our beliefs or change our opinion about how the process really works.
- Evaluate the functioning of the team during the performance of the work.

To make a visit to the gemba a success, follow these two important rules:

1. **Introduce yourself.** Introduce yourself and clearly state that the purpose for being at the gemba is to learn and understand how work is done. Make it clear that you are not there to judge people's performance or report their activities to

the boss. Once you have introduced yourself, silently observe the process for a period of time without speaking unless clarification is needed. Take notes.

2. **Get feedback.** At the end of your visit, ask to meet with key stakeholders. Engage them to validate your findings so everybody can get a common understanding of how "work is really done." This is best achieved by creating a graphic sketch of what you see and then use it to discuss each step with the stakeholders.

By spending time at the gemba and asking frontline stakeholders clarifying questions, *we uncover undisclosed information and conditions that might affect workflow efficiency and effectiveness.* By going to the gemba, we do more than just observe the process:

- We show respect for the people at the front line.
- We communicate that their opinion matters.
- We show we want to understand the conditions under which the work is being done.

AT THE GEMBA YOU SEE THE SYSTEM

What Is a System?

When we go to the gemba we see the frontline professionals doing their work in their natural work environment. What we see is the "system" at work. The clinical and operational outcomes we get in healthcare are the result of the "way we do things." The way we do things is a function of the people, structures, and processes with which we work. The people, structures, and processes form the system.

> **A System is a planned, organized, and purposeful structure with interrelated and interdependent elements that follow a set of detailed methods, procedures and routines to create and deliver a product, provide care, or achieve a goal.**

The results we get are the product of the interaction of all the components of the system that interplay to generate the output (outcome). **To improve an output (outcome), we must first understand the system that generates the output.** All systems have inputs, outputs, feedback mechanisms, and boundaries. They maintain (or aim to maintain) an internal steady-state. An analogy of a simple system and its interdependent elements is a team of four runners in a 4 × 100 meter relay race. The goal of the team is to win the overall race. Even if the team is made up of the four fastest runners in the world, it does not mean a certain victory. Those runners must have a plan, execute excellent hand offs of the baton between each other, as well as run a fast race. Runners need the appropriate equipment. Each runner is dependent on the next runner to actively engage in the baton hand off and not drop the baton.

> *Quotable quote: "Every system is perfectly designed to get the results it gets. If you want different results. . .you need to change the system."*
>
> *Paul Batalden*

System Components

In healthcare, as in other fields, systems are the sum of a number of components that combine to produce an output or outcome (see Figure 10-1). A system has the following interrelated and interdependent elements all combined to produce a specific outcome:

- **The vision, mission, and culture of the healthcare organization.** The vision is the reason for existence of the healthcare organization; the mission is the plan of how to achieve the vision; the vision, mission, and culture determine how the system is managed.
- **Healthcare organization's business principles.** These are foundational statements that guide the behavior of the healthcare organization, department, providers and staff.
- **The leadership structures.** Defines how workflow, accountability, and authority in an organization, department, or unit is structured.
- **Goals and targets**. These are the agreed-on statements of what the organization, department, or unit wants to achieve; with the goals and targets, leadership can establish the specific actions and steps required to achieve them.

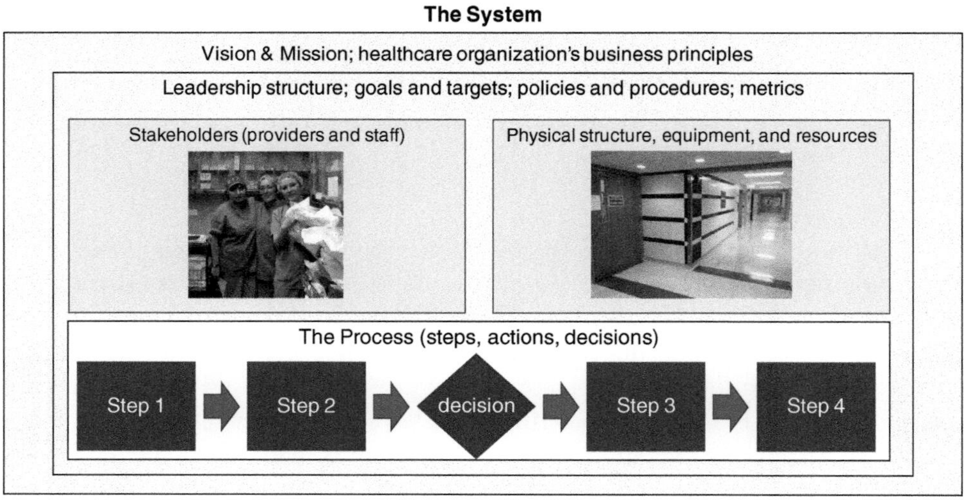

FIGURE 10-1   Components of the system.

- **Work processes.** A process is a set of interrelated or interacting steps, decisions, and actions that allow inputs to be transformed into outputs; a process is "how work is done." Leadership defines the work processes; the work processes in turn define the outputs or results that our customers (patients, providers, and staff) experience.

- **Policies and procedures.** Policies are the rules and guidelines formulated and designed to influence the activities carried out by the organization, department, or division. Procedures are specific methods used to operationalize the policies in the day-to-day operations. Policies and procedures assure goals and targets are translated into the steps that result in the outcome the organization, department, or unit desires.

- **The metrics used: measures of effectiveness and efficiency.** Metrics of effectiveness help us assess the extent to which we can meet or exceed the customer's needs or requirements. Metrics of efficiency help us assess the quantity of resources, including time, personnel, and money consumed in working to achieve effectiveness.

- **Stakeholders.** Stakeholders are the professionals with the subject-matter expertise and knowledge of the process who understand the system and do the work.

- **Physical structures and equipment.** What allows work (service, patient care, etc.) to be done.

"Systems Thinking"

To improve, we need to understand the system and follow a structured approach to uncover the root causes of the complex performance problem of the system. To improve we need **systems thinking.**

> **Systems thinking is a way to view a problem from a broad perspective that includes seeing the system and its overall elements, structures, cycles, feedback mechanisms, and handoffs as contributors to the problem of undesirable outcomes.**

Following the concept and logic of systems thinking, to improve we need to understand the system and the interaction of all its factors. To improve we need to follow a systematic approach with defined steps:

- Understand the mission, vision, and management of the system.
- Understand the leadership structure, goals, targets, policies, procedures, and the measurements used in the system.
- Define the outcome y we want to improve.

- Define the process(es) that is/are responsible for the outcome; to define the process we need the steps, actions, decisions, and handoffs that generate the outcome; we need to understand how work is done.
- Find possible causes, or x, of the outcome y.
- Filter and prioritize the most likely cause or critical x of the outcome y (the cause with the greatest impact). *Note:* There may be more than one critical cause x, and therefore we may need more than one solution.
- Find possible solutions, or s; filter and prioritize the best solution; pilot the best solution.
- Apply the best solution s to get the outcome we desire.

Quotable quote: To improve, you need to "deconstruct the conditions that created the problem." Bryan Stevenson

IT'S ALL ABOUT THE PROCESS

Improvement starts with the process. To improve an outcome, focus first on the process that generates that outcome. Healthcare improvement initiatives arise in an effort to deliver better patient care and provide the inputs and resources providers and staff need. Every outcome is the result of a system, and at the center of the system is the process (see Figure 10-2).

> **A process is defined as the collection of related steps, actions, decisions, and handoffs that are used to transform inputs into outputs.**

The degree to which we deliver care, positively impact our patients' experience, and provide the inputs and resources staff and providers need are the result of the performance of a process. When we talk about improving quality, what we usually mean is improving an outcome that is unsatisfactory in some way. This outcome, whether clinical, operational, or service-related, is the result of a process. The process is the way we do things. **It is often said that improvement is the science of "process improvement."** Some processes may need to be tweaked. Others will have to be redesigned to really improve the quality of care and the healthcare experience.

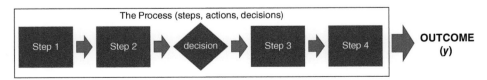

FIGURE 10-2   A process is a series of interrelated steps, actions, and decisions.

Thoughtful redesign, when necessary, will allow us to move beyond antiquated paradigms about how we plan, organize and provide care.

THE PROCESS MAP

The best way to understand how a process works is by creating a picture. The best picture in QI is a map. All processes that need to be improved should be first mapped to ensure our understanding of how work is actually being done.

> **A Process Map is a graphic representation of a process that shows the steps, actions, decisions, and handoffs that are used to transform inputs into outputs.**

A Process Map has several goals including

- Define the current state. That is, how is the work being done now?
- Graphically show the sequence of steps, actions, and handoffs that we routinely follow when performing a task.
- Build a common understanding of the entire process that enables everyone to get on the **same page**: the Primary Sponsor, QI team, and frontline stakeholders.
- Highlight areas in need of improvement by targeting **waste, workarounds,** and **bottlenecks.**
- Create a common vision for a future state (a better state!).

General Recommendations When Creating a Map

When creating a map

- Start by reviewing your Project Charter or SIPOC diagram to find the beginning and end of your process; this will determine the beginning and the end of your map.
- Decide what type of process map and desired level of detail works best for your project (see later for different mapping techniques).
- Go to the gemba to get an accurate and precise picture directly where work is done.
- It is best to **walk the entire process** from beginning to end, and see it for yourself.
- Use a **high-level map** when trying to define the boundaries of a process and scope of the project, or use **detail mapping** when you are interested in defining each step and action.
- Document the process title, dates, and authors on each version.

Schedule multiple observations, as not all work is done in the same manner every time. You will need to observe several frontline professionals performing the process at different times in order to get a sense of the most common way of performing tasks. Multiple observations will also allow you to see whether the performance of the task varies significantly from person-to-person. Like the Project Charter, maps are *living documents* that should be modified and updated when changes occur. Make sure your map is available for team meetings and refer to it frequently to understand the process.

Steps to Completing Your Map

- **Communicate your purpose.** The purpose of the mapping process must be clearly communicated to the frontline stakeholders (physicians, nurses, technicians, and staff working in that area) before you arrive at the gemba. Knowing the purpose will establish needed trust. Are you there to "see and report your observations to the boss"? Should they be concerned? Are they going to "get in trouble"? You should clarify the reasons for your presence and the goals of mapping while articulating that your primary interest is in the process, not the people who perform the process.
- **Create your first draft.** Draw a draft of the process steps using pen and paper or sticky notes. Draw first the major steps to accurately depict steps, actions, and decision points. Number each step in the order you see them. A good way to create a draft is to post the sticky notes on a Post-It 25×30 Easel Pad on the wall to visualize the entire sequence, and connect the steps with arrows in the direction work is being done.
- **Add additional information.** Check the flow, the sequence of steps, and the hand off points between each step. Add the steps of smaller sub-processes that flow into your main stream. Include information about each step as required. For each step you may want to add information about number of people performing the step, amount of time each step takes, equipment used, and any other information pertinent to that step. You can also add information on the movement of people, patients, material, or machines. List any problems you observe on a separate sheet of paper.
- **Ask questions.** Engage the key stakeholders in your process mapping. The stakeholders are the subject-matter experts working on the front line. Ask questions, clarify your observations, and seek their expertise as you are completing the map. Some good questions to start with may be: Who provides you the work? In what format does it arrive? What do you do with it? Who do you pass the work on to? In what format, and what do they do with it? What is the order of your tasks?
- **Create a common understanding of the process.** Meet with the team, process owners (the people responsible for the process), and stakeholders after completing the first draft of the process map. Validate it and revise it accordingly. Include customers and suppliers, if appropriate. If there are several ways

work is being sequenced, pick one to build your "current state" process map but note the different ways work is being done.

- **Create a digital copy.** Use any of the available software packages to create a digital copy of your map. Microsoft Visio® is a good alternative. Visio is part of the Microsoft Office Suite of products used to create layouts, diagrams, decision diagrams, flowcharts, and maps.

The Three Most Common Types of Mapping Techniques

There are several mapping techniques available. The choice depends on the type of problem you are trying to address and the goals you want to achieve. Consider these three as the more common mapping techniques:

1. **Basic Process Flow map.** This map will help you and your team understand the sequence of steps, actions, and decisions in a process.
2. **The Swim Lane chart.** This map will help you and your team focus on workloads and handoffs. It is a useful map for processes that cross functional boundaries.
3. **The Value Stream map**. This map shows the flows of information, work, and time in a process. It includes time and process efficiency metrics; it is a very valuable map to identify bottlenecks, constraints, steps and activities that do not add value to the process.

BASIC PROCESS FLOW MAP

Think of the Basic Process Flow map as an *algorithm* or a clinical pathway. Like an algorithm, a Basic Process Flow map is a graphic depiction of the sequence of steps, actions and decisions of the process or work that are being done.

> **A Basic Process Flow map is used to delineate the entire process in a graphical format, outlining the sequence of the individual steps, actions, and decision points used to provide a service.**

The goal of the Process Map is to provide an understanding of how work is performed by the front line. A Basic Process Flow map may also include the flow of documents involved in the process. However, it does not indicate the amount of time each step takes or any specific data pertaining to the process steps. Other types of mapping techniques are better suited to convey this type of information (see next). There are a number of basic shapes (symbols) commonly used when creating a Basic Process Flow map (see Figure 10-3).

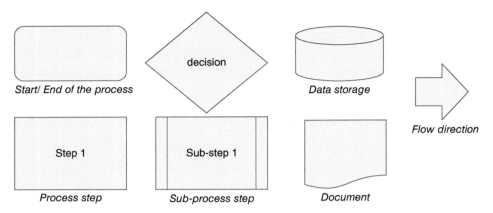

FIGURE 10-3   The Basic Process Flow map symbols.

Step to creating a Process Map:

- Determine the start and end-points of the process.
- Capture the steps of the process. Use paper and pencil or write each step of the process on a Post-it® note.
- Arrange the steps in the proper sequence.
- Identify the decisions points.
- Connect each symbol with arrows.
- Add any other pertinent information that will help you understand how work is done.
- Meet with the stakeholders to review and validate the process steps and sequence.

Create your draft using pencil and paper or Post-it® notes. Final versions can be made using Microsoft Visio® or Minitab Companion® (see an example in Figure 10-4).

"Must-haves" for all Basic Process Flow maps:

- Name of the process,
- Name of the authors,
- Date and revision level,
- Clearly identifiable start and finish points of the process,
- All the steps and decisions points with a consistent level of detail through-out the map, and
- Key of symbols and definitions.

You may also want to add photographs of key steps to enhance your understanding.

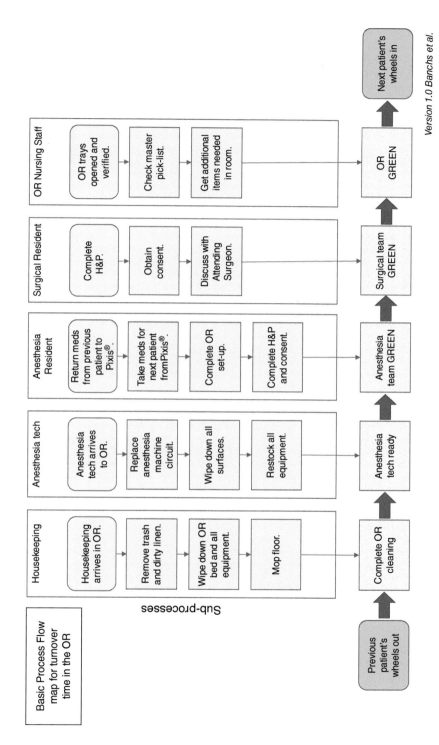

FIGURE 10-4   Basic Process Flow map for "turnover time (TOT) in the OR."

THE SWIM LANE CHART

The Swim Lane chart takes its name from the shape of a map because it mimics the swim lanes of an Olympic size pool. The Swim Lane chart is the preferred mapping technique for drawing processes with multiple departments, functions, and handoffs.

> **The Swim Lane chart is a Basic Process Flow map used to identify the sequential steps of the work flow as well as who is involved with each step.**

The Swim Lane chart is an excellent tool to

- identify **hand off points, and**
- identify **workloads.**

The benefit of this chart is the ability to identify workloads and all of the hand off points in the workflow (see example in Figure 10-5).

Hand off points are important because

- There is a transfer of knowledge, responsibility, or role at every handoff.
- Hand off points in a process are areas prone to problems, confusion, and mistakes.
- Defining each hand off point offers an opportunity to focus on ways of eliminating or minimizing the potential for problems at these junctures when redesigning the process.

THE VALUE STREAM MAP

What Is a Value Stream?

> **A Value Stream is the specific sequence of steps required to provide the service or care that customers expect.**

The Value Stream helps us understand the flow of information, sequence of work, and time required to provide value (service or care) to our customers. Understanding the Value Stream allows us to focus on the care process as a series of dependent, interconnected events. The Value Stream provides the transparency we need across the care continuum to identify problems and improve the patient experience. The Value Stream

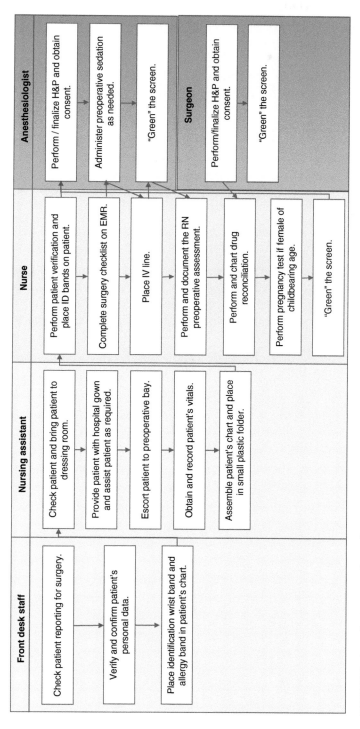

FIGURE 10-5 Swim Lane chart of "preoperative preparation."

- represents flow, not function;
- is variable for each service or care process; and
- moves across departmental boundaries.

As we often find, hospitals are organized according to departments and functions, instead of according to the flow of value-creating steps.

The Value Stream Map

> **The Value Stream map is a high-level view process map that shows the individual operational steps of a process, the time needed for each step, along with the flow of people, equipment, and information used to achieve the desired outcome.**

The Value Stream map (VSM) is always drawn from the customer's perspective and provides us with a visualization of the key steps and corresponding data needed to understand and improve a process. The VSM includes a representation and information of every step in the material and information flow. The VSM has three main flows (see Figure 10-6):

1. **Information flow.** The information flow shows the communication of process-related information and the transmission of data. Depending on the needs of the team, information collection and distribution points can include many levels of detail.

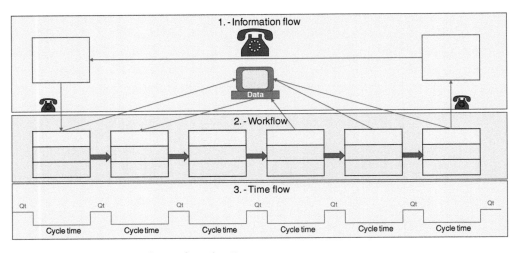

FIGURE 10-6   The three flows of a Value Stream map.

2. **Workflow.** This section of the VSM shows the steps of the process from start to delivery of the outcome. The VSM typically shows both the task and steps being performed (box) and the person or team performing the task. The workflow boxes include smaller fields that show key process data and pertinent step information. The VSM may include triangles showing the queue of features waiting at each stage of the process, and dotted arrows from one stage to the next called "push arrows." That show where the product or service is being pushed from one stage to the next vs. being pulled (more on this on Chapter 22 on improving flow).

3. **Time flow or Time Ladder.** The Time Ladder provides a simple visual representation of the value stream timeline. The upper portion of the Time Ladder represents the average amount of time that a product or service spends in the queue or waiting at each stage, and the lower portion of the Time Ladder shows the average amount of time that each product or service is actively being worked on. The time work is being done is considered value-added time.

Value Stream mapping is a great tool to give leaders and frontline professionals a picture of the entire care process, with both value and non-value-added activities. Once the value stream is identified and mapped, the ultimate goal is to eliminate the steps that do not create value in the process. Steps that are non-value-added are removed.

The VSM

- Shows the current state with the individual steps and operations drawn from the customer's perspective.
- Allows teams to really understand what patients experience helping us identify problems and discover the reality of the situation.
- Depicts three flows: information, work sequence, and time.
- Includes the duration of each step and the time between the steps in order to calculate process metrics which are very useful to identify and eliminate the various forms of waste. The first and most important role of the VSM is to highlight opportunities for improvement and the elimination of waste in the current process design.
- Provides a basis on which a QI team can create a future state VSM.

Steps to Create a Value Stream Map

- **Go to the gemba.** Go to the gemba and observe the process from start to finish (this may need to be done multiple times to get it right). Collect the necessary data for the major steps of the value stream as needed. Place the information in data boxes below the steps. Include process data and metrics for each process by gathering the following information (see the chapter on metrics):

- ○ Trigger: What starts the step? Is there any time spent setting up?
- ○ How long does the step take? This is called the **cycle time.**
- ○ How long does the entire process take? This is called the **lead time.**
- ○ How much time is spent in between steps? This is called **wait time.**
- ○ How many people are doing the work?
- ○ Collect process data for at least 30 samples, randomly distributed across shifts and days.

- **Record the first flow: the workflow.** Identify the beginning and the end of the value stream. Work up-stream to identify the five to seven main steps or activities. Identify the people who do the work for each step. Place the main activities in the proper sequence on the map. Add sub-processes, if required.

- **Add the second flow: time flow.** For each of the steps identified above, fill in the necessary data into data boxes below each major step. Document the valued added times, the non-value-added time between steps, and the totals for each on the bottom portion of the map. The time flow is also called the **Time Ladder.**

- **Document the third flow: information flow.** Map the information flow between activities. Document how the process communicates with the patient (customer), and the suppliers. Document how the information is gathered (electronic, manual, observation). Add the movement of materials (see example in Figure 10-7).

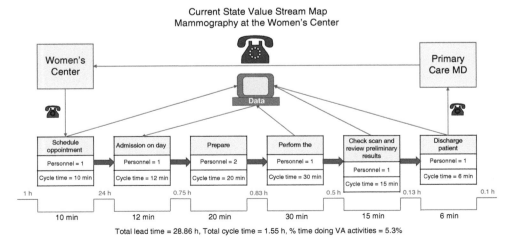

FIGURE 10-7   Current state Value Stream map for mammography at the Women's Center.

PROCESS DATA FOR THE VSM

The workflow boxes and the time ladder of the VSM can include key process data (see Figure 10-8):

- **Cycle time (CT).** This is the time it takes a healthcare professional to do the work of one step.
- **Total Cycle Time (tCT).** Usually refers to the sum of all steps. Cycle time is the number of working hours or minutes spent on process steps, not including waiting time and time in between steps.
- **Wait time (QT).** Time in between steps.
- **Total wait time (tQT).** Usually refers to the total wait time or sum of all wait times.
- **Lead time (LT).** Time it takes a single patient / object / information item to move all the way through a process or the entire Value Stream from start to finish. Lead time is the total time it takes to deliver the care, service, or product to the patient, provider, or staff. The lead time is also called total lead time or total process cycle time. Lead time = Σ cycles times + Σ wait times.

Additional time metrics are

- **Response time (RT).** The time it takes to react to a customer or patient request for a product, service, or care.
- **Process cycle efficiency (PCE).** Percent of time during the process or value stream that value-added work is done, or percent of time the customer (patient, staff, provider) is receiving the outcome the process was designed to produce. PCE is calculated by adding the time the process is doing value-added steps divided by the total time the process takes from start to finish. PCE= Σ VA steps / lead time

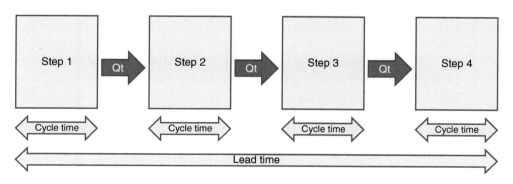

FIGURE 10-8   Common process metrics for the Value Stream map.

- **% complete and accurate (%CA).** Percent of times where a process step is completed without needing corrections or requesting missing items or information.
- **Rolled first pass yield (RFPY).** Percent of times where the entire process is completed without rework, or requesting missing items or information. The RFPY is calculated by multiplying all of the process steps' percentage complete and accurate ratings by each other. For example, $0.90 \times 0.92 \times 0.85 \times 0.79 = 0.56$, or 56% complete and accurate.

To collect time metrics, go to the gemba and observe the work being done. Then time each step of the process. Observe several cycles of the same process and calculate the average time it takes for each step and the time it takes in between steps. Record your findings.

EXERCISE: MAPPING "ORDERING BLOOD FROM THE BLOOD BANK"

A team has been chartered to improve how blood is ordered from the blood bank. There have been numerous complaints from the hemodialysis unit about the complexity of the process and the obstacles providers and nurses face when ordering blood from the blood bank. What follow are the steps of the current process for ordering blood from the blood bank, as described by several of the staff members. Following this description, draw a Basic Flow map of this process:

- *Log into the EMR and access the patient's chart.*
- *Under "orders", the physician places an order for a type and screen.*
- *The patient's nurse draws a sample of blood from the patient using a pink top tube; the blood tubing must be appropriately labeled with the patient sticker; date and time the sample was obtained must be clearly marked on the label.*
- *Nurse then sends the sample to the blood bank via the pneumatic tube.*
- *Once the sample is received in the blood bank, the blood bank technician will perform an initial ABO check and contacts the nurse for a second sample for an ABO re-check.*
- *The patient's nurse draws a second sample from a different site for an ABO re-check (pink top tube) and sends it appropriately labeled and timed to the blood bank.*
- *If blood is needed in the hemodialysis unit, a provider must place an order for crossmatch, indicating the number of units, and the need to release blood products.*
- *Once crossmatch is performed, the blood bank places the blood in a cooler and indicates in the computer that the number of units have been released.*
- *The provider must notify the clinic RN that blood has been released.*
- *A technician must be sent to the blood bank to get the blood.*

Record all the steps required to order blood; decide the start and end-points of your pro-cess. You may decide to write the steps of the process on sticky notes and place them on a wall surface prior to creating a digital version of your map. Identify the decisions points. Arrange the steps in the proper sequence. Connect each symbol with arrows. Add information as needed. Create a digital version if not done so already, and write the name of the process, and date, author, and version at the bottom of map.

REVIEW QUIZ

1. Which of the following IS NOT true regarding the gemba?
   A. Going to the gemba shows respect for the people "doing the work."
   B. The gemba is the place where work is done and value created.
   C. The goal in going to the gemba is to assess professional performance.
   D. Going to the gemba helps us understand the sequence and order of the steps of the processes.
   E. The gemba can be any area or unit in the hospital.

2. All of the following statements are true EXCEPT
   A. To improve an outcome, improve the process that generates the outcome.
   B. A process is a collection of related series of steps, actions, and decisions.
   C. The outcome of a process can be a product, service, or clinical care.
   D. A system refers only to one component, the group of people doing work.
   E. To understand a problem in y, we need to know the beginning and the end of the process that generates the outcome y.

3. Mapping a process
   A. builds a common understanding of the entire process,
   B. is not always needed,
   C. defines only the current state,
   D. is useful but cannot highlight areas of possible improvement, or
   E. is not needed when a project is addressing a clinical outcome.

4. A process map is a visual representation of "how the work is done."
   A. True
   B. False

5. All the following statements are true EXCEPT
   A. The gemba is the site where work takes place.
   B. It is always best to first get a very detailed map of the process when we go to the gemba.
   C. A map builds a common understanding of the steps and actions of the process among the QI team and all stakeholders.
   D. When mapping a process, it is important to communicate your intent to the front lines before arriving.
   E. A map can be drawn initially using only a pen and paper.

6. "Must-haves" for all process flow maps include
   A. the name of the process and authors of the map,
   B. the date and revision level,
   C. clearly identifiable start and finish points of the process,
   D. uniform and consistent level of detail throughout the map, or
   E. all of the above

7. What is the preferred map to show the steps, actions, and decision points in a process?
   A. Basic Process Flow map
   B. Swim Lane chart
   C. Spaghetti diagram
   D. SIPOC diagram
   E. Opportunity diagram

8. The symbol for a decision point on a basic process flow map is
   A. rectangle
   B. oval
   C. diamond
   D. arrow
   E. circle

9. In a Basic Process Flow map, which shape indicates the start and end points of a process?
   A. Rectangle
   B. Oval
   C. Diamond
   D. Arrow
   E. Circle

Key: 1c, 2d, 3a, 4a, 5b, 6e, 7a, 8c, 9b

CHAPTER 11

Get a Quick Win: Identify and Eliminate "Waste"

WASTE IS THE OPPOSITE OF VALUE

After going to the gemba and completing a process map we may be presented with an opportunity for an immediate improvement if we can identify and eliminate **waste**.

What Is Waste?

Waste is any step that does not add value. In the simplest of explanations, waste can be seen as the opposite of value. If something does not promote value, it is considered to be waste.

> **Waste is anything other than the minimum amount of equipment, material, technology, space, staff, and time that are essential to create or add value.**

While healthcare staff and providers do not typically contemplate the waste that occurs while providing patient care, patients do. Patients often keep track of the amount of time they had to wait to be seen by their providers; the time elapsed before they receive the results of their testing; the additional number of attempts required to start their intravenous line; or the times they have had to repeat the same information to different healthcare providers. **Once we understand how work is done, our next**

The Quality Improvement Challenge: A Practical Guide for Physicians, First Edition.
Richard J. Banchs and Michael R. Pop.
© 2021 John Wiley & Sons Ltd. Published 2021 by John Wiley & Sons Ltd.
Companion website: www.wiley.com/go/banchs/quality

task is to eliminate the steps that do not add value to the process. Identifying "what we are doing that doesn't need to be done" is a very important step.

Identifying waste is often harder than eliminating it because people resist change. People cling to "the way we have always done it." *Technically speaking, waste is not a cause but a symptom that helps identify the underlying issues within the system.* By identifying the underlying causes of waste, we can address them and improve the process and the resulting outcome.

How Do We Define Value?

> **Value is defined as any step or activity that is done right the first time; changes form, fit, or function of a product or service toward achieving what the customer expects; improves the course of a patient's disease; or provides what the patient is willing to pay for.**

Value in healthcare is defined as the health outcomes achieved per dollar spent, but in QI, value is defined in a more focused way. Value is defined in relation to the steps of the process that aim to achieve the outcome the customer expects.

Who Defines Value and Waste?

Value and waste depend on the outcomes achieved, and therefore should always be defined from the customer's perspective.

> **Value and waste are always defined from the perspective of the customer. The customer in healthcare is the patient, staff, or provider.**

WHY TARGET WASTE?

There are many reasons to target and eliminate waste in a process:

- Waste **increases the number of steps** in a process, making the process more burdensome toward achieving the outcome the customer (patients, providers, and staff) expects.
- Waste **decreases flow** (flow of people, information, material, patients), increasing the time it takes to perform the steps of a process. Decreased flow decreases efficiency, resulting in decreased quality.
- Waste increases the **workload** for our staff.

- Waste increases the amount of equipment, material, technology, space, and staff that are needed for performing the key activities that deliver value to our patients. Waste increases the cost of providing care.

> **The goal in identifying and eliminating waste is to reduce the workload of the staff and produce the highest-quality output for our customers (patients, staff, and physicians) with the right amount of work.**

- Waste results in decreased patient **satisfaction**, and increased staff and provider **frustration**.

By eliminating waste from processes, we improve the workflow and work environment for providers and staff. An optimized workflow and work environment results in quality care, improved patient experience, and a better work environment.

> *Quotable quote: "There is nothing so useless as doing efficiently that which should not be done at all." Peter Drucker.*

WHO IS TIM WOOD?

"TIM WOOD" is an acronym for the seven types of waste: transport, inventory, motion, waiting, overproduction, overprocessing, and defects (see Figure 11-1). Providers and staff that are familiar with the process might not notice wasteful steps because they are so used to them. TIM WOOD provides a framework for identifying all the wasteful steps in our processes so we can remove them. Our aim should be to identify and eliminate the seven wastes embedded in all processes. TIM WOOD is waste, and waste is responsible for defects, errors, lost productivity, increased costs and patient and provider frustration. **Have you seen TIM WOOD in your hospital?**

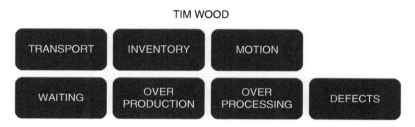

FIGURE 11-1   TIM WOOD and the seven types of waste.

Waste of Transportation

> **Transportation waste is the unnecessary movement of equipment, materials, or supplies to complete a task or the unnecessary relocation of patients to complete a treatment.**

Moving items, equipment or patients around incurs unnecessary effort, time, and cost that does not add value. Each time equipment is moved, it risks being lost or damaged. Transportation waste does not change: information, products, services towards delivering what the customer wants, or improving the course of the patient's health. Examples of transportation waste include

- moving items to and from an area where we are working because they have no clear drop-off location,
- moving items to several locations before reaching their final destination, and
- moving patients through multiple areas before they can reach their final destination.

Think of the movement of medications dispensed on the hospital wards. First, these medications arrive in large boxes at the hospital's loading docks. They are then transported to Central Pharmacy where they are taken out of the larges boxes and stored on shelves. These same medications are then placed in smaller containers and transported to the hospital ward where pharmacy personnel re-stocks the Omnicell® machines. Providers take these medications from the Omnicell® machines when administering them to their patients. Wouldn't it be easier to take these medications directly from the docks and store them in the Omnicell® machines in the patient care areas? It would surely avoid the extra work or handoff at each step, and decrease the risk of misplacing or mislabeling mistakes.

Waste of Inventory

> **Inventory waste is holding inventory (material, equipment, supplies) in excess of what has been planned or is needed in order to complete a task.**

Excess inventory decreases efficiency and makes it more difficult to perform a task and makes it difficult to find the items needed for the task. Inventory stored in excess of what we need is at risk of expiring, which will increase our costs.

Examples of waste of inventory are

- storing excessive equipment, supplies, or forms in the immediate work area and exam rooms;

- overstocking medications "just-in-case" a need may arise;
- overstocking in a clinic to avoid "running-out"; and
- overstocking a cart to have more items than what is needed.

Waste of Motion

Motion waste relates to the movement of providers or staff in excess of what is needed to complete a task. Waste motion is often related to problems with layout and workflow organization.

Examples of waste of motion are

- walking a distance to perform routine procedures because of inefficient work layout, such as weighing patients on one scale that is placed at the far end of a unit;
- placing charts, forms, and frequently used supplies outside of the immediate work area; and
- walking around a clinic looking for information, people, and materials outside of the work area.

Waste of Waiting

Waiting waste includes idle time created when people, information, equipment or materials are not available to perform the necessary functions.

In waste of waiting, providers and staff are waiting instead of performing at the pace of customer demand. Customers are waiting to receive a service or care.
Examples

- Providers and staff waiting for documents from the Surgeon's office to proceed with surgery.
- Staff waiting to verify a patient's insurance, lab results, tests, etc.
- Staff waiting for patients to arrive to start working.
- Patients waiting in the clinic to see their doctor.
- Patients waiting in line to register at the front desk.

Waste of Overproduction

Overproduction waste is doing more than is needed, making something in excess of what is needed, or repetitive steps that do not add value.

Doing more than what is needed for the patient is a form of overproduction. A wide variety of activities fall under this category, including repetitive testing, or filling out multiple registration forms.

Examples

- Ordering more tests than are needed "just-in-case."
- Working with batches (it is also a form of over processing, see next).
- Asking the patient to fill multiple forms that contain the same information.
- Preparing multiple intravenous infusions that will not be needed and will be discarded at the end of the day.

Waste of Overprocessing

Overprocessing waste consists of adding steps to a process or repeating the steps of a process while no value is added from the customer's or patient's perspective.

Examples

- Clarify unclear orders resulting in multiple calls to the physician's office.
- Use redundant charting with the same information entered by different sources.
- Duplicate regulatory paperwork.
- Review the chart multiple times by multiple clinicians to verify the same information with no clear role assignments.

Defects

A defect is work that contains errors or lacks something of value. A defect is any event, step, product, or care process that does not meet customer expectations for quality.

The customer (patient, staff, or provider) defines quality by

- identifying the needed (expected) outcome,
- the attributes of the outcome, and
- and the requirements that characterize the outcome.

The customer sets the *specifications for the attributes and requirements*. A defect is work that does not meet the specifications for the attributes and requirements expected by the customer.

Examples of defects are

- missing information on a patient's chart,
- lab results that are not accessible to the physician when needed and in the time frame needed,
- wrong information entered on an insurance form,
- medication errors,
- incorrect charges,
- surgical errors (complication), and
- failure to administer an anticoagulant in a timely manner.

How to Use TIM WOOD

- Map out your process from start to finish.
- For each of the wastes in TIM WOOD, ask yourself if you can find any examples of this waste in the mapped-out process?
- Make a note of each waste as you find it; on your map, color code each step as you identify waste. This will be useful as you move through the project.
- Ask yourself, why is this waste here? How is it possible? What is the cause?
- Get together with your team and brainstorm ways to eliminate the identified wasteful step.

TOOLS TO IDENTIFY AND ELIMINATE WASTE

Stand in the Circle

"Stand in the circle" is an observation technique that was first described and used by Taichii Ohno, considered to be the father of the Toyota Production System (TPS), the basis for Lean methodology.

> **The concept is simple: go to the gemba, pick a safe location and with a chalk draw a circle on the floor, then "stand in the circle" and just observe so you can identify the different forms of waste.**

Of course, you can practice stand in the circle without drawing a circle on the floor. Using chalk on the floor of an ICU or an OR is going to be frowned upon. The goal is not the circle but, using your eyes and ears, to see and understand the process in order to uncover the waste.

To practice "stand in the circle" in the traditional way described by Taichii Ohno, follow these steps:

- Introduce yourself, explain the purpose of your visit; be polite but try not to engage in any conversation at this time.
- Spend at least 30 minutes watching the work process.
- Record on a sheet of paper as many items of waste as you observe, ideally 30.
- Record all forms of waste, including energy and time.
- Record any abnormalities or atypical things you notice.
- Then record any ideas you may have to improve the process.

"Waste Rounds"

> **Waste Rounds are conducted in patient care areas, clinics, and supporting units to provide an informal method for a team to "walk the process" and "see the waste."**

Waste Rounds provide

- a way to "see" the process,
- an informal forum to discuss waste,
- an opportunity to uncover problems,
- a way to engage frontline professionals about better ways of doing things, and
- a method for achieving greater success in changing the culture of the organization.

When you are ready to "Waste Round," make sure you are in the right frame of mind and ready to see things with new eyes. The point is not to see the process as the subject-matter expert (SME) that you are but to see the process as a "waste detective." Walk the entire process to see and identify waste. Identify waste by asking yourself some of these questions:

- Are we wasting movements? Are we searching for things?
- Are we hand-carrying items regularly?
- Are supplies and equipment in the right place?
- Are we preparing things we don't need, such as spiking bags of IV fluids in advance?
- Are we asking repetitive questions? Are we duplicating work?
- Are there excessive supplies? Are there items that are obsolete? Where are the delays?

The goal of Waste Rounds is to ultimately make the process easier, simpler, and faster for those who actually do the work.

MAPPING TECHNIQUES TO IDENTIFY WASTE

The "Spaghetti" Diagram

Mapping techniques can provide you with valuable information when looking for ways to remove waste from a process. One of the most useful ways is the Spaghetti diagram.

> **The Spaghetti diagram is a mapping technique that shows movement or physical flow of people, staff, providers, work, and materials in a process and it is used to decrease wasted motion of the front lines as they perform their jobs.**

The Spaghetti diagram is also called the **transportation or workflow diagram**. As the name indicates, the final product looks like a bowl of pasta (see example in Figure 11-2). Data regarding the distance traveled, the amount of time expended during the movement, and the number of trips required to perform the process can also be compiled to complete the information provided about the process.

The Spaghetti diagram is often used to improve the physical layout of a work space and the sequence of work. If lines repeatedly converge in one location, assess the situation to determine if the work can be done in a different way, a different sequence, or tasks can be performed at the same time to avoid backtracking and

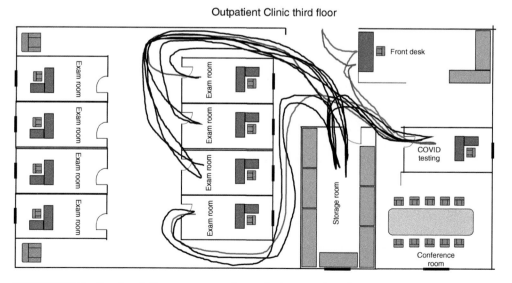

FIGURE 11-2   Spaghetti diagram: a mapping technique to identify waste.

unnecessary movement. Lines that crisscross often depict too many hand offs and signal that significant delays may occur.

The Opportunity Flowchart

From the Lean methodology perspective, there are three types of steps in every process (see Figure 11-3):

1. **Value-added steps (VA).** These steps are critical toward achieving the outcome the customer (patients, staff, and physicians) expects. Value-added steps are defined from the customer's perspective. These steps transform inputs into next steps toward completion of the outcome the customer expects, are done right the first time, and the customer cares for them. An example of a value-added step is administering p.o. medication to treat pain.
2. **Business value-added steps (BVA).** Steps the customer may not perceive as value but are required to allow the performance of the value-added steps, or to maintain compliance. They are also steps required for the survival of the business. An example would be collecting insurance information when arriving at an emergency department (ED).
3. **Non-value-added steps (NVA).** These are the steps that do not value, and therefore are considered waste.

> **The opportunity flowchart is a basic process mapping technique that categorizes process steps into three categories: value-added (VA), non-value-added (NVA), and business value-added (BVA) steps.**

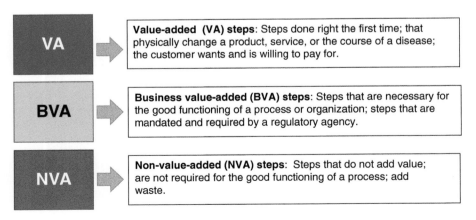

FIGURE 11-3   Three types of process steps.

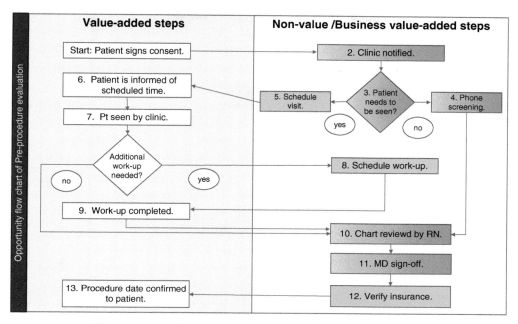

FIGURE 11-4   The opportunity flowchart: a mapping technique to identify waste (Non-value-added steps).

The focus is on eliminating and/or reducing steps that do not add value in order to improve the process. To build an opportunity flowchart (see example in Figure 11-4)

- Divide the page into two sections.
- Draw the process steps with time flowing down the page.
- For each step, ask the following questions: From the perspective of the customer, is this a VA or NVA (BVA) step? If the work process was optimized, would we need this step? Does the customer need this step?
- Place each step (VA, NVA, BVA) and decision point in the corresponding column.
- Join steps with arrows.
- Number each step.

EXERCISE: IDENTIFYING WASTE IN THE PEDIATRIC UNIT

Early yesterday, an improvement team spent one hour walking the hallways and speaking with the front line. They interviewed medical students, physicians, nurses, and staff working in the pediatric unit. The team made a number of observations and recorded their findings on a sheet of paper. Your task is to create a completed summary table assigning each of the team's finding to the corresponding waste classification.

For each observation, mark with an "x" the corresponding type of waste (remember TIM WOOD!). The team noticed the following:

- Items are being moved to and from an area with no clear drop-off location.
- Patients and their families are waiting in the room to be discharged.
- Duplicate charting and entries in the EMR are made by three different teams.
- Nurses and staff must look for needed items outside of the work area.
- Calls placed to residents for clarification of unclear orders that then had to be rewritten.
- Nursing staff prepares multiple intravenous infusions discarded at the end of the day.
- There is missing information on patient's chart (demographic info).
- Supplies for dressing changes are moved to several locations before reaching their final destination.
- Excessive supplies are stored in cabinets.
- Physicians look at the computer multiple times waiting for test results to appear.
- Staff wait for patients to arrive from the ER.
- Physicians' orders are placed in the computer all at once after rounds.
- The wrong medication is given to a patient.

Summary table

Observation	T	I	M	W	O	O	D
1							
2							
3							
4							
5							
6							
7							
8							
9							
10							
11							
12							
13							

REVIEW QUIZ

1. A Spaghetti diagram is often used to
   A. improve the physical layout of a space,
   B. figure out what to eat for dinner,
   C. show the hand offs between hospital and suppliers,
   D. identify value-added (VA) and non-value-added (NVA) steps, or
   E. revise a SIPOC diagram.

2. All of the following are true regarding mapping techniques EXCEPT
   A. A basic process flow map is the preferred tool to show waste.
   B. A basic process flow map helps us understand the process steps, actions, and sequence.
   C. An opportunity flowchart shows value-added and non-value-added steps.
   D. A Value Stream map shows the flow of information, work, and time in order to identify activities that do not add value to the final outcome.
   E. Swim Lane charts can be used to identify workloads.

3. Value is
   A. anything done right the first time,
   B. a step that improves the condition of the patient,
   C. a step the customer is willing to pay for,
   D. work that changes or transforms something in the process toward the final outcome, or
   E. all of the above

4. All of the following are true regarding waste EXCEPT
   A. Waste is the opposite of value.
   B. Waste is anything in excess of the minimum amount of equipment, personal, staff, time, and resources needed to create value.
   C. Waste is a symptom of an underlying problem, not a cause.
   D. Waste results in an increased process flow.
   E. Eliminating waste improves the work environment.

5. Which of the following is a waste of transportation?
   A. Storing excessive equipment, supplies, or forms in the immediate work area and exam rooms
   B. Placing charts, forms, and frequently used supplies outside of the immediate work area
   C. Ordering a test "just-in-case"
   D. Moving items to and from an area because they have no clear drop-off location
   E. Redundant charting with the same information entered by different sources

6. Which of the following is a waste of overproduction?
   A. Asking the patient to fill multiple forms that contain the same information;
   B. Transporting patients through multiple areas of the hospital
   C. Looking for information and material outside the work area

    D. Waiting for patients to arrive

    E. Overstocking medications "just-in-case" a need arises

7. Which of the following is a waste of overprocessing?

    A. Waiting to see the results of an X-ray

    B. Walking each patient to a distant scale to record their weight

    C. Reviewing the chart multiple times by multiple clinicians to verify the same information

    D. Waiting for physicians to finish a patient's exam

    E. Storing a lot of supplies in the immediate work area

8. All of the following statements are true EXCEPT

    A. "Stand in the circle" is a tool to identify waste.

    B. "Waste rounds" can uncover sources of waste and is a way to engage the frontline professionals.

    C. The goal of "stand in the circle" is to see, understand, and uncover waste.

    D. The opportunity flow chart is a mapping technique that stratifies steps into value-added and non-value-added.

    E. The best way to identify waste is to analyze data from a report.

9. The Spaghetti diagram

    A. provides valuable information regarding the flow of work, material, and people;

    B. is the preferred technique to show motion and physical flow;

    C. is a tool for defining the number of process steps;

    D. is often used to assess workloads; or

    E. is the preferred mapping technique to calculate the time spent in each process step.

10. "Preparing more IV solutions than needed" is an example of which type of waste?

    A. Transport

    B. Inventory

    C. Motion

    D. Wait

    E. Overproduction

11. "Overstocking supplies in the ICU cabinets to avoid running out" is an example of which type of waste?

    A. Overproduction

    B. Overprocessing

    C. Inventory

    D. Transport

    E. Motion

12. "Completing a surgical consent form without a time or date" is an example of which type of waste?

    A. Defect

    B. Overproduction

    C. Overprocessing

D. Inventory

E. Motion

13. "Walking across the unit to get charts, forms, or supplies" is an example of which type of waste?

A. Inventory

B. Motion

C. Wait

D. Transport

E. Defect

Key: 1a, 2a, 3e, 4d, 5d, 6a, 7c, 8e, 9b, 10e, 11c, 12a, 13b

CHAPTER 12

Measure What Matters: Choose the Right Project Metrics

MEASUREMENTS

Measurements Are Everywhere

HCAHPS surveys, key performance indicators, Press-Ganey scores, clinical performance indicators, complication rates . . . we all know measurements are important and driven by consumers, third-party payers, regulatory agencies, and the needs of our healthcare organizations. While we may not be absolutely convinced about their usefulness, nevertheless, measurements provide actionable information critical to our improvement efforts. In the world of QI, data are critical elements for the success of the project.

What Are Measurements, and Why Do We Need Them?

> **A measurement takes a concept and describes it in terms of a number, usually referred to as data.**

If we don't measure what we do, we cannot objectively know our level of performance. Measurements define the present, the future, and guide our decisions regarding ways in which we need to improve. In QI we need measurements to answer three basic questions:

The Quality Improvement Challenge: A Practical Guide for Physicians, First Edition.
Richard J. Banchs and Michael R. Pop.
© 2021 John Wiley & Sons Ltd. Published 2021 by John Wiley & Sons Ltd.
Companion website: www.wiley.com/go/banchs/quality

1. **How is our process behaving?** Can we meet our customer's needs?
2. **Are we meeting the needs of our customers?** Are we achieving what our patients, staff or providers expect?
3. **How often are we meeting their needs?**

Our performance cannot be judged anecdotally based on opinions, past experiences, or contextual factors unrelated to the actual process. These influences become entangled in our memory and often contribute significantly to the formation of positive or negative opinions of performance prior to the consideration of actual objective data. Problems arise when we try to maintain the status quo based on our subjective positive feelings about our performance despite unfavorable objective data that highlight opportunities for improvement. To improve, we need a measurement of the current state so we know *"where we are and where we need to go."*

> *Quotable Quote: "If you can't measure something, you can't understand it. If you can't understand it, you can't control it. If you can't control it, you can't improve it." H. James Harrington*

METRICS

What Is a Metric?

> A metric represents a measurement of the relationship of one or more dimensions in our process used to understand, compare, or track performance.

A metric is

- a numerical value that represents a measurement that can be expressed with data,
- a quantifiable measure that is used to track and assess the status of a specific process, and
- the key indicators of our QI project's progress and benefits.

Metrics define our present and guide our decisions regarding our improvement priorities. Metrics allow us to understand performance, identify problems, establish causal relationships, and demonstrate success. Metrics are the drivers of the QI project because they help define what we need to measure and the goals we need to achieve for customer satisfaction. When we say "number of hospital admissions per day," then "number of hospital admissions" is the measure, "per day" is the dimension, and "number of hospital admissions per day" is the metric. Because metrics represent a measurement of the relationship of one or more dimensions in our process, they are often expressed as a proportion or percentage.

Metrics are used in QI initiatives to do several things:

- Estimate current performance.
- Determine how well a work process is performing over time.
- Identify causes of poor performance.
- Find opportunities for improvement and delineate goals.
- Understand the effects of changes we make on a work process.
- Continuously monitor the effectiveness of improvement efforts.

Data and Metrics

> **Data is the set of numbers or calculations that are gathered for a specific metric.**

Data integrity is vital to ensuring our metrics are accurate. We use data to create statistics that will help us make better decisions. Walter Shewhart, the father of statistical quality control, observed that we use data for basically two reasons:

1. **To obtain quantitative information.** In other words, to see how we are doing and make a judgment on the past.
2. **To obtain a causal explanation.** Basically, data allows us to predict the future based on past performance.

Concepts, measurements, data, and metrics are interrelated and lead us to making decisions about our processes (see Figure 12-1).

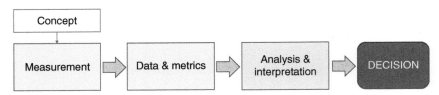

FIGURE 12-1   From concept to decision: concepts, measurements, data, and metrics are interrelated.

WHO DECIDES WHAT WE NEED TO MEASURE?

The decision of what to measure and what metric/s to use in our QI project is influenced by three factors: the needs of the customer, the requirements of our stakeholders, the QI team's expertise:

1. **The needs of the customer.** Patients, providers, and staff are the customers of our healthcare processes. They expect an outcome. The outcome customers expect must have certain attributes and must be delivered within certain requirements (the Voice of the Customer, VOC). The customer must also define the specifications for both the attributes and requirements of the final product (the CTQs) (see Chapter 8). Metrics represent these specifications and are the vital signs of our QI projects. Project metrics are key to evaluate the success of the project in meeting the patients' or customers' expectations. The VOC and the Critical-to-Quality (CTQ) tree are the basic tools used to define the project metrics (see Figure 12-2).

2. **Critical Needs of the stakeholders.** Achieving customer's requirements and the ability of the stakeholder to fulfill their expectations are interrelated. In order to be able to deliver the services that customers expect, the resource needs of the frontline stakeholders must be met. How can we provide quality care if the front line doesn't have what they need? CTQs are the specifications that define customer's expectations and the primary project metrics. Critical Needs (CN) are the attributes and requirements (specifications) of the stakeholders that define frontline performance and the ability to deliver the outcome customers expect. Measuring how often the needs of the stakeholders are met is important, and adds a needed dimension in our understanding of the problem (see Figure 12-3).

3. **The QI team's expertise.** Customers define the outcome/s they need, but may not have the required knowledge to know how to achieve it. When this is the case, staff and providers on the QI team may need to define the steps, actions, decisions, and **process metrics** needed to achieve the desired outcome. Patients may want a specific outcome but might not know what steps are needed or how

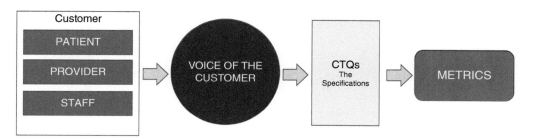

FIGURE 12-2   The Voice of the Customer (VOC) defines what to measure.

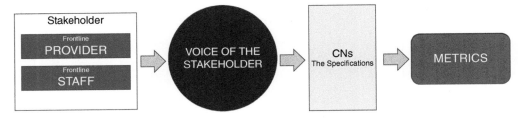

FIGURE 12-3   The Critical Needs (CN) of the front line can also define what we need to measure.

this is achieved. The specific metrics should be set by subject-matter experts following their experience and available best-practice recommendations. For placement and maintenance of a central line for example, patients want "safe care without complications." Experts must set requirements (CTQs) for central line placement and maintenance that will lead to no complications. A bundle use (CDC 2011) has been recommended to avoid central line–associated bloodstream infection (CLABSI). The bundle includes among others: hand hygiene, full-barrier precautions, chlorhexidine skin antisepsis, optimal catheter site selection, and early removal of lines that are not needed. "Safe care without complications" is the Voice of the Customer. The CTQs and metrics ("percent compliance with each item of the CLABSI bundle") are derived from expertise of providers following current recommendations (see example in Figure 12-4).

Example: Improving STAT Chest X-rays in the ICU

At the request of hospital leadership, you have assembled a QI team to improve the quality of service provided for STAT chest X-rays in the intensive care unit (ICU). You first order of business is to understand what "quality of service" means to the customer. Quality is not set by your team but by the customers who, in this case, are the ICU ordering physicians. After several face-to-face interviews, you are able to get the VOC, define the drivers, and drill down to develop the CTQ attributes and requirements of customer satisfaction. Armed with the CTQs, you can now set your project metrics (see Figure 12-5).

> **Quotable quote: "Not everything that counts can be counted and not everything that can be counted, counts." Albert Einstein**

THE TWO TYPES OF METRICS USED IN QI PROJECTS

In the healthcare environment, there are two types of processes: clinical and operational (support processes for clinical care). A clinical process refers to the steps, actions, and decisions used to provide clinical care. A support process refers to the steps,

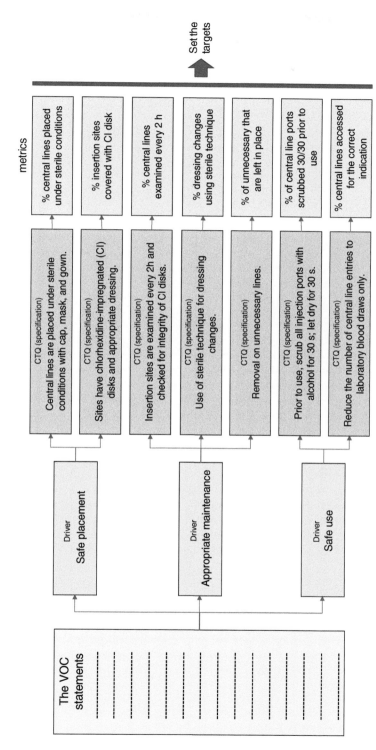

FIGURE 12-4 The decisions of what to measure may need to be driven by stakeholders' experience in achieving the expected outcome.

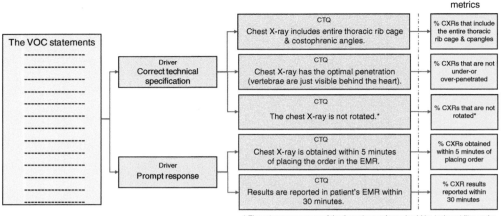

FIGURE 12-5   Project metrics to improve STAT chest X-rays in the ICU are derived from VOC, CTQs and ICU providers' expertise.

actions, and decisions used to provide a service or product that is required to deliver care. The type of process we are targeting will define the type of metric we need. For clinical processes, the metric may be the "rate of surgical site infections." For a support (operational) process, the metric may be "time from order to arrival of antibiotics." Independent of the type of process, metrics are used to assess the performance of a process and can be classified as either metrics of effectiveness or metrics of efficiency:

1. **Metrics of effectiveness.** These metrics provide a quantitative assessment of what the process delivers (outcome) and help us answer the question: Is the process delivering what the customer needs? Metrics of effectiveness assess our performance in *meeting the requirements of our customers in relation to the specifications for both the attributes and requirements of the final outcome* (see Figure 12-6). Examples of metrics of effectiveness are: percentage of correct antibiotics administered; percentage of EMR charts with the correct information; percentage of accurately scheduled appointments. Metrics of effectiveness assess the output of the process and are sometimes called **outcome metrics** or **lagging indicators**.

2. **Metrics of efficiency.** These metrics provide a quantitative assessment of **time and resources used to deliver the outcome** the customer needs. Examples of metrics of efficiency are: percentage of time prophylactic antibiotics are administered within 60 minutes; percentage of stroke patients that receive antithrombotic therapy within 60 minutes of hospital arrival (door to needle time for tissue plasminogen activator).

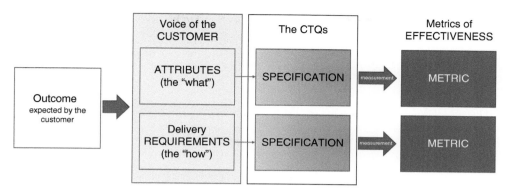

FIGURE 12-6 Metrics of effectiveness assess our performance in meeting the specifications for both the attributes and requirements of the outcome.

Metrics can also be classified according to the target or outcome the QI project is trying to improve:

1. quality,
2. safety,
3. productivity, or
4. cost.

WHAT DOES A "GOOD" PROJECT METRIC LOOK LIKE?

A good project metric measures what is important:

- to the customer (the VOC and the CTQs),
- to the stakeholder (the VOS and CN), and
- in achieving the goals of the project.

In addition to measuring what is important, a good project metric must be:

- practical and reasonably obtained;
- sensitive and specific;
- able to have a set and agreed upon standard definition;
- operationally defined: everybody understands how the measurements are obtained; and
- validated and accepted by the customer (people receiving the work product) and the key stakeholders (people doing the work).

From the perspective of a provider, metrics need to be relevant to clinical care and a reliable indicator of quality. If providers can't make the connection between what they do every day and the metric used to define their performance, the metric will not be seen as a useful tool to improve quality.

How Many Metrics Do We Need in Our QI projects?

Metrics need to measure what is important to the customer:

- Choose a small number of metrics that characterize the attributes and requirements of the outputs the customer expects.
- Narrow your selection to a maximum of two or three metrics you want to improve. However, you may need additional measurements of the performance of the process that will help you in the search of the cause(s) of the problem.

Projects are more successful when there are fewer metrics, when the metrics have been properly defined, and when there is a realistic possibility to achieve the targets.

METRICS ARE EXPRESSED AS TWO TYPES OF DATA

Data can be quantitative or qualitative (nominal and ordinal). Metrics are expressed as quantitative data and are either continuous or discrete. Discrete data can be further broken down into count (summary) and attribute or (categorical) (see Figure 12-7):

1. **Continuous data** are measures that reside on a divisible continuum or scale that can take on any value on that scale. Continuous data can be subdivided into an infinite number of smaller values. Examples of continuous data are time, height, and length. An hour can be broken down into minutes, minutes into seconds, and seconds into tenths of a second, and so on. Common summary statistics are the average (mean) and standard deviation.

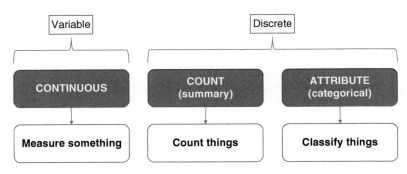

FIGURE 12-7   Three types of data.

2. **Discrete data** measures the occurrence of events or characteristics. Discrete data can be sorted into distinct, separate, nonoverlapping **categories** (e.g., good/bad, male/female, types of injury), or **counts** (e.g., on-time surgeries, number of patients in the waiting room). Discrete data has finite values and cannot be subdivided into smaller increments and still have any useful meaning. First surgery of the day can either start on time or not. We can count the number of on-time surgeries, but we cannot divide them to get an average. That is, 3.5 on-time starts does not have any useful meaning as we cannot have "half" a surgery. QI teams need to be wary of some common pitfalls:

   a. Discrete data can sometimes look like continuous data. For example, 38.6% of patients live between 0 and 2 miles from the hospital. Just because you have a number and decimals does not necessarily mean you are working with continuous data. The number 38.6 is actually a descriptive statistic of a specific category, 0–2 miles. The number came from a proportion. The patient either is in this category or is not. Therefore, this is discrete data. When considering whether the team is working with continuous versus discrete data, think about the unit of measure. Ask yourself if cutting the value in half makes any sense.

   b. Sometimes continuous data is converted to discrete data. For example, delivery time can be measured in days, hours, or minutes (continuous data) or it can be measured as on-time or late (discrete categories).

Each type of data has specific characteristics, advantages and disadvantages (see Table 12-1).

TABLE 12-1   Pros and Cons for Each Type of Data

		Pros and Cons of Continuous vs. Discrete data
Continuous data	Pro	Continuous data has more statistical tools available; a smaller sample size is usually required; graphs can display both distribution and variation in the data, which can help to see trends and patterns.
	Con	Continuous data needs an accurate and precise measurement system; Measurement System Analysis (MSA) is key to assure the reliability of the measurement process and instruments before obtaining data.
Discrete data	Pro	Discrete data is usually readily available; typically, discrete data does not require any measurement instrument.
	Con	Discrete data requires a large sample size compared to continuous data; needs a clearly defined area of opportunity (AOO) to assure all groups have the same representation before any meaningful comparison can be made; occurrences need to be independent of each other.

COMMON METRICS USED IN QI PROJECTS

Defects and the Defect Rate (Metrics of Effectiveness)

> **A defect is any event, step, product, or care process that does not meet customer expectations for quality.**

A defect is work that contains errors or lacks something of value. Customers define quality by identifying the attributes and requirements of the outcome they expect. With a defect, customer expectations are not met. Defects generate

- re-work and an additional cost in time and money,
- customer complaints,
- frustration of the people doing the work, or
- patient harm.

A complication is a defect; it is not what the patient (customer) wants. A complication is a failure to meet the patient's expectations for quality care.
Examples of defects are:

- missing information on a patient's chart (the customer is a provider),
- lab results that are not in the computer (the customer is a provider),
- wrong information on an insurance form (the customer is a third-party payer),
- a medication error (the customer is the patient), and
- incorrect charges (the customer is the patient).

> **A defect rate is a metric of effectiveness that represents the percent of outcomes that fail to meet the customer's specifications for quality.**

A defect rate is the percentage of output that fails to meet a quality target. Defect rates can be used to evaluate both clinical and operational (healthcare delivery) processes. The defect rate is also called the failure rate. The complication rate is also a defect rate. Examples of complication (defect) rates are: percentage of postoperative MIs; percentage of patients readmitted for congestive heart failure; percentage of patients with an acquired hospital pneumonia. Other examples of defect rates are: percentage of defective prescription per month; percentage of pain medication not administered within 30 minutes of patient request; number of inaccurate EMR demographic information per 1000 charts; number of supplies not delivered on time to the ICU per week; or the percentage missed diagnosis.

Time (Metrics of Efficiency)

> **Time can be used as a metric of efficiency to represents how long a step or process takes to deliver the care, product, or service that patients, providers, or staff expect.**

Time metrics can also be used to assess how much time is spent adding value or in activities that do not add value. As discussed in Chapter 10 with the value stream map, time metrics include cycle time (CT), total cycle time (tCT), wait time (QT), total wait time (tQT), and lead time (LT). Additional time metrics include response time (RT), process cycle efficiency (PCE), percentage complete and accurate (%CA), and rolled first pass yield (RFPY).

Cost (Metrics of Efficiency)

> **Cost can be used as a metric of efficiency to assess the financial resources used to provide quality care.**

Cost answers the questions: What are the financial resources used to deliver care to our patients, or products and services to our staff and providers? What are the operational costs relative to what we provide? The most common cost metrics are

- **Total process cost (TPC).** Total costs of providing care including labor, material and overhead, to produce the service, product, or to deliver care.
- **Cost per transaction (CPT).** Total process cost divided by number of services/products produced or patients seen.
- **Cost per item.**

Additional Terms

There are some additional terms used to refer to a metric you should be familiar with:

- **Key driver (KD).** A metric or key performance indicator for the processes that have the maximum impact on the desired goals.
- **Quality indicator.** A metric, key performance indicator, or key driver of processes linked to outcomes used to define quality.
- **Indicators.** Indicators are calculated measures of performance and may consist of a set of different metrics. Indicators are commonly known as **Key Performance Indicators,** or **KPIs.** A KPI is a metric that is tied to a target. KPIs are usually shown as a ratio of the actual measurement to the target.

The KPIs can also be called primary metrics (PM). Here is an example: If we need to see 100 patients per day to meet our demand, "patients" is the number, "patients per day" is the metric, and 100 is the target. If we see 80 patients on day one, our KPI is 80%.

REFERENCE

1. CDC. (2011). Guideline for prevention of intravascular catheter-associated bloodstream infections. https://www.cdc.gov/infectioncontrol/guidelines/bsi/index.html.

CHAPTER 13

Practicalities for Planning and Collecting Baseline Data

WHY DO WE NEED TO COLLECT DATA?

As discussed in Chapter 12, data is an essential part of every improvement effort. In QI, we need measurements to answer three basic questions:

1. **How is our process behaving**? Can we meet our customers' needs?
2. **Are we meeting the needs of our customers?** Are we achieving what our patients, staff, or providers expect?
3. **How often are we meeting their needs**?

We collect data to

- estimate current performance and find how well a process is performing over time,
- identify causes of poor performance,
- find opportunities for improvement and delineate our goals,
- understand the effects of changes we make on work processes, and
- continuously monitor the effectiveness of improvement efforts.

Quotable quote: "In God, we trust. All others bring data." often attributed to W. Edwards Deming

The Quality Improvement Challenge: A Practical Guide for Physicians, First Edition.
Richard J. Banchs and Michael R. Pop.
© 2021 John Wiley & Sons Ltd. Published 2021 by John Wiley & Sons Ltd.
Companion website: www.wiley.com/go/banchs/quality

WHERE CAN I FIND THE DATA THAT I NEED?

Before you go and collect data, you need to know what kind of data you need and where to find it. A well-written **Project Charter** will help you focus on the primary metric; a robust **data collection process** will help you make data collection effective, efficient, repeatable, and reproducible. Once you decide the type of data you need, you may find yourself in one of these three situations:

1. The data you need is part of a scheduled report or dashboard the hospital, department, or unit publishes. The information is being collected as part of regulatory compliance, QI initiatives, audits, professional performance, and others.

2. The data you need for your project is not routinely reported but information that is being entered into the hospital's information system by staff and providers is available upon request. You may need IT to generate a new report or the help of an expert who knows how to get data out from your EMR's data warehouse.

3. The data you need for your project is not entered into the hospital's information system; you may have to create your own collection forms and find ways to collect the data directly from the field. Another option is to focus on an existing metric that you can get, and use it as a surrogate of your project's primary metric.

Epic, Cerner, CareCloud, Athena health, GE Centricity, eClinicalWorks, Nextgen, and Allscripts are top vendors of electronic medical records (EMRs) in the US. For every hospital's information system, healthcare organizations store data in their **enterprise data warehouse** (**EDW**). An EDW is a central repository of integrated data from one or more disparate sources that stores current and historical data in one single place. These data are used to create the analytical reports needed by the healthcare organization. Data stored in the EDW is uploaded from operational systems such as patient EMRs, clinical care platforms, and billing.

The most relevant sources of data for your QI project are:

- **Your EMR and other digital sources.** The EMRs (electronic medical records) are a rich source of information that has made data more accessible and much simpler to get than in the past. However, it is difficult for providers to directly access and extract the reports they need. The assistance of staff from the hospital's IT department is often needed, and it is not unusual for trained ancillary staff to have to manually extract this information. Also included in this source is data coming from hospital reports, risk management, QI committees, morbidity and mortality reports, etc.

- **Administrative data.** Patient data can be gathered from claims, enrollment, insurance, and others. These data include demographic information, diagnosis, procedures codes, type of service, length of stay (LOS), location of services, and charges, among others. The data is readily available and reasonably standardized, but offer a limited amount of clinical information and often lack accuracy.

- **Patient surveys.** Patient surveys are often used in QI projects. Surveys are typically administered to a sample of patients by mail, by telephone, or via the internet. Surveys contain information about the healthcare experience, reports on the care, service, or treatment received. Surveys have well-established best-practices but are costly and have a number of inherent biases when administered. Also, patient survey results can often either be misleading or not representative of the sampled population.
- **Third-party registries.** Third-party applications provide a single platform for hospitals and healthcare organizations to acquire, manage, and analyze data using proprietary analytic technologies. Examples of third party registries are Surgical Compass and Press Ganey Associates LLC.
- **The gemba.** At times, data needed for a QI project can only be obtained directly at the point of care, or gemba, by the improvement team.

WHAT MAKES DATA SO HARD TO GET?

Each team in each healthcare organization must determine the availability of data for their project, and then decide what data they must obtain directly from the field. In any case, getting data requires planning, hard work, and an investment of time. Getting data in the healthcare environment is difficult due to several reasons:

- Data collection, storage, and management are complex and convoluted.
- Data is often collected using intake forms, evaluation forms, administrative files, and others and then manually entered in the electronic medical record to be shared among staff and providers. This manual process is fraught with error and missed information, leaving QI teams with incomplete or inaccurate data.
- Data is collected in multiple formats, such as text, digital, and pictures.
- Much of the data is located in multiple places, coming from different EMR platforms, different sites, not all of which are synchronized.
- Diseases, processes, and procedures have inconsistent and variable definitions, and may have different coding.
- The data you need is sometimes just not collected by your healthcare organization. This is often the case with operational data. For example, we know when the patient arrived at our clinic, we know when the patient left, but we do not record the exact time a patient spent with the physician!

THE KEY TO DATA COLLECTION IS TO START WITH A GOOD DATA COLLECTION PROCESS

A data collection process should follow the four steps of a PDSA Cycle (Plan-Do-Study-Act). The PDSA cycle is a learning and testing process used in pilots. Chapter 21 has more about the PDSA cycle with respect to testing and piloting the best solutions. For now, just remember these four logical steps for all data collection:

1. **Plan.** What do we want to know? The team must first agree on what is the goal of collecting data. In other words, what is the purpose? They must also agree on what type of data is needed, the location(s) of where to initiate the collection, the start and end times, and the operational definitions (see next section). If continuous data is needed, the team must also agree on whether a measurement system analysis (MSA) is needed to ensure both the accuracy and precision of the measurement instruments. Accuracy refers to any bias the instrument may have relative to a target. For example, a weight scale may have a bias when a certified 100 lb weight is placed on the scale and on average it reads 102 lbs. This would indicate a 2 lb bias. Precision refers to the consistency of the measuring instrument, in other words, the ability to duplicate readings when multiple readings are taken of the same unit(s) of work. We want minimal variation of the readings. If discrete data is to be collected, then the team must agree that the areas where data will be collected have the same area of opportunity (AOO). Finally, the team must decide what factors or conditions will be used to stratify and analyze the data.

2. **Do.** By what method? Once the goal of the data collection is established, we must then determine the collection methods. Can we get the data directly? Do we need the help of IT? As applicable, the team should consider developing and using templates or forms to make the data collection easier for those involved in the data collection. Collecting data incurs costs in both time and money; it is not free. Avoid being data rich and information poor: ensure the data we are collecting will actually answer the question(s) we want to know.

3. **Study.** How are we doing? How do we know? Once data collection has started, periodically check the progress of the data collection efforts, including accuracy and precision of the efforts. Remember that data collection needs to be repeatable and reproducible. Be there at the beginning to make sure data collection is done correctly and data collectors can ask questions and get feedback. You don't want to put all these efforts in collecting data only to realize there are missing items or flaws in the data collection process.

4. **Act.** Do we need to modify the way we are collecting data or can we continue? The team will also need to decide how the data is to be analyzed, and what graphic formats should be used to communicate it. Remember that looking at the data as a time series can be one of the best methods of analyzing data, as it allows for the identification of any trends or patterns. Agreement on how to present the data should be established by the team during the data collection process.

To learn more about how to organize your data collection process, check the Data Collection Planner at the end of the chapter.

THREE RULES OF DATA COLLECTION

Good data collection should follow three important rules:

1. Collect data using an operational definition.
2. Use the Principle of Stratification.
3. Collect data in a time-ordered sequence.

Rule # 1: Collect Data Using an Operational Definition

An operational definition is a simple statement that provides a clear and concise explanation of each metric and how the data must be collected.

> **An operational definition is a concise statement that clearly defines the data collection criteria, gives a communicable meaning to the metric, and makes the data collection process both repeatable and reproducible.**

When collecting data, we want the results to be **repeatable**, which means if we were to measure the same unit of work multiple times, our results would be consistent. We also want our data collection efforts to be **reproducible**, meaning if we were to have more than one person measure the same unit of work, the results would be consistent. This is especially important if we will be collecting data at different locations and on different shifts, for example.

Utilization of operational definitions is the key to good data collection. An operational definition puts communicable meaning into a concept. It is a definition everyone can work with. With an operational definition, a measurement or metric means the same today, tomorrow, next week, or next month, no matter who is utilizing it. Without an operational definition, a specification or a standard can be meaningless, making the investigation of a problem or improvement efforts costly and ineffective. Without an operational definition, teams, Primary Sponsors and key stakeholders may get embroiled in arguments and controversy.

A good operational definition meets these three criteria:

1. It is **specific** and **measurable.**
2. It is both **repeatable** and **reproducible.**
3. It has been **agreed upon** by both the stakeholder (staff or providers who do the work) and the customer (patient, staff, or provider who receives the work product). This criterion assures a common understanding of the way data is to be collected with a higher likelihood that all parties will accept the result and the ensuing conclusion.

The operational definition should include the following:

- The **name and definition** of what is being measured. The specifics of what is being measured can also be described using a picture.
- The **measurement instrument** to be used.
- The **assessment method** or specific test measurement to be performed.
- The **decision criteria** used to determine the measurement.
- The **inclusion and exclusion** criteria.
- The **sample size**.
- The **sample frequency**.

Example: Temperature Management on Arrival to the ED

Project: *"Improve temperature management in the ED"*
   Primary Project Metric: "Temperature on arrival to the ED"
   Operational definition

- *Metric name = Temperature on arrival to ED*
- *Measurement Instrument = Digital thermometer*
- *Assessment method = Assess temperature using tympanic membrane*
- *Decision criteria= Collect temperature of patient within 5 minutes of arrival*
- *Inclusion / Exclusion criteria = exclude children under 8 years of age, drowning victims, and victims found under hypothermic conditions*
- *Sample Size = 150 patients over 6 months*
- *Sample Interval / Frequency = Every shift, 15 randomly assigned patients*

Sample size: How much data should we collect? The amount of data you need to collect depends on the magnitude of the change you want to detect and the error you are willing to accept. The sample size calculations allow you to know how much data you need in order to be able to say with confidence whether the improvements you are making are significant.

- **For continuous data.** Sample size is calculated by estimating the **standard deviation** and deciding on the **precision required.** A very basic approach to estimating the standard deviation when there is no baseline data is to look at the historical range of a process and to divide by 4. Dividing the difference between the highest and lowest value by four is a safe bet and a good rough estimate.
- **For count and attribute data.** To estimate the proportion needed to help estimate the sample size, we can use the historical range divided by 100 as a rough estimate. For a more effective calculations, use the sample size formulas.

Sample interval: When should data be collected? Data must be collected on a regular, consistent basis, at a prescribed and planned frequency. When looking at a process during an improvement initiative, the frequency of sampling should occur at least four times every cycle. This will ensure that expected changes will be observed during the course of the data collection. For example, if we are observing a process that lasts an hour, collect the same metric every 15 minutes.

Rule # 2: Use the Principle of Stratification (Rational Subgrouping)

> **Stratification refers to collecting and organizing data according to specific subcategories in order to identify patterns and trends that will allow us to observe the independent variables affecting the outcome we want to improve.**

When data can be subdivided by a factor, condition, or grouped by some category, it is easier to interpret and uncover the source of variation (causal mechanisms) that underlie patterns. Data can be stratified by time periods, demographics, treatments, providers, etc. Stratification is important in understanding the causes of variation in the data. Stratification occurs on the basis of specific category or layers, a specific condition, or factors. When analyzing data, the goal should be to stratify in such a way that there is minimal variation within a subgroup and maximum variation between the groups.

The QI team needs to know their "business" well in order to decide on which possible independent variables they need to collect data that may have an impact on the dependent variable (outcomes) we are trying to improve. A number of tools or methods may be used to identify specific subcategories of data that must be collected, including

- brainstorm sessions: brainstorm diagram or tree diagram;
- the Five Ws (Who, What, When, Where, Why); or
- the 3 Hs (How, How much, How long).

See more about these tools in the chapters on the "Right Solution."

Example: Stratification Factors for "Time from Order to Arrival of TPN Bag"

A QI project aims to improve the delivery of total parenteral nutrition (TPN) to the surgical floors. The primary metric for this project is "time from order to arrival of TPN bag to the surgical floor." To determine how data was going to be stratified (the sub-categories of data that we are going collect), the QI team met for a brainstorming session and agreed on the following categories:

- *By time of day; by day, by month;*

- *By ordering physician; by level of training of the ordering physician;*
- *By patient's primary diagnosis; by patient ICD-10 code; and*
- *By pharmacist; by level of training of pharmacist.*

If you routinely use a Microsoft Excel spreadsheet to collect data, and you organize data in columns, the name on the first column should be your primary metric; subsequent columns can be organized according to your stratification or sub-categories.

Time	Date	Day	MD	MD level	DRG	ICD-10	Pharmacist	Training	Unit

Rule # 3: Collect Data in a Time-Ordered Fashion

> **The time order may be an essential context for data collection that should be preserved in order to make interpretations meaningful.**

Time may be the variable (x) that affects the outcome metric (y) that we are trying to improve.

Data collected in a time-ordered fashion is very useful:

- to track and visualize the current performance of a process,
- to understand the type of variation and identify patterns that provide insight into the nature of the causes of the problem, and
- to monitor the status or performance of improvement work.

MAKE YOUR DATA COLLECTION MORE EFFECTIVE WITH A DATA COLLECTION PLANNER

> **The Data Collection Planner is a tool used to prepare and guide our data collection, and to assure the data is reliable and relevant to the key questions our project is looking to answer.**

A Data Collection Planner will help make your data collection process effective, repeatable, efficient, and reproducible.

A Data Collection Planner includes the following items:

- the rationale for data collection,
- the metrics and their operational definitions,

- the stratification factors, and
- a checklist of steps to assure the data collection is effective and efficient.

TABLE 13-1   A Data Collection Planner Makes Our Data Collection Process Effective, Repeatable, Efficient, and Reproducible

The Data Collection Planner			

Why are we collecting data?

- To obtain a baseline so we can understand the process we are trying to improve
- To pilot a change and test a hypothesis with a PDSA cycle
- To assess performance after implementing a change
- To continuously monitor an improved process

Operational definition	Metric #1	Metric # 2	Metric #3
What is the name of the metric?			
How is the metric defined?			
What is the data source?			
Who will collect data? Where? When?			
By what means? With what instruments?			
How often will data be collected?			
What are the inclusion and exclusion criteria?			
What is the sample size and sample frequency?			

Stratification	Metric #1	Metric # 2	Metric #3
What factors, categories, or conditions should we consider when collecting data?			

Checklist

- An operational definition has been validated, and agreed on by all parties.
- Sample size, sampling frequency, and subgroup sizing has been addressed.
- Stratification factors have been considered (rational subgrouping).
- All personnel involved in data collection have been properly trained.
- Clearly defined procedures/methods for recording data are available.
- Units of measurement have been identified.
- Location of data collection has been identified (where are we going to collect the data).
- If data collection requires instruments, these have been calibrated.
- Measurement System Analysis (MSA) has been considered and performed as required.
- Data collection forms/templates have been prepared, communicated, and implemented.
- A go-live date has been set.

REVIEW QUIZ

1. Rules for effective data collection include the following:
   A. Data should be collected in a time-ordered fashion.
   B. Data should be collected according to an operational definition.
   C. Data should be collected using principles of dissemination.
   D. All of the above
   E. A and B only

2. The operational definition should fulfill all the following conditions EXCEPT
   A. be specific,
   B. reserved only for large-scale projects,
   C. be measurable,
   D. agreed upon by customers and stakeholders, or
   E. be repeatable and reproducible.

3. The operational definition includes the following items:
   A. name and definition of the metric;
   B. name and definition of the metric, the measurement instrument, the decision criteria;
   C. name and definition of the metric, the measurement instrument, the decision criteria, sample size, and sample frequency;
   D. name and definition of the metric, the measurement instrument, the decision criteria, sample size; or
   E. measurement instrument, the decision criteria, sample size.

4. Regarding the principles of stratification, all of the following are true EXCEPT
   A. Stratification refers to collecting and organizing data according to specific subcategories.
   B. Stratification can be used to identify patterns and trends in the data.
   C. Data should be stratified according to the needs of the individual that will collect data.
   D. Stratification is also called rational subgrouping.
   E. Brainstorming sessions and Five Ws can be used to make decisions on how to stratify data.

Table 13-1 shows the Data Collection Planner template our QI teams use. In this example we have three project metrics.

Key: 1e, 2b, 3c, 4c

CHAPTER 14

Define Baseline Performance: Is the Process "Stable"?

HOW DO I ASSESS A PROCESS'S BASELINE PERFORMANCE?

In Chapter 12, we said we need measurements (data) to answer three basic questions:

1. **How is our process behaving**? Can we meet our customer's needs?
2. **Are we meeting the needs of our customers** (Are we achieving what our patients, staff or providers expect)?
3. **How often are we meeting their needs**?

The first question addresses **Process Stability**. *Process Stability is a measure of* **consistency**, *or the ability of a process to repeatedly generate values of a specific key measure within a range, or in other words, variation limits. If the process is stable, it will produce predictable results over time.*

Before we can use our data to answer these three questions, we are going to have to process it to get the information and knowledge it contains. Data cannot be used as it has been collected from the field because it is in a "raw" format (Wheeler 2000). This means data needs to be organized, summarized, and then transformed to provide the most accurate and insightful depiction of the true performance of the process.

The Quality Improvement Challenge: A Practical Guide for Physicians, First Edition.
Richard J. Banchs and Michael R. Pop.
© 2021 John Wiley & Sons Ltd. Published 2021 by John Wiley & Sons Ltd.
Companion website: www.wiley.com/go/banchs/quality

> To assess how our process is performing in meeting the needs of our customers (process stability), we are going to need two summary statistics (numbers) and two graphs (pictures).

- **Two summary statistics (numbers).** Summary statistics are descriptive statistics. They are used to summarize a single property of the data into a single value; they help us understand without the need to see all of the data at once. We are going to need two summary statistics: **a measure of central tendency** (mean, median, or mode), and a **measure of dispersion** (range, variance, or standard deviation). Summary statistics assume data is homogenous and comes from a single process (the same universe!).
- **Two graphs (pictures).** To understand and assess the performance of our process, we are also going to need two graphs: a **snapshot**, and a graph of **time-ordered data** showing performance over time.

Different types of data require different types of summary statistics (see Figure 14-1):

- Mean: Sum of all individual values divided by the total number of values (middle by weight).
- Mode: The most frequently occurring value in a data set.
- Median: The middle value when data is arranged in the ascending or descending order. Half of the values will be above, and half will be below.
- Range: Difference between the highest and the lowest value.
- Standard deviation: The square root of the sums of the differences of the values from the mean, squared, divided by the sample size minus one.

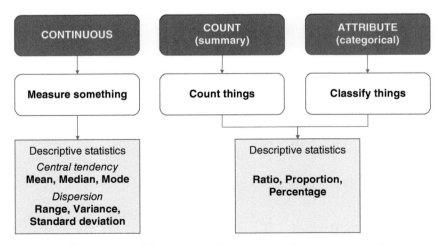

FIGURE 14-1   Different types of data require different types of summary statistics.

- Variance: The standard deviation squared.
- Ratio: A proportional relationship between two different units of measure.
- Proportion: A relationship between two different units of measure, where the denominator is constrained by the numerator. The value can be expressed as a number between 0 and 1.0.
- Percentage: A proportional relationship between two same units of measure or numbers expressed as a unit of 100.

WHY DO WE NEED A COMBINATION OF NUMBERS AND PICTURES?

To understand the performance of your process, like for all data analysis, you need to answer the **description question** and the **homogeneity question**.

- Summary statistics answer the **description question** of data analysis: given a sample of data, what arithmetic value/s summarize the information contained in those numbers (Wheeler 2012)? Summary statistics are built on the assumption that we can use a single value to characterize the property of a data set because all data comes from a single process (universe).
- The **homogeneity question** of data analysis tests the assumption all data comes from a single process (universe). If the data set comes from different processes, or a process that is operated under different conditions, then we cannot use one value to "describe what is, in effect, not one property of the process but the summary of different processes" (Wheeler 2012).

Therefore, before we can use a summary statistic to interpret data and assess the performance of a process (the description question), we will need to examine our data for evidence of homogeneity (the homogeneity question), which is implicitly assumed by the use of a summary statistic. A lack of homogeneity in our data will therefore prevent us from making any assessments about the performance of our process. How can we know how the process is performing if data comes from two different processes (or more) or a process operated under different conditions?

While the implicit assumption of homogeneity is part of everything we do in **clinical research**, homogeneity cannot be assumed whenever we analyze process data obtained in the field for **quality improvement** (Wheeler 2012). Clinical research uses experimental data. Quality improvement uses observational data. Because of the specific way we set the conditions of our experiments and data collection, homogeneity is implicit in clinical research but it is not in quality improvement.

Clinical research	Quality improvement
Experimental data	Observational data
Homogeneity implicit	Homogeneity needs to be determined

- **Experimental data** is specifically collected under controlled conditions where the purpose of the experiment is to detect the differences between the conditions studied. Since part of performing an experiment is taking the effort to assure homogeneity within each treatment condition, the assumption of homogeneity is implicit.
- **Observational data** is directly collected from the field. Homogeneity cannot be inferred and needs to be determined and managed. Since most of our QI data is not experimental, we risk making a serious mistake if we do not give the question of homogeneity careful consideration.

> **Before we can use a Summary Statistic (number) to assess the performance of our process, we must assess the data for homogeneity. Graphs (pictures) are the preferred tools to provide the answer to the homogeneity question.**

The focus, methodology, statistical tools, and goals of data analysis are clearly different between clinical research and quality improvement (Daniel 2010) (see Table 14-1).

TABLE 14-1   Differences between research and quality improvement work.

Differences between Clinical research and Quality Improvement (QI)	
Clinical research	**Quality improvement (QI)**
Focus: Study populations; the aim is to generate **new** clinical knowledge.	Focus: Study processes; the aim is to improve using **existing** knowledge.
The methodology is **experimental** (deductive); uses a **limited** amount of data over a defined period of time; compares **aggregate** data from population A versus population B.	The methodology **is observational** (inductive); uses an **unlimited** amount of data over time; compares **each point** to the previous data point trying to determine if a change has occurred.
Goals of the analysis: looks for **signal difference** in a finite amount of data under research conditions.	Goals of the analysis: Looks for **signal versus noise** in the data obtained under operational conditions.
Statistical tools: uses probability models, regression analysis, confidence intervals, and hypothesis testing.	Statistical tools: uses run charts and control charts to characterize the natural variability of the process.
The aim is to generate **new clinical** knowledge.	The aim is to improve using **existing** knowledge.

GRAPHS ARE THE BEST TOOLS TO INTERPRET DATA

The Anscombe's Quartet

Francis John Anscombe was a British statistician known among other things for his work on the importance of data graphing. To illustrate this point, Anscombe created a table with four data sets that have nearly identical simple descriptive statistics, yet have very different distributions and show significant differences when graphed. These data sets are known as the "Anscombe's Quartet" (See Table 14-2). For each data set, summary statistics are as follows: Mean of x for each data set: 9; Mean of y for each data set: 7.50; Sample variance for each data set: 11; Sample variance of y for each data set: 4.122 (4.127); Correlation between x and y for each data set: 0.816; Linear regression line for each data set: $y = 3.00 + 0.500x$ (see Table 14-3).

As you can see, the mean of x and y, the variance of x and y, and the correlation and linear regression are the same for the four data sets. Given these results, we may erroneously conclude these four data sets come from the same population and follow a similar statistical model. However, if these four data sets are graphed, a different conclusion can be drawn (see Figure 14-2).

- The first scatterplot (top left) appears to be a simple linear relationship, corresponding to two variables that are correlated. A linear regression fits the model.

TABLE 14-2 The Anscombe's Quartet data set.

The Anscombe's Quartet data set							
I		II		III		IV	
x	y	x	y	x	y	x	y
10.0	8.04	10.0	9.14	10.0	7.46	8.0	6.58
8.0	6.95	8.0	8.14	8.0	6.77	8.0	5.76
13.0	7.58	13.0	8.74	13.0	12.74	8.0	7.71
9.0	8.81	9.0	8.77	9.0	7.11	8.0	8.84
11.0	8.33	11.0	9.26	11.0	7.81	8.0	8.47
14.0	9.96	14.0	8.10	14.0	8.84	8.0	7.04
6.0	7.24	6.0	6.13	6.0	6.08	8.0	5.25
4.0	4.26	4.0	3.10	4.0	5.39	19.0	12.50
12.0	10.84	12.0	9.13	12.0	8.15	8.0	5.56
7.0	4.82	7.0	7.26	7.0	6.42	8.0	7.91
5.0	5.68	5.0	4.74	5.0	5.73	8.0	6.89

TABLE 14-3   The Anscombe's Quartet summary statistics.

Anscombe's Quartet data set summary statistics		
Variable	**Property**	**Value**
X	Mean of x for all data sets	9
	Sample variance of x for all data sets	11
Y	Mean of y for all data sets	7.50
	Sample variance of y for all data sets	4.122
X & Y	Correlation between x and y in each case	0.816
	Linear regression line in each case	y = 3.00 + 0.5x

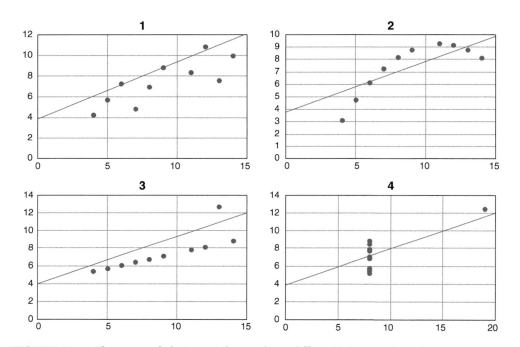

FIGURE 14-2   The Anscombe's Quartet data set has a different interpretation when graphed.

- The second graph shows a relationship between the two variables that is not linear. In this case the Pearson correlation coefficient cannot apply and the data set does not fit a linear regression model.
- In the third graph the distribution is linear; however, there is an outlier that should be further investigated before any valid conclusions may be made. The regression is offset by the one outlier that lowers the correlation coefficient from 1 to 0.816.
- The fourth graph shows an example where one outlier is enough to produce a high correlation coefficient, even though the other data points do not indicate

any relationship between the variables. Clearly, a linear model does not fit the data set.

What Can We Learn from the Anscombe's Quartet?

- **A table makes interpreting data very difficult.** A table is an easy, familiar, and common way of displaying information. However, tables have an abundance of detail that often obscures the patterns that can emerge from data as well as the relationships between numbers and variables. A table may offer the complete data set, but makes it difficult to summarize, analyze, and interpret the information contained in the numbers. Furthermore, because a table is not usually accompanied by the context under which data was obtained, it is difficult to draw any conclusions from the data. Data presented as a table cannot be used alone to provide an assessment of the performance of the process.
- **Using aggregate or summary statistics to understand your data can be misleading.** Data presented in the aggregated or summary form is very useful to summarize a single property of the data into a single value. This method is frequently used in healthcare organizations to report key metrics, assess performance, and progress towards strategic objectives. Summary statistics include **measures of central tendency** (mean, median, and mode) and **measures of dispersion** (range, variance, and standard deviation). Summary statistics are useful to describe a single property of the data but you must be aware the summarized data reflects only a **single property** of the process. It does not show all of the data at once, giving only a **snapshot view** of the process's performance at a single point in time. As a result, used alone, summary statistics do not provide enough information to either completely understand the performance of a process over time, or compare the performance of the process at different times.
- **Data presented as a graph is best for interpretation.** The Anscombe's Quartet highlights the importance of graphing data to ensure a robust analysis and to avoid inaccurate and misleading interpretations, such as those that may occur when we only use a table or a summary statistic to assess the performance of our process. A graph displays data in a visual format that makes it easier to understand. *Graphs provide the context for interpreting a value because they include all the relevant values and the time order where appropriate.* A graph is the preferred format to present data when trying to assess the performance of a process (process stability).

DO I NEED TO HAVE DATA NORMALLY DISTRIBUTED?

In general, normality is a data distribution pattern associated with continuous data. Count and attribute data are not expected to be normally distributed. Some statistical tools and techniques rely upon the assumption of a normally distributed set of data to yield valid and reliable results.

Continuous data is said to be normally distributed when it resembles the **Normal Theory model**, which is a theoretical distribution. The key property for a normal distribution is the relationship between the mean and the standard deviation, where 99.73% of the area under the bell-shaped curve is contained between −3 and +3 standard deviations from the mean.

Several tools can be used to check if the data is normally distributed, including

- The **histogram.** It has a bell-shaped curve for normal data.
- The **probability plot or fat pencil test,** which plots sequentially ordered data. It is approximate a straight line when the data is normally distributed.
- **Anderson-Darling test**. The p-value is greater than 0.05 for normally distributed data, assuming an alpha error of 0.05.

If we test our data for normality, we should be aware that

- The **null hypothesis** (H_o) is that the data is normally distributed. Hence, the alternative hypothesis (H_a) is that the data is not normally distributed.
- In the case of hypothesis testing, we are looking to **reject the null hypothesis**.
- In the case of normality testing, we are looking to **accept the null hypothesis**; hence, if the p-value is less than 0.05, we can conclude that the data *is not* normally distributed. If the p-value is greater than 0.05, we can conclude that the data *is* normally distributed.

Continuous data that is not normally distributed can signal non-homogeneous conditions and should direct us to question the context and conditions of the original observations rather than engage in statistical gymnastics to transform the data to a normal distribution. Normality is not a prerequisite for statistical analysis.

Non-normally distributed data **should not** be converted to normally distributed data because it will hide the signal for non-homogeneous conditions. Non-normally distributed data should prompt us to question and investigate what is the real cause of the lack of homogeneity of the data.

When data is not normally distributed, we should ask ourselves

- Does the data come from multiple or different processes?
- Is the data being collected under different conditions that render the conclusions of the analysis invalid?

> **Checking data for homogeneity is of much greater importance than testing for normality. Since the histogram and the control chart (see later) are the preferred tools to check the data for homogeneity, testing data for normality is not necessary.**

THE GRAPHICAL ANALYSIS

After data collection, the first step in data analysis is exploring the data using graphs and summary statistics to assess the performance of the process. The kind of graph will depend on the type of data and the goal of the analysis (see Figure 14-3).

For continuous data, the first question is always the homogeneity question. For attribute data, it is about comparing data across categories and identifying the most common attributes.

THE HISTOGRAM: A TOOL TO GET A SNAPSHOT WITH CONTINUOUS DATA

A histogram, also called a **frequency plot**, is the preferred tool to graph **continuous data** when we have at least **50 points** in the data set. A histogram displays bars representing the count within different ranges or intervals.

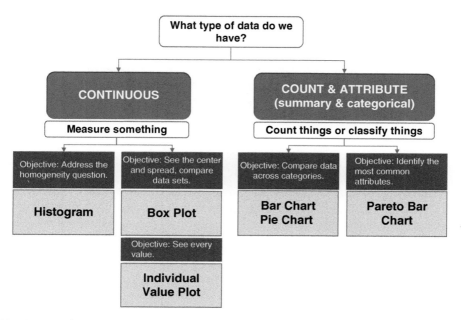

FIGURE 14-3   The Graphic Analysis for different types of data.

> **A histogram provides a "snapshot" in time of our data. It shows the basic properties, shape, and distribution of the data, and helps us assess the data for homogeneity.**

- The histogram provides a visual depiction of the **center** and **distribution** of a data set.
- The histogram helps assess data for homogeneity (the control chart is the preferred tool; see next chapters).
- Patterns can be graphically illustrated to help understand, reduce, and eliminate variation.

A histogram displays data in bars representing the count within different ranges of non-overlapping data. These ranges are often called **bins**. Each group, class, or bin represents a different segment in the range of data. In the most common presentation for the histogram, the variable of interest is presented on the x-axis and the frequency of occurrence or counts is on the vertical axis.

Types of Histograms

There are four common histogram shapes (see Figure 14-4):

1. **Bell-shaped histograms**. For these histograms, the data is loosely aggregated around the mean. A bell-shaped histogram can help confirm data is **homogeneous**, and typically suggest that the process is performing as we would expect. A bell-shaped histogram allows us to use the mean and standard deviation as a single value to describe a single property of the process or process performance. *Be aware that while the process may perform as expected, the outcome of the process may not be the one we are looking for.*

2. **Histograms with outlier data points**. These histograms usually indicate that the process is unstable and unpredictable (see unstable process in the chapter of analysis of variation). Further investigation of the process with the development of a special cause action-plan is frequently warranted because the process is not performing at the expected level.

3. **Skewed histograms with data polarizing in one end of the diagram.** This type of histogram represents data from a process that is operating under changing conditions and necessitates a probe of the reasons for the skewness at the gemba.

4. **Bimodal histograms with two peaks**. For these histograms, the existence of two data sources and two distinct pathways through the process are revealed. Data is not homogeneous. This pattern requires an evaluation of the process conditions at the gemba since it appears as if there are two separate ways in which the process is being performed. This histogram may also indicate that

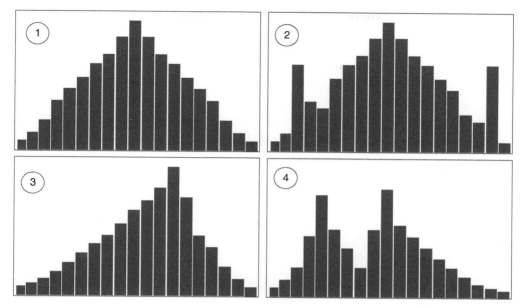

FIGURE 14-4   Types of histograms.

two different types of data that should not be combined have been combined or that data has been collected under two different conditions. The number of bars should be appropriate to avoid hiding bimodal distributions and the signal for data that is non-homogeneous. A good rule of thumb is for the number of bars or bins to equal approximately the square root of the total number of data points. For example, a histogram with 100 data points should have approximately 10 bars or bins. *When a histogram shows a bimodal distribution, conclusions about the performance of the process should not be drawn until further investigation has been done to understand and address the bimodal distribution.*

How to Create a Histogram

To create a histogram, follow these steps:

- Count the total number of observations in your data set.
- Take the square root of the total number of observations. This will give you the approximate number of bins (bars) you will need.
- Determine the width of each bin (bar) by calculating the range (highest value – lowest value) and divide it by the number of bars. Round up if necessary.

- Calculate the value range for each bin (bar). Choose the minimum value in the data set. Using the bin width, establish an interval that contains the minimal value. Create subsequent bins in increasing order until the last bin contains the largest value in the data set.
- Create a table of frequencies. Make a table with three columns: first column is for the bins in increasing order; second column should have the tally (frequency) for each bin; the third column keeps the cumulative frequency. Tally the number of observations in each bin keeping track of the frequencies.
- Chose a scale for the *y*-axis that will accommodate the class with the highest frequency.
- Construct bars for each class. The height of each bar corresponds to the frequency of the bin class.

Alternatively, you can plot your data on a histogram, by using one of the standard software packages available such as Microsoft Excel ®, Minitab®, or SPSS® Predictive Analytical Software.

ADDITIONAL GRAPHS YOU CAN USE WITH CONTINUOUS DATA

The Box Plot

The box plot provides a quick look at the distribution of a set of data, and presents an

> **A box plot or box-and-whiskers plot (or diagram) is a method for graphically depicting groups of numerical data through their quartiles.**

assessment of the variation and dispersion of data. The components of a box plot are divided into the **"box"** area and the **"whiskers"** outside the box. The box plot displays the data in **quartiles,** with lines extending vertically from the box that indicate variability outside the upper and lower quartiles (see Figure 14-5).

The "box" of a box plot diagram

- Is divided by a line that corresponds to the median of the data set.
- Shows the range of data values comprising 50% of the data set. The lower edge of the box corresponds to the first quartile. The upper edge of the box corresponds to the third quartile; hence the box represents the second and third quartile of data.
- The width of the box is called the interquartile range (IQR).

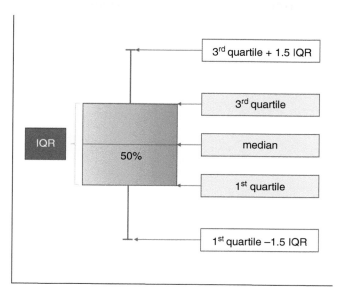

FIGURE 14-5   The "box" and "whiskers" of a box plot.

The "whiskers" of a box plot diagram

- Extend from the upper edge of the box or third quartile + 1.5 times the inter-quartile range (IQR).
- Extend from the lower edge of the box or first quartile – 1.5 times the interquar-tile range (IQR).
- A value is considered an *outlier* if it is above the upper or below the lower "whiskers."
- The whiskers can also represent the minimum and the maximum value of the data set.

The box plot is used to assess the distribution and variation of a continuous data set or to compare performance of multiple data sets. Be sure to include the total number of observations used to create the box plot. There is no distinguishing factor that can differentiate between a box plot that was created with three data points versus 300 data points.

The Individual Value Plot

The individual value plot is a graph that shows a dot for the actual value of each observation in a group.

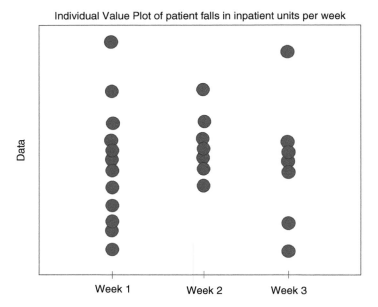

FIGURE 14-6   The individual value plot of patient falls in inpatient units per week.

The individual value plot (also called the **dot plot**) is a graph used with **continuous data** to assess and compare sample data distributions. The individual value plot shows graphing of separate values, which is especially valuable when you have relatively few observations (less than 50 data points) or when it is important to assess the effect of each observation (see example in Figure 14-6).

When to use the individual value plot:

- to see the individual distribution of the data set,
- to see distribution and spread of all the data,
- to spot outliers,
- to see the location and spread of the dependent variable y at each level of the independent x variable, or
- to make group comparisons.

THE BAR CHART: A TOOL TO GET A SNAPSHOT WITH DISCRETE DATA

A bar chart is a way to summarize categorical data using rectangular bars with heights or lengths proportional to the values they represent.

The purpose of the bar chart is to

- show the different values for each category of data;
- show the relationship between categories on one axis and discrete values on the other axis;
- show changes or differences in data among groups;
- compare the number, frequency, or other measure between discrete categories of data; and
- display causes, and the contribution of each cause to a problem.

The bar chart is a graph for discrete data. Discrete data needs a clearly defined **area of opportunity** (AOO), which means

- The different discrete categories are independent.
- Data have the same opportunity to appear.
- Data is generated by a process operated under the same conditions.

There are different types of bar charts with the bars plotted vertically or horizontally:

- **Vertical bar charts** are the most common type of bar graphs. They are very useful when presenting categories of data. One disadvantage of vertical bar graphs is that they don't leave much room at the bottom of the chart if long labels are required (see example in Figure 14-7).
- **Horizontal bar charts** are best used to depict time issues or when long labels are better placed horizontally.
- **Stacked bar charts** are used to convey information about more than one variable, cause, or factor. One of the disadvantages of a stacked bar chart is that it may not show data in as clear of a manner as intended.

To create a bar chart

- Decide on the type of bar chart you need.
- On the y-axis, place the measured values.
- On the x-axis, place the specific categories being compared. Some bar graphs present bars clustered in groups of more than one, showing the values of more than one measured variable.
- Arrange the values in order if desired.

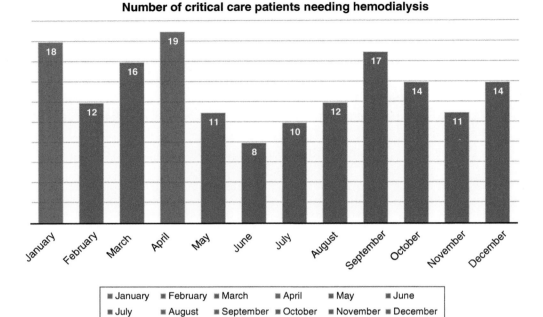

FIGURE 14-7   A Bar chart of "Critical care patients needing hemodialysis."

ADDITIONAL CHARTS YOU CAN USE WITH DISCRETE DATA

The Pie Chart

Pie charts represent data in a circular graph divided into a number of sections, each of which designates a proportion of all the data collected.

Use pie charts to represent percentages for categorical data. Pie charts are ideal for giving a quick idea of the proportional distribution of the data and are very useful for data stratified in a small number of categories; see Chapter 18, Figure 18-7.

Limitations

- Pie charts can only show a small number of categories or segments of data. As the number of segments increase, the size of each segment/slice becomes smaller. This makes them unsuitable for large amounts of data with lots of segments.
- Pie charts take up more space than some of the other graphic alternatives. This is mainly due to their size and need for extra space for a legend.

- Pie charts are not the ideal graph to make accurate comparisons between groups of data. It is harder to distinguish the size of an item by comparing the areas of a graphs.

The Pareto Bar Chart

> **The Pareto bar chart is a specialized bar chart used with count and attribute data that presents a graphical visualization of the frequency of the individual causes displayed in decreasing order using cumulative percentages.**

The Pareto bar chart displays the ordered frequency data according to their cumulative percentages. It is often use to filter and prioritize the most likely cause of a problem. For more information on the Pareto charts, see Chapter 18 on filtering and prioritizing the most likely cause.

CASE STUDY: IMPROVING RTA TIME AT ST. MICHAEL'S HOSPITAL

Nursing leadership at St. Michael's Hospital is concerned about the time it takes a nurse on the wards to administer medication to a patient in pain. The time from patient request (push of the call button) to administration of medication is called the RTA (Request To Administration) time. RTA has been followed for several months. This February, the average RTA was 30 minutes. In January, the average RTA was 26 minutes. In February last year, the average RTA was 34 minutes. While February's performance shows an improvement when compared to February last year, the average RTA time in February has increased compared to January. Cohort benchmark performance (data in similar hospitals around the country) for RTA is 21 minutes. This is well below the current RTA time average at St. Michaels. What actions, if any, should nursing leadership take at St. Michaels? Is February getting better, worse, or is the change not significant? How is the process overall performance?

January (average)	February (average)	February (year before)	Year to date	% Yearly difference	Cohort Benchmark
26 min	30 min	34 min	28 min	−12%	21 min

To answer these questions, there are three possible options:

Compare February to the Cohort Benchmark. The average RTA for February is 30 minutes, which is higher than the cohort benchmark. We may be inclined to conclude that performance is getting worse. However, there are two problems if we use this option to make a decision:

1. As explained before, using an average assumes data is homogeneous, has been obtained under similar conditions, and the process is influenced by factors that are similar or uniform in nature. This may not be the case. This assumption (homogeneity) needs to be tested.

2. There is a limited amount of information obtained from comparing one number to another (February to the cohort benchmark). Comparison between two values doesn't provide sufficient evidence to be conclusive. It only allows a "binary" assessment where performance may be judged as being either good or bad (Wheeler 2000).

Compare the averages. February's RTA is higher (worse) than January, but is improved when compared to February last year. This option, too, has problems if used alone to assess the performance of the process:

1. Averages are high-order descriptive statistics (summary statistics) that are globally computed and assume data is homogeneous.

2. When comparing two averages (numbers), both numbers may be subject to normal variation. It may be difficult to determine just how much of the difference in value is due to normal variation and how much is due to improvement or deterioration (change) in the process.

Request more data to make a decision about the performance of the process. Would it be sufficient to get more data? Are we going to be able to assess process performance? That depends! Consider the average "request-to-administration" (RTA) time graph with data for the previous two years (see Figure 14-8). Is the process getting better? Can you say conclusively that the "request-to-administration" (RTA) time is improving or deteriorating?

What Can We Learn from the **RTA Time at St. Michael's Hospital?**

- Summary data reflects only a single property of the process. It does not show all the data at once, giving only a snapshot view of the process's performance at one point in time. As a result, it does not provide enough information to make decisions on how the process is performing **(the example of the Anscombe's Quartet).**

- Using summary or aggregate data such as an average to interpret performance is a problem because higher order descriptive statistics (summary statistics) are globally computed and assume data is homogeneous. This might not be the case **(the homogeneity question).**

- Averages are derived from the values generated by the process. It is the "voice of the process," which gives us some insight into the outcome. However, the average is only a summary of the data and, as such, can only give a

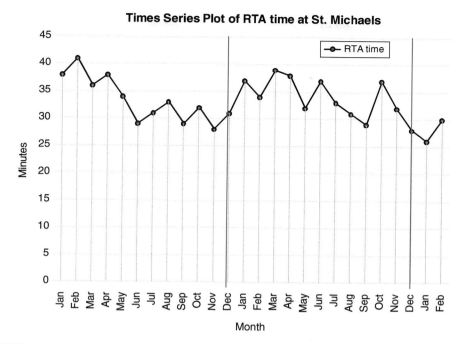

FIGURE 14-8   Time series plot of "Request To Administration (RTA) time at St. Michael's Hospital."

snapshot view, or single picture of the process's performance. This snapshot view shows us where we are but it does not tell us where to go or what to do (Wheeler 2000)

- When comparing two averages (numbers), both numbers may be subject to normal variation. It may be difficult to determine just how much of the difference in value is due to normal variation and how much is due to an improvement or deterioration of the process i.e. a change in the process (**the Problem with Variation**).

- We may believe there has been a drop in performance, which may prompt us to change the process to get better performance when in reality, the higher RTA value may just be random variation.

  - Changing a process because we assume the process is deteriorating when nothing has changed is called **tampering** and creates a **type I or alpha error** (false alarm). As we keep tampering, results will get worse, variation will increase, and we will not improve the process's performance.

  - If, on the other hand, we believe the higher RTA values are just due to random variation, but in reality, the process is deteriorating and we fail to act, then we incur a **type II or beta error** (failure to alarm).

THE ANSWER TO THE PROBLEM OF VARIATION IS A GRAPH OF TIME-ORDERED DATA

> **A graph of time-ordered data should be used to examine the process for signs of homogeneity and interpret variation.**

Using a graph of time-ordered data to examine the process for signs of homogeneity and interpret variation has been called the **process-centered approach** to data interpretation (Wheeler 2000). The process-centered approach focuses on the **process behavior** rather than on a single value (Summary Statistic) to assess process performance. The process-centered approach considers **variation** in the values as the critical piece of information:

- If the process shows a type of variation that results from homogeneity, we can proceed to make statistical inferences about the performance of the process and determine the best course of action based on the results.
- If the process shows signs of non-homogeneity, we need to first find out why this is happening before making any changes to the process.

The process-centered approach focuses on the **Voice of the Process (VOP)**, rather than on the outcome (target, average, or percentage). The process-centered approach is the best method to avoid making a type I or type II error.

The process-centered approach needs **time-ordered data**. Data comes from a process, and processes are dynamic and constantly changing. Time-ordered data needs to be collected on a regular consistent basis, such as hourly, daily, weekly, etc.; needs to be collected at a known and planned frequency. Time-ordered data is then used to

- visualize actual process performance,
- identify patterns in the data as well as the amount of variation, and
- track and evaluate how the changes (improvements) made to the process are performing over time and if any additional changes may be necessary.

Understanding the Types of Variation

If we record our systolic and diastolic pressures, not all measurements will be the same even when they are obtained within seconds from each other. The same can be said about the tidal volume (TV): each breath may yield a slightly different value but that doesn't mean there is a problem. Actually, we expect small differences in values. When we observe a large change in values, however, we may need to ask ourselves whether something is wrong. So, the question is: what change in value is significant? How do we establish a threshold when comparing two data points? At which point do we know a value is different and indicates that something has changed? The answer is by **characterizing the variation** in the data. Understanding the type of variation can help us understand what type of action(s) may be needed. Time-ordered data helps us understand the type and magnitude of the variation and alerts us to when a change in the values are indicative of non-homogeneity and a changing (or deteriorating) process.

Walter Shewhart identified two sources of process variation (variation in the process data):

1. **Chance variation,** caused by factors that are inherent and belong to the process; and
2. **Assignable variation,** due to factors that are not part of the process and produce unpredictable results.

W. Edwards Deming later relabeled these two causes of variation as Common Cause Variation instead of chance variation, and Special Cause Variation instead of assignable variation.

What Is Common Cause Variation?

Let's use an example: Imagine you collect data on the total time a patient spends in the outpatient asthma clinic. We will call this the *lead time*. A patient's lead time in the clinic is determined by a number of factors, for example: the time of the day; the day of the week; the total number of patients scheduled; the appointment schedule interval; the number of staff and physicians working; the time staff and physicians take to see each patient or complete their tasks; and patients' DRGs. These factors are always present and should exert a random influence on the lead time. As long as nothing substantial changes in the design of the process (the way the clinic schedules and see patients, and the type of patients seen), lead time will vary within a range.

Factors that affect the clinic's lead time

- are intrinsic components of the process design (the way the clinic is designed to run),
- are always present, and
- exert a random effect on the outcome (the lead time).

A process under the influence of these factors (intrinsic)

- generates values that are expected within a predictable range of process performance; data is said to be **homogenous** (the homogeneity question);
- shows variation among values that is **random**, does not have a **pattern**, and this variation is called **"noise"** or **Common Cause Variation.**

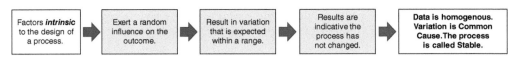

FIGURE 14-9　Relationships for Common Cause Variation.

When a process experiences Common Cause Variation, the process is said to be "stable." When a process is stable, higher and lower values should not be interpreted as evidence the process is either improving or deteriorating, rather values to be expected given the design of the process (see Figure 14-9).

Common Cause Variation is also called routine or random.

Factors that are intrinsic to the design of a process exert a random influence on the outcome, generate values that are expected within a range, and therefore, belong to a process that has not changed and is performing as designed (stable process).

Because the process is essentially the same and has not experienced a change, past results can be used to **predict future results,** within a certain range. No specific action is required on a stable process as long as the results are acceptable. See below for further details.

What Is Special Cause Variation?

Let's return to the outpatient asthma clinic lead time example. What would happen if, at certain irregular and unpredictable intervals, patients requiring emergency asthma treatment were sent to the clinic from the ED (Emergency Department)? How would the arrival of these patients affect lead time for the rest of the patients waiting to be seen? Specifically, how would it affect daily and weekly lead time averages? If patients were allowed to come up from the ED at unpredictable intervals, we could no longer say lead time in the clinic is driven by factors that are predictable and intrinsic to the design of the system. Lead time would be significantly increased by the random arrival of patients requiring emergency treatment.

In addition to factors that are always present and exert a random influence on patients' lead time, lead time would be influenced by factors that are extrinsic components of the process design (the way the clinic is designed to run), are not always present, and are unpredictable. That is, we don't know when they appear and the effect they will have on lead time.

A process under the influence of these factors (extrinsic factors) generates values that are unexpected, and outside of a predictable range of process performance. Data is considered to be non-homogenous (the homogeneity question). Variation is **non-random,** may follow **trends** or **patterns,** and is called a **signal** or **Special Cause Variation.**

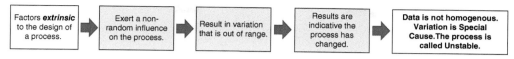

FIGURE 14-10   Relationships for Special Cause Variation.

When a process experiences Special Cause Variation, the process is said to be **unstable.** Special Cause Variation is alerting us that the process **has changed** and is not performing as designed. Special Cause Variation should prompt us to investigate the cause of poor process performance (see Figure 14-10).

Special Cause Variation is also called assignable or exceptional.

> **Factors that are extrinsic to the design of a process exert a dominant influence on the outcome, generating values that are unexpected and out of range. This variation belongs to a process that has changed and is not performing as designed (unstable process).**

Because of the unpredictable influence extrinsic factors may exert on the process, the outcome is either difficult or impossible to predict and past results will not predict future results.

Technically speaking: A stable process is a process that is within **statistical control,** meaning the outcomes can be predicted within a statistical range, whereas an unstable process with Special Cause Variation is a process that is "out of statistical control" and the outcome cannot be predicted.

VARIATION GUIDES THE IMPROVEMENT STRATEGY

The type of variation defines the improvement strategy (see Figure 14-11).

With Common Cause Variation and a Stable Process

There is **noise.** Common Cause Variation is caused by the influence of factors that are intrinsic to the process design. Common Cause Variation tells us the process has not changed and is performing as designed. There are two options:

- If a stable process is generating satisfactory results, nothing else needs to be done, although we should be constantly looking for improvement opportunities and therefore **continue to monitor.**
- However, if a stable and predictable process is not producing the desired outcomes, or there is significant variation, we should consider improving it as it will continue to produce the same, suboptimal results. To improve a stable

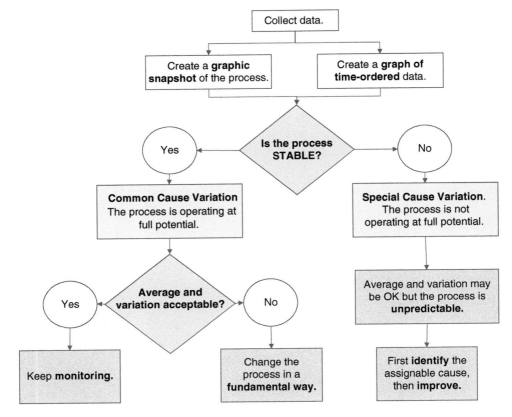

FIGURE 14-11   The improvement strategy.

process, we must **fundamentally change the process,** by redesigning it or by changing the conditions under which it operates so that a different mix of factors affect the output. As Donald Wheeler states, "Unless and until the underlying process is changed in some fundamental way, you will continue to see values that are unsatisfactory. Looking for differences between the good days and the bad days will simply be a waste of time" (Wheeler 2000).

To improve a stable process

- Stratify data to look for patterns or trends.
- Investigate the cause of the problem.
- Select the most likely causes.
- Hold a brainstorming session to generate a list of possible solutions to address the causes.
- Select and prioritize the best solution.

With Special Cause Variation and an Unstable Process

There is a **signal**. A signal in the data is indicative of non-homogeneity and the existence of an external factor that is affecting the process. This factor is usually unpredictable, dominant and responsible for Special Cause Variation. A process that is unstable and exhibits Special Cause Variation has changed. Therefore, to improve, we must **first track down the assignable cause** of variation and try to eliminate it before further improvement can occur. We should not try to improve an unstable process. When Special Cause Variation exists, improvement efforts should focus on tweaking the current process by eliminating the unpredictable causes of variation. When a process shows Special Cause Variation

- Go to the gemba and examine possible causes of variation.
- Find and remove the assignable causes of variation.
- Correct the output, improve the process, and the system that created the output.
- Develop a mitigation plan to address signals that cannot be eliminated.

The Bottom Line

To understand and assess process performance, first address the question of homogeneity. You will need two numbers and two graphs. Then consider variation. The **process-centered approach** considers variation in the data as the critical piece of information to explain the behavior of the process, and to determine if there are signs of non-homogeneity indicative of a process change. The type of variation will determine the improvement approach (see Table 14-4).

TABLE 14-4   Analysis of Variation: the bottom line.

Analysis of Variation: the bottom line	
Common Cause	**Special Cause**
What does it mean?	
The variation is random and expected. Variation shows **noise.**	The variation is unexpected and shows patterns and trends. Variation shows a **signal.**
How are the expected values?	
Results are predictable and data is **homogenous.**	Results are unpredictable; data is **not homogenous.**
How is the process?	
The process has not changed and therefore is **stable.**	The process has changed and therefore is **unstable.**

(Continued)

TABLE 14.4 (Continued)

Analysis of Variation: the bottom line	
Common Cause	**Special Cause**
Are results predictable?	
Yes, results are predictable within a range.	No, results are unpredictable.
What are the most common mistakes?	
Type I error: We interpret noise as a signal and make changes to the process that doesn't need it; the results get worse.	**Type II error**: We interpret a signal as noise, we fail to intervene, and results continue to deteriorate.
What is the preferred improvement strategy?	
If the results are acceptable, continue to monitor; if the results are not acceptable, change the process in a **fundamental way.**	Whether the results are acceptable or unacceptable, we need to intervene; first look for assignable causes of variation and eliminate them; **tweak** the process; we can further improve the process when stable.

Getting Back to the RTA Time at St. Michaels

The average RTA time from month to month is variable. Differences between averages may not represent a change in the process. Variation may just be "noise." On the other hand, variation may be a signal that something in the process has changed and we may need to intervene to prevent further deterioration. How do we know if we have noise or a signal? How do we know when to intervene? How can we decrease our chance of making a type I or type II error? The answer is by using tools to analyze variation (see next chapter).

To assess the performance of the RTA time at St. Michaels, we need

- Data.
- The context (How was data collected?).
- A **snapshot graph.** This shows the data and includes a summary statistic of the findings.
- An analysis technique that filters the noise from the signal. This is a graph of **time-ordered data** showing performance over time and variation.

The use of summary descriptive statistics alone, such as the mean, washes out the individual data points that reflect the true nature of the process's functionality and guide meaningful improvement actions. A better way to display data involves using time-ordered data and an analysis technique that filters the noise from a signal such as a run chart or a control chart. See these tools on the next chapters.

TIPS WHEN PRESENTING DATA

When presenting data, it is important to consider how to clearly and effectively communicate your results to the audience. With an effective presentation, you will gain credibility and project buy-in. Here are some recommendations

- **Start by explaining the "why" of the project.** Remind your audience about the nature of the problem, why we collected data, and what is the goal of the project.
- **Present data with the necessary context.** Data must be presented with the necessary context to ensure that the original assumptions are understood. Context should include: the raw data and a full description of the conditions under which the data was collected (who, what, when, where, how, and how much).
- **Show a graph.** A graph displays the data in a visual format that makes it easier to understand and communicate the message. A graph provides the context for interpreting a value because it includes all the relevant previous values.
- **Avoid complexity.** Make sure your graphs are appropriate to the audience. Don't just show any graph; the goal is to communicate the message that is imbedded in the data.
- **Don't forget the title**. Make sure your graph has a clear title. Do not use the type of graph as the title of the slide, rather make sure the title is the explanation of what your data is trying to communicate.
- **Don't forget the labels.** Make sure the labels on the x- and y-axis have the correct units of measure and bear clear names.
- **Make it visual.** Display big graphs that are clear and unobstructed by other images; preferably one chart or graph per page/slide unless you are making group comparisons.
- **Include a chart with time-ordered data.** Summary data and graphs of the snapshot of a process must be accompanied by time-ordered data. Summary graphs and data give only a snapshot view of the process's performance, which is not enough to completely understand the process behavior over time. Summary graphs and data may hide the time-order of the data, which may be the clue to identifying patterns and trends in the data.
- **Summarize your findings**. Help your audience understand what the data (graph) means; with each slide/page or chart, summarize the findings; provide a concise summary of the results.

REVIEW QUIZ

1. To understand a process, you need
   A. a metric,
   B. summary statistics,
   C. summary statistics and two graphs,
   D. a snapshot of the process, or
   E. a graph of time-ordered data only.

2. Quality improvement work is characterized by all the following EXCEPT
   A. Collection of observational data.
   B. Data needs to be examined for homogeneity.
   C. The methodology is experimental.
   D. An unlimited amount of data can be collected over time.
   E. Data analysis aims to separate noise from a signal.

3. Continuous data can be displayed using a
   A. histogram
   B. box plot
   C. individual value plot
   D. bar chart
   E. A, B, and C

4. Attribute data should be displayed preferentially using a
   A. Control chart
   B. Run chart
   C. Bar chart
   D. Box plot
   E. Histogram

5. Which is true of a histogram?
   A. It is a graphic tool used for attribute data.
   B. It displays bars representing a single count.
   C. A bi-modal histogram suggests that data are non-homogeneous with the existence of two data sources, or a process operated under two different conditions.
   D. It is recommended to use with less than 50 data points.
   E. A bell-shaped histogram suggest data are non-homogeneous.

6. Regarding the box plot
   A. The "box" shows the first and second quartile of data.
   B. The box plot shows dispersion of the data around the mean.
   C. The box plot is a useful tool to show data in quartiles.
   D. Has "whiskers" that extend from the first to the fourth quartile of the data set.
   E. Shows a "box" that contains 75% of the data set.

7. Variation is
   A. an intrinsic component of all data sets,
   B. always present in the data,
   C. usually predictable within a certain range,
   D. considered to be Common Cause Variation when variation is caused by factors that are always present and a part of the process, or
   E. All of the above

8. Which of the following is TRUE?
   A. Factors affecting Common Cause Variation are external to the process.
   B. With Special Cause Variation, there is a factor that dominates over other random factors and distorts the results.
   C. There is always a small amount of Special Cause Variation in every process.
   D. With Common Cause Variation, there is always an assigned and unpredictable specific factor.
   E. Common Cause Variation means the process is unstable.

9. Regarding a robust improvement strategy
   A. When data shows noise, we should investigate the root cause of the problem.
   B. With Common Cause Variation, you must change the process in some fundamental way to change the results.
   C. Special Cause Variation requires going back to the gemba.
   D. With Special Cause Variation, you must find and remove the assignable cause of the problem.
   E. All of the above

Key: 1c, 2c, 3e, 4c, 5c, 6c, 7e, 8b, 9e

REFERENCES

1. Daniel M. Improving quality in anesthesia: where are we starting from and how are we going to get there? *Pediatric Anesthesia* 2010. 20:681–683.
2. Wheeler D. Myths about data analysis. Manuscript 238. International Lean Six Sigma Conference 2012.
3. Wheeler D. *Understanding Variation. The Key to Managing Chaos.* SPC Press 2000. Second Edition

CHAPTER 15

Tools to Characterize the Type of Variation: The Run Chart

WHAT IS A RUN CHART?

Common Cause Variation is characterized by **random variation** in the data, called **noise**. A run chart is used to identify **nonrandom patterns** of variation in the data called **signals** that are indicative of the presence of special cause variation.

The run chart is an analysis technique that filters **noise** from a **signal**. The run chart

> **The run chart or time series plot is a graphical display of time-ordered data used to detect signals or nonrandom patterns of variation that are indicative of the presence of Special Cause Variation.**

shows data points in the order in which they occur and reflects changes in the process and process performance over time. A run chart can be used to

- Define the **performance** of a process.
- Identify **special cause variation** (nonrandom patterns) in a data set.
- Show an **improvement** as nonrandom patterns of variation.
- Monitor improvement intervention and assess whether gains are maintained.

An advantage of the run chart is that it can quickly identify special cause variation in data sets with less than 50 points.

The Quality Improvement Challenge: A Practical Guide for Physicians, First Edition.
Richard J. Banchs and Michael R. Pop.
© 2021 John Wiley & Sons Ltd. Published 2021 by John Wiley & Sons Ltd.
Companion website: www.wiley.com/go/banchs/quality

MAKING A RUN CHART

The run chart is a simple tool that can be used in the field with just a pencil and paper. A quick run chart can be created while on rounds, at the bedside, or while looking at data trends on an ICU monitor. To make a run chart in the field, follow these steps:

- Create the horizontal axis (x) and scale using time in hours, days, weeks, or months according to your data.
- Create the vertical axis (y) and scale using the metric you are going to plot. Estimate the range of the data points by looking at the largest and smallest values. Make sure most of the data lies around the center of the vertical axis and label the vertical axis accordingly.
- Plot each value on the chart and connect the data points with a line.
- Calculate the median of the data and use it to place a center line on the chart. The median is the number in the middle of the data set when data is sequentially ordered. If the number of observations is odd, use the middle value; if the number of observations is even, use the average of the two middle values. Using the median is advantageous because it is not influenced by extreme values in the data.
- Place a title at the top of the page to clearly define the process data or metric you are graphing.
- Use the run chart rules to interpret the results (see next).

INTERPRETING THE RUN CHART

A run chart is used to identify nonrandom patterns in the data indicative of the presence of special cause variation. There are four rules or circumstances that indicate a nonrandom pattern:

> **Rule 1: Presence of a shift.** A shift is characterized by six or more consecutive points either above or below the center line (the median). Values located on the median can be disregarded because they don't add to or break the shift (see example in Figure 15-1).

A shift is based on a probability of an event happening six times in a row. The probability of six points being either above or below the line is $p = .03$, which is below the standard accepted threshold level of significance of $p < .05$ (Provost 2011).

> **Rule 2: Presence of a trend.** A trend is characterized by the presence of **five** or more consecutive points all going up or all going down.

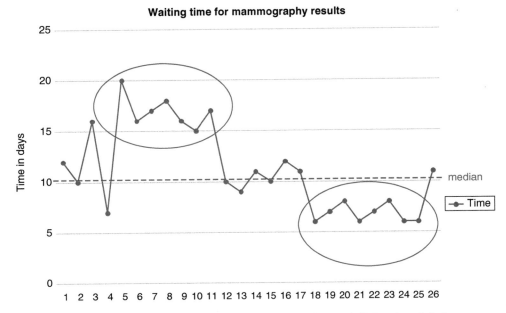

FIGURE 15-1   Run chart of "Waiting time for mammography results" showing violation of rule 1.

The decision to take five points as trend comes from experience and accepted best-practice (Provost 2011). Values that are the same are counted as one, and values on the center line do not make or break a trend (see example in Figure 15-2).

Rule 3: Too few or too many runs. A run is defined as a series of consecutive values on either side of the center line. Points on the center line do not break a run.

After counting the number of runs, a table is referenced for comparison of the number of actual runs to the number of expected runs (see Table 15-1). The run chart table uses the total number of data points on the run chart that do not fall on the median to establish the minimum and maximum number of expected runs. Too few or too many runs are indicative of a nonrandom pattern of variation. The probability of the number of runs being above or below the predicted number and not being a non-random pattern of variation is less than 5% and hence meets the threshold of accepted level of significance of $p < .05$ (Provost 2011).

Rule 4: Presence of extreme points. This rule is based on the simple observation of an outlying value that is above or below the others and that is obviously different from all values.

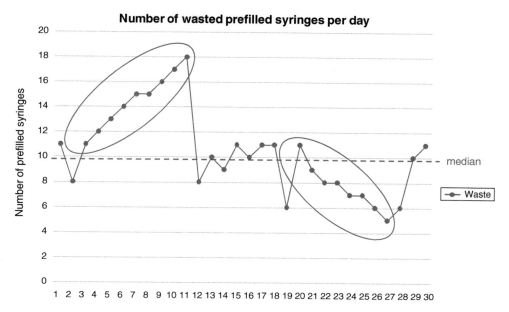

FIGURE 15-2   Run chart of "Number of wasted prefilled syringes per day" showing violation of rule 2.

TABLE 15-1   The Run Chart Table for Interpretation of the Number of Runs

Run chart table for interpretation of the number of runs					
# of points not on the median	Lower limit	Upper limit	# of points not on the median	Lower limit	Upper limit
10	3	8	34	12	23
11	3	9	35	12	23
12	3	10	36	13	24
13	4	10	37	13	25
14	4	11	38	14	25
15	4	12	39	14	26
16	5	13	40	15	26
17	5	13	41	16	26
18	6	14	42	16	27
19	6	15	43	17	27
20	6	16	44	17	28
21	7	16	45	17	29
22	7	17	46	17	30

(Continued)

TABLE 15.1   (Continued)

Run chart table for interpretation of the number of runs					
# of points not on the median	Lower limit	Upper limit	# of points not on the median	Lower limit	Upper limit
23	8	17	47	18	30
24	8	18	48	18	31
25	9	18	49	19	31
26	9	19	50	19	32
27	9	19	60	24	37
28	10	20	70	28	43
29	10	20	80	33	48
30	11	21	90	37	54
31	11	22	100	42	59
32	11	22	110	46	65
33	11	23	120	51	70

We need a minimum of 10 total data points to apply Rule 1 (presence of a shift) or rule 3 (too few or too many runs) because these two rules are probability-based.

Example: Order-to-Result (OTR) Time at Mercy Hospital

A QI team was launched at Mercy Hospital to improve the order-to-result (OTR) time for stat ABGs (arterial blood gases) in the MICU (Medical ICU). On average, the chemistry lab takes 37 minutes to report a result for a STAT ABG. Random weekly values were recorded and are shown for a period of 20 weeks (see Table 15-2). Given these results, what can you say about the performance of the process? Are there nonrandom patterns of variation in the data suggestive of special cause variation? What should the improvement team do?

  When applying the four rules of a run chart to the data set from Mercy Hospital, no clear evidence of nonrandom patterns of variation appear (see Figure 15-3). The four rules for data interpretation on the run chart show:

- *Rule 1: no shifts.*
- *Rule 2: no trends.*
- *Rule 3: there are a total of 20 values that are not on the median. The run chart table indicates that, for a data set with 20 values, the lower limit for the number of*

TABLE 15-2 OTR Times for STAT ABGs at Mercy Hospital

OTR times for STAT ABGs at Mercy Hospital			
Week	Time	Week	Time
1	29	11	34
2	32	12	36
3	33	13	41
4	38	14	38
5	36	15	35
6	41	16	32
7	38	17	36
8	36	18	39
9	46	19	44
10	47	20	41

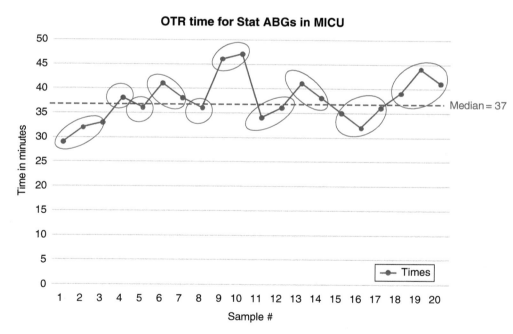

FIGURE 15-3 Run chart of "OTR times for STAT ABGs at Mercy Hospital's MICU" showing the number of runs.

runs is 6 and the upper limit is 16. The run chart at Mercy Hospital shows a total of 10 runs, which is within the expected upper and lower limits.

- *Rule 4: no extreme points.*

Interpretation: There are no shifts, trends, extreme points, or an unusual number of runs. Therefore, we can conclude data is homogeneous and variation is random (noise) or common cause. The process is stable and has not changed. Current and future results are predictable.

Strategy: If we feel the performance of the process (order-to-result time for stat ABGs in the MICU) is acceptable (median of 37 minutes, minimum 29, maximum 47), we should continue to monitor the process. If the process performance is unacceptable, the QI team should launch a QI project to redesign the way STAT ABGs are handled in the chemistry lab.

Example: Narcotic Discrepancies at Chicago Med

Data provided in Table 15-3 depicts the average number of weekly narcotic discrepancies (ND) identified by pharmacy at Chicago Med (see Table 15-3). Data was collected over a period of four weeks. Using a time-series plot (run chart), analyze the data for non-random patterns of variation. What does the data suggest? What are your conclusions? What should the QI team do?

When applying the four rules of a run chart to the data set from Chicago Med, no clear evidence of nonrandom patterns of variation appear (see Figure 15-4). The four rules for data interpretation on the run chart show:

- *Rule 1: no shifts.*
- *Rule 2: no trends.*
- *Rule 3: a total of 20 values that are not on the median. The run chart table indicates that, for a data set with 20 values, the lower limit for the number of runs is 6 and the upper limit is 16. The run chart at Mercy Hospital shows a total of 11 runs, which is within the expected upper and lower limits.*
- *Rule 4: no extreme points.*

Interpretation: There are no shifts, trends, extreme points, or an unusual number of runs. Therefore, we can conclude data is homogeneous and variation is random (noise) or common cause. The process is stable and has not changed. Current and future results are predictable.

Strategy: Leadership at Chicago Med felt that a median 20.5 narcotic discrepancies was not acceptable. A QI team was charted to redesign the process. After creating a Problem Statement, Project Charter, and Process Map, the team focused on finding the most common causes of narcotic discrepancy. After several meetings and pilots, a more reliable way to document narcotics by front line staff was rolled-out.

Example: C-section Rate at London Memorial

*Data provided in the accompanying table shows the monthly **C-section rate** over a 24-month period at London Memorial (see Table 15-4). The Chair of Obstetrics &*

TABLE 15-3   Number of Narcotic Discrepancies at Chicago Med

Narcotic discrepancies at Chicago Med					
	Mon	Tues	Wed	Thurs	Fri
Week 1	16	25	21	31	22
Week 2	18	20	19	27	20
Week 3	18	21	20	23	21
Week 4	17	20	23	21	19

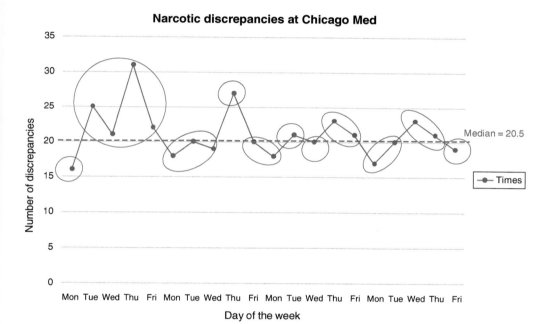

FIGURE 15-4   Run chart of "Narcotic discrepancies at Chicago Med" showing the number of runs.

Gynecology is concerned that the average C-section rate is too high. Using a time-series plot (run chart), analyze the data for nonrandom patterns of variation. What does the data suggest? What are your conclusions? What should the Chair of Obstetrics & Gynecology do?

When applying the four rules of a run chart to the data set from London Memorial, no clear evidence of nonrandom patterns of variation appear (see Figure 15-5). The four rules for data interpretation on the run chart show:

- *Rule 1: no shifts.*
- *Rule 2: no trends.*

TABLE 15-4 C-section Rates at London Memorial

C-section rate at London Memorial							
Jan	Feb	Mar	Apr	May	Jun	Jul	Aug
12	9	15	10	18	11	17	15
Sep	Oct	Nov	Dec	Jan	Feb	Mar	Apr
14	13	16	12	16	9	15	17
May	Jun	Jul	Aug	Sep	Oct	Nov	Dec
10	12	13	9	18	11	14	12

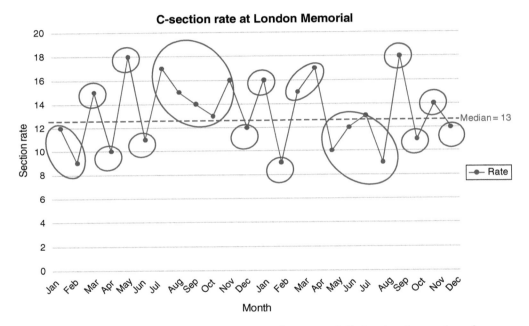

FIGURE 15-5 Run chart of "C-section rate at London Memorial" showing the number of runs.

- *Rule 3: There are a total of 22 values out of 24 are not on the median; the run chart table indicates that, for a data set with 22 values, the lower limit for the number of runs is 7 and the upper limit is 17. The run chart at London Memorial shows a total of 15 runs, which is within the expected upper and lower limits.*
- *Rule 4: no extreme points.*

Interpretation: *There are no shifts, trends, extreme points, or an unusual number of runs therefore we can conclude data is homogeneous, and variation is random (noise) or common cause. The process is stable and has not changed. The Chair of Obstetrics &*

Gynecology can expect future results to be predictable, with a median range around 13%. C-section rate shows significant variability.

Strategy: *The average C-section rate at London Memorial is within the recommendations of the Royal College of Obstetricians and Gynaecologists (RCOG), however the Chair of Obstetrics & Gynecology felt action was needed to decrease the current month to month and provider variability. A team composed of junior and senior faculty was assembled to launch a QI project with the goal of decreasing the variability and possibly the C-section rate.*

REFERENCE

1. Provost L, Murray S. *The Healthcare Data Guide. Learning from data for improvement.* Jossey-Bass, 2011.

CHAPTER 16

Tools to Characterize the Type of Variation: The Control Chart

THE CONTROL CHART

The Control chart, also called the **process behavior chart**, was first described by **Walter Shewhart**. The Control chart is a graphical display of process-based, time-ordered data used to detect trends and patterns that provide clues about the type and source of variation.

> **A Control chart is a graphical display of data used to characterize variation and understand the process behavior over time.**

The Control chart is better suited than the run chart to characterize variation and to understand the process performance. A Control chart (process behavior chart) is the preferred tool to

- Examine a collection of values for homogeneity.
- Characterize variation.
- Define process stability and performance.
- Assure a process is stable, allowing predictability of results.
- Monitor a process over time.
- Find evidence of improvement.

The Quality Improvement Challenge: A Practical Guide for Physicians, First Edition.
Richard J. Banchs and Michael R. Pop.
© 2021 John Wiley & Sons Ltd. Published 2021 by John Wiley & Sons Ltd.
Companion website: www.wiley.com/go/banchs/quality

The results of the analysis of data using a Control chart are key when deciding whether an improvement should focus on making fundamental changes to the process or on modifying/tweaking the current system. When common cause variation is present and the results are suboptimal, a process should be changed in a fundamental way, by redesigning it or changing the conditions under which it operates. When special cause variation is present, we should instead go to the gemba and find the factor(s) or causes of poor performance. To use a Control chart, two conditions must be met:

1. Data must have been collected and organized in a time-series order manner.
2. There needs to be a minimum of **30** consecutive data points for the I-mR chart (see later), or a minimum of **100** data points of consecutive subgroups if data is organized in subgroups (for the X-bar and R chart; see later).

The normal distribution is not assumed or required to use a Control chart.

THE INDIVIDUALS AND MOVING RANGE (I-MR) CHART

The I-mR process behavior chart combines two charts:

1. Individuals chart, abbreviated I or X-chart
2. Moving range chart, abbreviated mR chart

The Individuals and Moving Range chart, abbreviated I-mR or X-mR chart, is the preferred Control chart to characterize variation and determine process stability with continuous data collected as single values (see example in Figure 16-1).

The Individuals Chart (I or X-Chart)

The Individuals chart shows time-ordered data of the variable we are studying. This chart has three lines (see Figure 16-2):

1. **Center line**. The center line is referred to as the **process location**. The center line is the calculated **mean (average)** of the dataset (x). It is used as a visual reference for detecting shifts, trends, and patterns and helps us characterize the type of variation present;
2. **Upper and lower control limit (UCL and LCL) lines**. The upper and lower control limits are commonly referred to as the **natural process limits** for the Individuals and Moving Range chart (see next). They are calculated from the data and plotted equidistant to the center line or mean (more about this in the next sections);

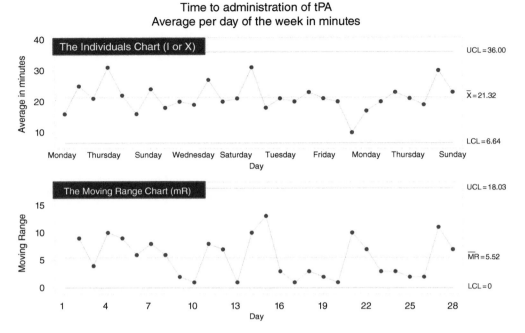

FIGURE 16-1   The Individuals and moving range (I-mR) chart. Chart created with Minitab®
Software package. Printed with permission of Minitab, LLC. All rights reserved.

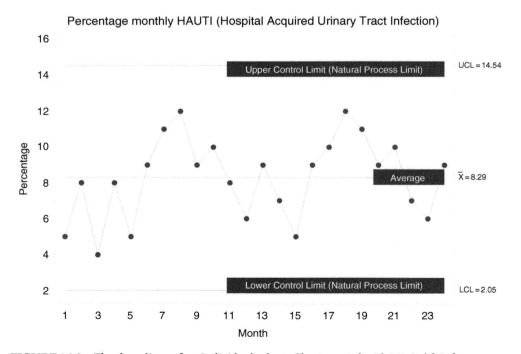

FIGURE 16-2   The three lines of an Individuals chart. Chart created with Minitab® Software
package. Printed with permission of Minitab, LLC. All rights reserved

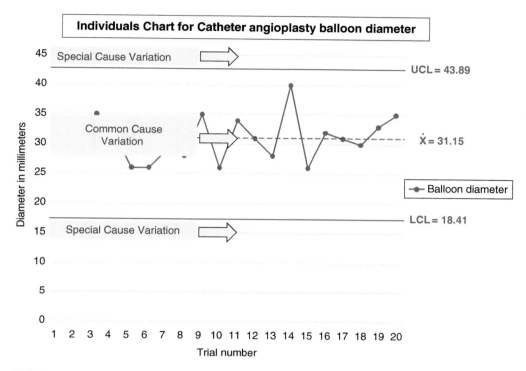

FIGURE 16-3   Individuals chart for "Catheter angioplasty balloon diameter" showing the two areas of an Individuals chart.

These three lines define two areas (see Figure 16-3):

1. **Area inside the control limits.** The limits indicate the **process threshold,** or points at which the process output is considered unlikely. The area between the upper and lower control limits (upper and lower natural process limits) is referred to as the **process dispersion or natural process variation.** It is the area where results are expected to be if the process is stable and shows only common cause variation. The probability of a value to be in that area in a stable process (common cause variation) is 99.73%.

2. **Area outside the control limits.** The area outside of the control limits is where results are not expected and typically result from an unstable process (special cause variation). The probability of a value to be in that area in a stable process is 0.27%.

The Moving Range Chart (mR chart)

The Moving Range (mR) chart is a chart that shows the **dispersion** of the data. The mR chart plots the moving range over time using the values from the Individuals chart. Each value in the mR chart is obtained by subtracting the previous value from each new individual observation in the Individuals chart (I/X). The moving range values have no positive or negative sign. The mean of the moving range is calculated and plotted as the center line. The mean for the moving range is obtained using the following formula: $MR = \sum mR / n - 1$ (there are $n - 1$ ranges). The mR chart has only an **upper control limit** (the lower control limit is zero).

THE UPPER AND LOWER CONTROL LIMITS OF THE INDIVIDUALS CHART

All Control charts (process behavior charts) require the calculation of the upper and lower control limits (UCL and LCL), also called **upper and lower natural process limits.** These limits and the area contained within these limits help us separate common cause from special cause variation.

> **The I-mR chart uses both a measure of location and a measure of dispersion to create empirical limits based upon the existing data. These empirical limits are used to assess the homogeneity of the data, characterize variation, and define process stability and performance.**

How to Calculate the Control Limits on the Individuals Chart?

Control limits are calculated based on the **variation** present in the data in the Individuals chart. The formulas to calculate the upper and lower control limits (UCL and LCL) are

UCL = MEAN of the data + K * Estimate of the dispersion of the data,
LCL = MEAN of the data – K * Estimate of the dispersion of the data

where K is a constant with a value that varies according to the type of Control chart used. The estimate of the dispersion of the data is obtained using an **estimated standard deviation.**

Why Use an Estimated Versus a Globally Computed Standard Deviation?

Why not use a globally computed standard deviation to calculate the dispersion of the data? To compute the standard deviation, calculate the mean (the simple average of the numbers); then for each number subtract the mean and square the result. Work out the mean of those squared differences, and then take the square root of that result.

The problem with using the mean (average) to calculate the global standard deviation and assess dispersion of the data is that the mean is a **summary statistic**. As we said in previous chapters, any summary or high-order descriptive (summary) statistic that is globally computed assumes **homogeneous** data and, therefore, originates from a process that has not changed. The problem is that what we assume is precisely what we don't know and are trying to find. Using a formula to calculate the empirical limits (upper and lower control limits) of the process on the Individuals chart that includes the calculated mean is basically wrong.

To avoid the problem associated with using a globally computed standard deviation as the natural process variation limit, the I-mR Control chart uses the **Jennett's "method of successive differences"** or **average two-point moving range** to calculate the dispersion of the data set. Jennett's method uses the average of the differences between a current value and the one before to determine the spread, or **estimated standard deviation,** of the data.

In 1942, W. J. Jennett proposed the **method of successive differences** as a measure of dispersion instead of a globally computed standard deviation to find the dispersion of the data (natural process variation). By using the average of the differences between successive values as a measure of dispersion, Jennett effectively created the chart for individual values and moving range, or XmR chart. In the 1950s, Neumann, Hartley, and Kamat provided the mathematical evidence that established that the average two-point moving range can be reliably used in the calculation of the dispersion of a data set avoiding the problems associated with calculating the standard deviation using the mean of the data set. The estimated standard deviation used by Control charts to characterize the dispersion of the data is called **sigma.**

The Formula for the Upper and Lower Control Limits

The most common way to compute the upper and lower control limits for the Individuals chart is to compute the average for the data set and combine it with the average of the moving ranges multiplied by a scaling factor. Using this approach, the formula for the upper and lower control limits are:

> UCL = MEAN of the data + (2.66 × average of the moving range),
> LCL = MEAN of the data − (2.66 × average of the moving range).

The number 2.66 constant is a scaling factor, or **bias correction factor** that provides the adequate value to convert the average moving range into the appropriate amount of spread for individual values. The Control chart uses an estimation of the standard deviation called sigma multiplied by three to calculate the **process dispersion or natural process variation** or area between the upper and lower control limits. Hence, 3 × sigma = 3 × average mR / d2, where d2 is the bias correction factor for a two-point moving range. For the Individuals chart, d2 = 1.128, which gives us 3/1.128

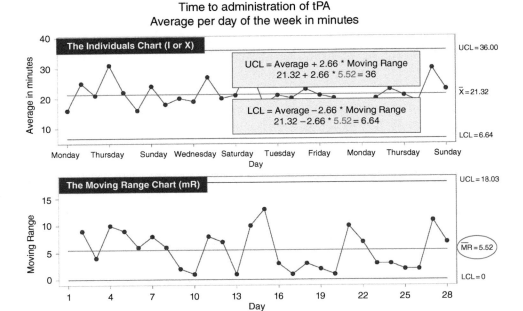

FIGURE 16-4   The upper and lower control limits of the Individuals chart. Chart created with Minitab® Software package. Printed with permission of Minitab, LLC. All rights reserved.

or 2.660 as the constant K to multiply to the average moving range to obtain the limits of the natural process variation (see Figure 16-4).

When we use the successive difference between two points to compute the limits of the Individuals chart, we must make sure that successive values are logically comparable, sequential in time, and differ only because of routine variation. We cannot place values that we know are from different processes in the same chart and compute the limits based on their differences. *When the process changes, new limits must be calculated.*

Why Is the Area Inside the Control Limits Three Sigma from the Mean?

The natural process limits, or expected variation in the data, are **three sigmas** (estimated standard deviation) on either side of the average of the data set (X). The moving range is used as a local measure of dispersion, multiplied by 2.66 (constant scaling factor, or bias correction factor) rather than the Standard deviation to compute the natural process limits. **The limits indicate the process dispersion, or natural process variation, and the points at which the process output is considered unlikely.** The area inside the control limits is where results are expected to be if the process is stable and has only **common cause variation**. The area outside of the control limits is where results are not expected and typically result from an unstable process with **special cause variation**.

Walter Shewhart, the father of statistical process control, set the natural process limit to be three sigma (sigma = estimated standard deviations) based on prevailing statistical principles and **strong empirical evidence**; "the strongest justification of three-sigma limits is the empirical evidence that the three sigma limits work well in practice – that they provide effective action limits when applied to real world data" (Wheeler 2004). The choice of three sigma is supported not only by strong empirical evidence, but by Tchebysheff's theorem and the Vysochanskii–Petunin inequality probability distribution model.

- **Tchebysheff's theorem.** Pafnuty Tchebysheff, a Russian statistician, stated that the probability that a random value differs from its mean by more than K standard deviations is less than or equal to $1/k2$. Stated in another way, given a population of n measurements, at least $1 - (1/X2)$ of measurements will lie within X standard deviations. This means that for any data set, 99.7% of the data is captured by the curve within 3 standard deviations from the mean. It also implies that there is only a $100 - 99.7\%$, or 0.3%, chance of finding a value beyond three standard deviations that does not belong to the data set (homogenous data).

What Does It All Mean?

Three sigmas is the natural **process variation**.

> **When calculating the standard deviation using Jennett's method of successive differences, any value contained within three estimated standard deviations (sigma) is probably the result of common cause variation and belongs to a process that is stable. Any value outside the process behavior limits is probably the result of special cause variation and alerts us the process is unstable.**

Values inside the natural process variation limits (control limits) are considered to be influenced by factors intrinsic to the system and show common cause variation while values outside the limits are the result of factors that are extrinsic to the system and show special cause variation. Data is not required to follow a normal distribution in order to use a process behavior chart. However, data should be time-ordered. The three-sigma limit will filter out virtually all of the routine variation regardless of the shape or the probability model used (Wheeler 2009).

There is a difference between three standard deviations and the three sigma upper and lower control limits. Standard deviation is a measure of dispersion of the data; the upper and lower control limits are the range of natural variability of the process. *Standard deviation and the control limits do not always coincide.*

The Problem with Relying on a Target to Set the Process Performance

*Establishing a target without knowing the **natural process variation limits** (upper and lower control limits) is a common mistake. The target, which is the voice of the customer (VOC), is what we demand of the process. The natural process variation limit is what the process generates, independent of what we want (the voice of the process, or VOP). If we set a target without understanding the process performance and the range of variation, i.e. the upper and lower control limits, our attempts at achieving an unrealistic target will only encourage a distortion of the process or a distortion of the way data is collected in order to conform to the external demands.*

UPPER CONTROL LIMIT OF THE MOVING RANGE (MR) CHART

The formula to compute the upper limit of the moving range chart is

> Upper limit for moving range chart = Average moving range × 3.268

3.268 is the constant or scaling factor for the mR chart. It is the value required to convert the average range into an appropriate upper bound of ranges. The lower limit of the moving range is not computed because the value is 0. The mR chart is a valuable addition to the Individuals chart for several reasons:

- **Checking calculations.** It helps to validate the limits of the Individuals chart. By using the center line of the mR chart, you can check to see if the limits have been correctly computed.
- **Early warning.** The mR chart can detect sudden shifts (variation) even when the individual values are still within the control limits on the Individuals chart (X chart).
- **Detects false special cause variation.** When too many values are the same, the excessive number of zero ranges that result will deflate the average moving range and tighten the limits. The process behavior chart will have many false alarms. Only the mR chart can alert us to this condition (Wheeler 2010).

Other Option to Calculate Limits for the I-mR Chart

There are only two measures of dispersion to use when creating a chart for individual values: the average moving range and the median moving range. Other options to calculate the limits should not be used (Wheeler 2010).

- **Average moving range.** Explained above.
- **Median moving range.** Used only when some large moving ranges may have inflated the average moving range. This approach should not be used as the default approach because of the lower efficiency of the median in computing the dispersion of the data (Wheeler 2000). Limit for Individuals (I) chart = Average of the data ± 3.145 × Median of the moving range, where 3.145 is the constant or scaling factor. Upper limit for mR = 3.865 × Median moving range.
- **Using the global standard deviation** to calculate the limits on the I-mR chart is incorrect, as described before. The computation of the global standard deviation assumes the data to be homogeneous, which is precisely what the Control chart is designed to check. Whenever the data is not homogeneous, the computation of the limits will result in overinflated upper and lower control limits that will not be able to detect special cause variation (Wheeler 2000).

HOW TO DETECT SPECIAL CAUSE VARIATION WITH THE I-MR CHART

Rules

There are several rules for detecting special cause variation that simplify the analysis of Control charts. The most commonly used method to detect special cause variation is the identification of a value located outside the control limits (see example in

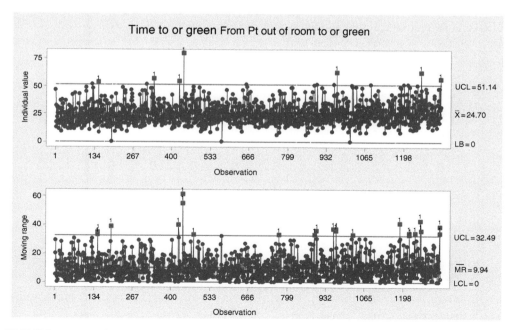

FIGURE 16-5   Individuals chart showing violation of rule 1. Chart created with Minitab® Software package. Printed with permission of Minitab, LLC. All rights reserved.

Figure 16-5). This is "Rule 1" and provides the strongest evidence to conclude there is a nonrandom variation in the data that signals special cause variation.

Rule 1   A **point outside of either upper or lower control limit** is the most commonly accepted rule to detect a nonrandom pattern of variation in the data indicative of special cause variation.

A point exactly on the control limit is still considered to be indicative of common cause variation. Several additional rules can be used to characterize the variation found in a data set when using a I-mR control chart. These rules are used to differentiate the noise of common cause variation from the signal of special cause variation.

Three additional rules are based on detecting the presence of runs, trends, and patterns. The chance of these three rules occurring in combination is the same as the chance of Rule 1 (Provost 2011).

Rule 2   **2 out of 3 successive points** in a row are both on the same side of the center line and are more than 2 sigma units away from the average.

Rule 3   **4 out of 5 successive points** in a row are both on the same side of the center line and are more than 1 sigma unit away from the average.

Rule 4   **8 consecutive points** are less than 1 sigma unit from the center line (on either side).

*Sigma = Standard deviation calculated with the method of successive differences

The four rules maximize the detection power of the control chart. Additional rules are available but should be used with caution so they do not increase the chance of false alarms:

- Rule 5: 9 or more points in a row above or below the center line.
- Rule 6: 6 points in a row all decreasing or increasing.
- Rule 7: 14 points in a row, alternating up and down.
- Rule 8: 15 points in a row within 1 sigma from the center line, above or below.

Using Zones

Divide the Individuals (I) chart in three zones (see example in Figure 16-6):

1. **Zone A** is the zone from 2–3 sigma above the average – as well as below the average.
2. **Zone B** is the zone from 1–2 sigma above the average. There is a corresponding Zone B below the average.
3. **Zone C** is the zone closest to the average. It represents the area from the average to 1 sigma above or below the average.

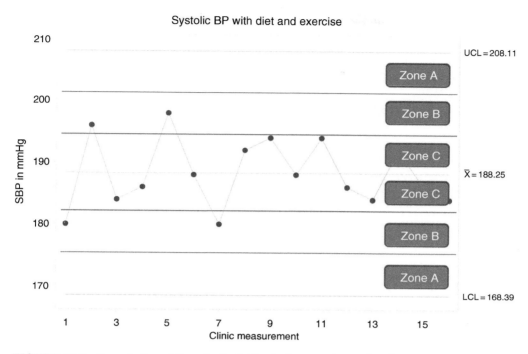

FIGURE 16-6   Zone A, B, and C on the Individuals chart can be used to detect special cause variation. Chart created with Minitab® Software package. Printed with permission of Minitab, LLC. All rights reserved.

Then apply the following rules:

- Rule 1: 1 or more points beyond control limits.
- Rule 2: 2 out of 3 points in Zone A or beyond.
- Rule 3: 4 out of 5 consecutive points in Zone B or beyond.
- Rule 4: 7 consecutive points in Zone C.
- Rule 5: 7 consecutive points trending up or down.
- Rule 6: 8 consecutive points with no points in Zone C.
- Rule 7: 15 consecutive points in Zone C.
- Rule 8: 14 consecutive points, alternating up and down.

THE I-MR CHART GUIDES THE IMPROVEMENT STRATEGY

When the I-mR Chart Shows Common Cause Variation

- With common cause variation and a stable process (process in **statistical control),** the output is predictable within a range (the natural process variation between the upper and lower control limits). The Control chart will show **no**

violation of rule 1 (all the data is between the upper and lower natural process or control limits), 2, 3, or 4 (no runs, trends, and patterns).

- If a stable process produces satisfactory results, continue to monitor.
- A process may otherwise be stable but produce unacceptable results or great variability, in which case we must make a **fundamental change** in the process design or **change the conditions** so that a different mix of factors affect the output.
- When an I-mR chart shows common cause variation but either the average, the limits, or the total amount of variation are unacceptable:
  - Investigate the root cause of the problem.
  - Stratify data to look for patterns.
  - Brainstorm solutions; pilot the best ideas.
  - Change the process in some fundamental way (see Chapter 14, Figure 14-11).

When the I-mR Chart Shows Special Cause Variation

- With special cause variation, the process is **unstable** and can be said **not to be in statistical control.** The output of this process is not predictable.
- The control chart will show either a **violation** of rule 1 (data above or below the upper and lower natural process or control limits), 2, 3, or 4 (presence of runs, trends, and patterns).
- Whether an unstable process produces satisfactory results or not is irrelevant. The process has changed and the results are unpredictable.
- To improve the process's average and/or reduce the process variation, the specific data points that are out of statistical control will need to be evaluated independently, and the factors that contribute to the special cause variation eliminated before further improvement can be made.
- When a control chart shows special cause variation, the appropriate strategy is to
  - Go to the gemba and examine the possible causes of variation.
  - Find the assignable causes.
  - Remove the causes.
  - Fix the output, the process, and the system that created the output.

Is Special Cause Variation Ever Desirable?

Finding special cause variation or the existence of a signal in your data is not always bad. This may point to a change that is due not to a drop in process performance but to **an improvement**. A control chart showing special cause variation only alerts you of a change in the process, but does not provide any clues as to the reasons for the change. With special cause variation, we must go back to the gemba (or review data) to understand the reason for the change. In some cases, the change comes as a result of an improvement. We can also use the rules for special cause variation to provide evidence of an ongoing improvement in a process. This will be true as long as the signal shows data going in the right direction.

Example: The Individuals and Moving Range (I-mR) Chart of a Patient's SBP

The Individuals and moving range (I-mR) chart of a patient's systolic blood pressure (SBP) shows special cause variation after two changes in blood pressure (BP) medication (see Figure 16-7). Because the process has changed (there are different conditions that affect the blood pressure, i.e medication) the I-mR chart is detecting values above and below the upper and lower control limits indicative of special cause variation. Data above the upper control limit is indicative of the patient's blood pressure on diet and exercise. Data between the upper and lower control limits is indicative of the patient's blood pressure on an ACE inhibitor. Data below the lower control limit indicates the patient's systolic blood pressure on a double regimen of medication (ACE inhibitor plus a beta-blocker). The presence of special cause variation is alerting us of a change, but not necessarily to the reason for the change. It is up to us to figure it out. In this example, the change is positive, the SBP trend is downwards, and is the result of medication. Computing different limits for each phase and separating the data in three different phases (processes) shows a clearer picture of the improvements detected initially by special cause variation on the first I-mR chart (see Figure 16-8).

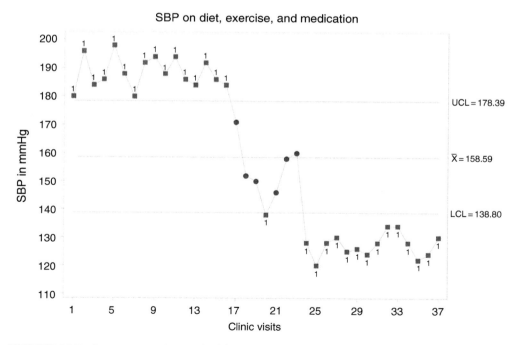

FIGURE 16-7   Improvement in systolic blood pressure management appears as special cause variation. Chart created with Minitab® Software package. Printed with permission of Minitab, LLC. All rights reserved.

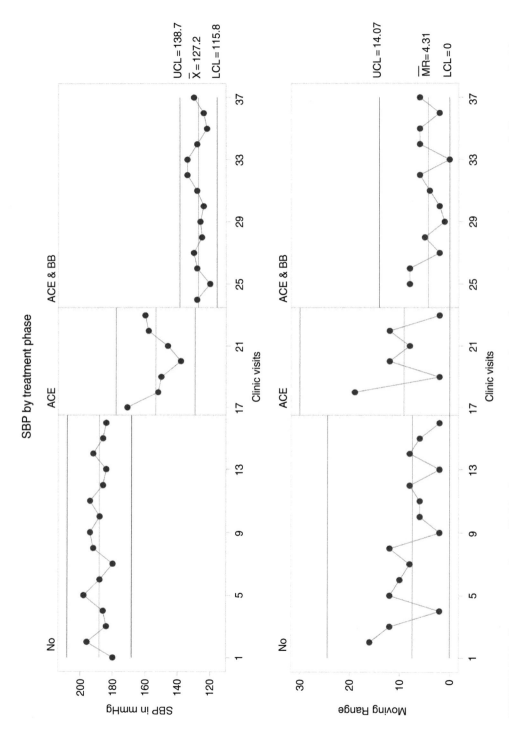

FIGURE 16-8   Improvement in systolic blood pressure management is clearer when new limits have been computed. Chart created with Minitab® Software package. Printed with permission of Minitab, LLC. All rights reserved.

ADDITIONAL CONTROL CHARTS

Additional Control charts are sometimes used for continuous and discrete data (see Figure 16-9).

Charts for Continuous Data

The X-Bar and R Chart. The X-bar & R chart is used for continuous data. The X-bar & R chart is used for continuous data collected in **samples < 10**. The X-bar and R charts use a theoretical model, not the measure of location and a measure of dispersion to create the empirical limits (upper and lower control limits). While the I-mR chart works well for many different cases, this is a specialized chart that can be used under certain conditions that are more sensitive to process shift. It is sometimes common to produce large volumes of one same item. When this is the case, we can collect multiple measures within a very short time frame – one after the other. Because this sample is collected under the same conditions, we can put them together into a subgroup and use the average and range of the subgroup to track process performance over time. When the conditions require it, using the X-bar and R chart may give you better sensitivity to assess performance of the process. With tighter control limits, the average chart will be more sensitive to process shifts than the I-mR chart. For this to be true,

- We cannot subgroup things that are inherently different.
- The internal homogeneity of the subgroup must be maintained and is critical.
- Variation within the subgroup must represent the appropriate random variation for the process.

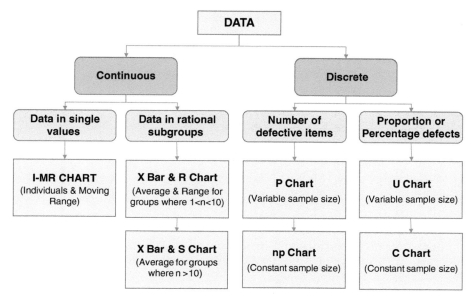

FIGURE 16-9   Types of Control charts for continuous and discrete data.

The X-Bar and S Chart. The X-bar and S chart is used for continuous data collected in **samples > 10**. Like the X-bar and R chart, the X-bar and S chart uses a theoretical model, not the measure of location and a measure of dispersion to create the empirical limits (upper and lower control limits).

Charts for Discrete Data

Continuous data is optimal because it provides information on the center and dispersion of the data distribution using a smaller sample size. However, there will be times when an improvement team must collect count and attribute data that describes qualitative characteristics that cannot be measured on a continuous scale. Count and attribute data are used to evaluate whether a service or product conforms or does not conform to specifications or the number of errors or defects that occur during the process. For example, count and attribute data include the number of patient safety events, the number of IV infiltrations, or the number of patients who left without treatment from the emergency department (ED).

Control charts for discrete data are the P chart, U chart, np chart, and C chart. All use theoretical models to create limits based on their assumed probability model and a measure of location. The assumed probability model for the P and np charts is a **binomial distribution** (pass/fail, yes/no, treated/not treated, etc.). For the U & C charts, the model is a **Poisson distribution** (count data such as the number of errors and proportion or percentages).

- **P Chart.** The P chart assumes data follows a binomial distribution with only two attributes for the data (occurrence versus nonoccurrence, defective vs. not defective), there is the same area of opportunity, the sample size is variable, and the occurrence of the attribute is independent from unit to unit.
- **U Chart.** The U chart assumes data follows a Poisson distribution, compares percentages and proportions, and the sample size is variable. The U chart counts occurrences, with the probability of an occurrence being relatively rare. Occurrences are independent of one another.
- The np chart is like the P chart but for constant sample sizes. The C chart is like the U chart but also for constant sample sizes.

The Preferred Control Chart

For both continuous or discrete data, the I-mR chart (X-mR) is the preferred chart **to characterize variation and understand the behavior of the process over time.**

CASE STUDY: DOOR-TO-INFUSION (DTI) TIME AT HURON MEDICAL CENTER

Huron Medical Center is a community hospital that became certified as a Comprehensive Stroke Center three years ago. With this new accreditation came the requirement to track several metrics to measure performance and the quality of care. Tissue plasminogen activator (tPA) is the only clot-busting drug approved by the FDA for treating ischemic strokes, and is effective only when given within a few hours after onset of a stroke. The "percentage of ischemic stroke patients identified as eligible for tissue plasminogen activator (tPA) who are treated within 60 minutes of arrival to the ED" is one of several metrics that is being followed as a comprehensive QI effort.

The interval between patient arrival and treatment with tPA is known as the "door-to-infusion time" or DTI time. The performance for the door-to-infusion time for all "stroke codes" over the last six weeks is presented here (see Table 16-1). To assess the current performance of the process (process stability) an I-mR chart should be created. To create an Individuals chart of door-to-infusion time,

- *Calculate the values for the moving range by subtracting each DTI time from the previous value; there is no value for the moving range assigned to the first DTI time (see Table 16-2).*
- *Calculate the average moving range (Average mR = 7.91).*
- *Calculate the average "door-to-infusion time" (Average X = 35.36).*
- *Calculate the upper control limit (UCL = 35.36 + 2.66 × Average moving range = 56.40).*
- *Calculate the lower control limit (LCL= 35.36 – 2.66 × Average moving range = 14.31).*
- *Create the Individuals chart (see Figure 16-10).*

The Individuals chart for *door-to-infusion time for all "Stroke Codes"* shows *common cause variation and therefore a stable process. While the average is acceptable, the Individuals chart shows significant variability (from 14.31 to 56.40 minutes). A QI project should be launched to improve the ED team's performance.*

TABLE 16-1 Door-to-Infusion Times for All Stroke Codes at Huron Medical Center

Door-to-infusion times for all "stroke codes" at Huron Medical Center (time in minutes)

#1	34	#7	34	#13	30	#19	41	#25	27	#31	45
#2	31	#8	40	#14	34	#20	34	#26	34	#32	30
#3	38	#9	34	#15	41	#21	27	#27	27	#33	30
#4	39	#10	36	#16	38	#22	30	#28	45	#34	45
#5	44	#11	34	#17	38	#23	34	#29	25	#35	25
#6	38	#12	41	#18	30	#24	41	#30	34	#36	45

TABLE 16-2 Calculation of Moving Range for Door-to-Infusion Times at Huron Medical Center

Calculation of moving range values					
Value	Previous value	Moving Range	Value	Previous value	Moving Range
34	no	none	30	41	11
31	34	3	41	34	7
38	31	7	34	27	7
39	38	1	27	30	3
44	39	5	30	34	4
38	44	6	34	41	7
34	38	4	41	27	14
40	34	6	27	34	7
34	40	6	34	27	7
36	34	2	27	45	8
36	34	2	45	25	20
34	41	7	25	34	9
41	30	11	34	45	11
30	34	4	45	30	15
34	41	7	30	30	0
41	38	3	30	45	15
38	38	0	45	25	20
38	30	8	25	45	20

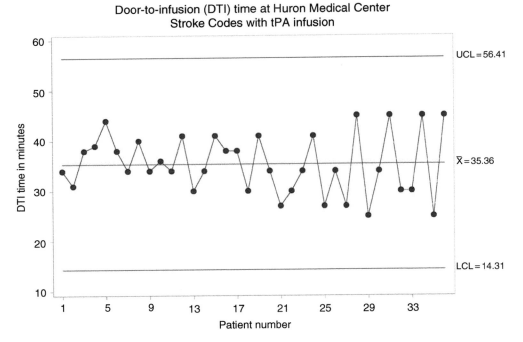

FIGURE 16-10 Individuals chart of "door-to-infusion time" for all "stroke codes" at Huron Medical Center. Chart created with Minitab® Software package. Printed with permission of Minitab, LLC. All rights reserved.

REFERENCES

1. Provost L. (2011). *The Healthcare Data Guide. Learning from Data for Improvement.* Jossey-Bass.

2. Wheeler D. (2004). *Advanced Topics in Statistical Process Control.* SPC Press.

3. Wheeler D. (2009). Do you have Leptokurtophobia? The abnormal need for normal distribution. *Quality Digest.*

4. Wheeler D. (2010). Individual charts done right and wrong. How does your software rate? *Quality Digest.*

CHAPTER 17

Define Baseline Performance: Is the Process Capable?

IS THE PROCESS MEETING THE NEEDS OF THE CUSTOMER?

With our work and the design of our processes, we strive to meet our customers' (patients, staff, and physicians) requirements. We also want our processes to meet these requirements now as well as in the future. The process design must be able to continue to deliver the results our customers expect. To assess the performance of our process design (the way we work), we need to answer these three questions (see Chapters 12 and 14):

- **How is the process behaving? Can we meet our customer's needs**? Is the work process stable and predictable? Is the process reliable?
- **How is the output? Are we meeting the needs of our customers?** Is the output compliant/conforming to customer's needs and expectations?
- **How often are we meeting their needs?** How often is the process output meeting customer requirements and specifications?

The first question addresses **process stability**. Process stability is a measure of **consistency**, or the ability of a process to repeatedly generate values of a specific key measure within a range, or in other words, variation limits. If the process is stable, it will produce predictable results over time. To make predictions about future performance using past data, we must first characterize the type of variation using **histograms**, **Run charts**, and **Control charts**.

The Quality Improvement Challenge: A Practical Guide for Physicians, First Edition.
Richard J. Banchs and Michael R. Pop.
© 2021 John Wiley & Sons Ltd. Published 2021 by John Wiley & Sons Ltd.
Companion website: www.wiley.com/go/banchs/quality

The second and third questions address **process capability**. Process capability is a measure of **conformity,** or how well the process is delivering what the customer needs and/or requires and how often does it accomplish this. To answer this, we are going to have to compare the performance of the process to the specific performance requirements expressed by the customer.

The answer to these three questions provides a **roadmap to assess process performance** (see Table 17-1). A stable process will behave consistently within limits. Therefore, the output will also be consistent and predictable. An unstable process will

TABLE 17-1   Roadmap to Assess a Process's Performance

Steps, Actions, and Tools to Assess Process Performance			
Steps	**Goal**	**Actions**	**Tools**
Step 1 **Analyze data.**	Characterize the data generated by the process.	Continuous data: See the center and spread, compare data sets. Use summary statistics.	Histogram, Box plot, Individual Value plot
		Discrete data: Compare data across categories. Identify the most common attributes.	Bar chart, Pie chart, Pareto chart
Step 2 Answer the **Homogeneity** question.	Test the assumption data comes from a single universe (single process, same conditions).	A characteristic found only in continuous data. When interpreting discrete data, make sure data have been collected under the same Area of Opportunity (AOO).	Histogram Run chart and Control chart
Step 3 Is the process **Stable?**	Make sure the process is consistent and predictable.	Collect time-ordered data (continuous or discrete). Characterize the type of Variation.	Run chart and Control chart
Step 4 Is the process **Capable?**	Make sure the process output conforms to the needs of the customer.	Compare the "Voice of the Customer" (VOC) to the "Voice of the Process" (VOP) to assess and quantify how well the process is meeting customer demands (specifications).	Capability Analysis Sigma level
		For discrete data use Parts Per Million (PPM) defective to compare the "Voice of the Customer" to the "Voice of the Process"	Parts Per Million (PPM) defects Sigma level

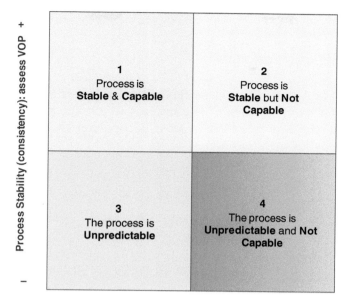

FIGURE 17-1   There are four possible scenarios when evaluating a process's performance.

not behave consistently, and the output will not be consistent or predictable. Before assessing process capability, we must determine process stability. Considering both process stability and capability, we have four possible scenarios (see Figure 17-1):

1. The process is stable (consistent) and capable (conforming) and is performing optimally.

2. The process is reliably producing results (the process is stable) but not all the results meet customer satisfaction. In this case, a QI team must either change the process, or change customer expectations, i.e. the CTQ specifications.

3. Regardless of the results, the process is unstable (the performance is unpredictable). It's a dangerous place to be because special cause variation is present. The results may seem OK now, but we cannot reliably trust that the outcome of the process will meet customers' needs in the future. Before we can do anything, we must go to the gemba and identify and eliminate the causes of special cause variation.

4. The process is unstable and not capable of producing the results the customer expects. Eliminate the special cause variation first; then redesign or fundamentally change the process so it can deliver what the customer needs.

PROCESS CAPABILITY

What Is Process Capability?

> **Process capability compares the voice of the customer (what the customer wants, or VOC) to the voice of the process (what the process delivers, or VOP) to quantify how well the process is consistently meeting the needs (specifications) of the customer.**

- **Voice of the Process (VOP).** The results delivered by the process are called the Voice of the Process (VOP). The VOP is the process output. This output can be characterized by an average value (data needs to be homogenous) and the total variation of the values (hopefully only common cause variation).
- **Voice of the Customer (VOC).** From the voice of the customer we develop Critical-to-Quality (CTQ) attributes and requirements of services. The CTQs are the key measurable characteristics of the product or process whose **specification limits** must be met in order to meet the customers' demands. The specification limits are what the customer expects from the healthcare product or service (see Chapter 8). Specifications are usually set by the customers (patients, staff, or providers), but can also come from other sources such as best-practice advisories, regulatory agencies, or third-party payers. There is usually an **upper** and **lower specification limit**. Examples of specifications limits include: completing a clinic visit between 15 and 30 minutes; the joint commission requires all class B and C ambulatory operating rooms to have 20 to 30 room air exchanges per hour; administering prophylactic antibiotics between 30 and 60 minutes before incision; setting the door-to-injection (DTI) time of tPA (tissue Plasminogen Activator) within 60 minutes (upper specification limit).

> **The customer (patient, staff, or provider) defines quality by identifying the needed outcome, the attributes of the outcome, and the requirements that characterize the outcome. Customers also define the specifications for both the attributes and requirements.**

A defect is any failure to meet the specifications set by the customer. Process capability determines the percentage of defects or the percentage of work where customer expectations are not met.

- A **process is capable** when the range of values for a specific measure of interest (CTQ) consistently falls entirely within the customer required specification limits.
- A **process is not capable** when the process variation is greater than the VOC. Process capability can only be obtained for processes that are stable (in statistical control).

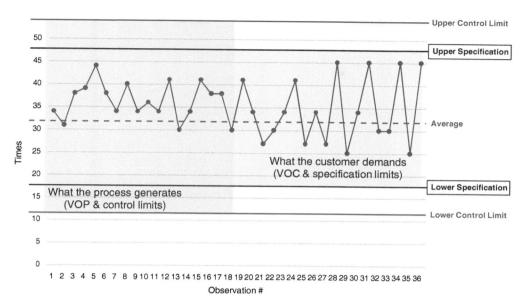

FIGURE 17-2   The relationship between specifications (VOC) and control limits (VOP).

Specification limits are the targets set for the process output by the customer or expert. **Control limits** are the indicators of the variation in the performance of the process (the natural process behavior limits) and are the actual values the process is operating on. Essentially, process capability compares the process's specifications to the process's variation or control limits (see Figure 17-2). In this example (Fig 17-2), the VOP (control limits or natural process behavior) is greater than the VOC (specifications set by the customer), and the process may generate values that do not meet the specifications set by the customer (defects).

Conditions to Calculate Process Capability

Three conditions must be met to assess the capability of any process:

1. The **process** (VOP) is **stable** and **predictable** and therefore exhibits only common cause variation.
2. The **specifications** (VOC) are known, have been operationally defined, and have been mutually agreed-upon by the customer and the stakeholder. If this is not the case, it may be very difficult to agree on what is a defect. Front line professionals, stakeholders, and the customer may have different views of what is acceptable performance and, therefore, what constitutes a "defect."
3. The **measurement system** is accurate, and the measurement system variation is minimal compared to the process variation. In other words, the

variation observed in the data is due to process performance and not due to a measurement system that is unreliable.

Process Capability for Continuous Data

For continuous data, the simplest and easiest method to determine process capability is to plot a histogram of the individual values taken from the Control chart and compare them to the specifications (VOC). The width of a histogram shows the total variation of the process values (VOP); what the customer needs is the VOC or specifications.

Data that falls outside the upper and lower specification limits is considered to be

> **Process capability establishes a ratio of the width of the histogram (VOP) to the width of the specifications (VOC) as a measure of process performance, and quantifies the amount of data outside the specification limits that is considered to be a defect.**

nonconforming with the performance requirements of the process or specifications, and is referred to as a defect (see Figure 17-3).

CASE STUDY: THE NEW BALLOON ANGIOPLASTY CATHETER AT UIC

A new balloon angioplasty catheter for interventional radiology has been designed by a bioengineering team at the University of Illinois. When deployed, the balloon diameter

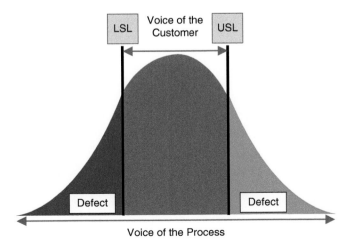

FIGURE 17-3   Data outside the upper and lower specification limits are considered defects.

needs to have a minimum of 1.2 millimeters, and a maximum of 1.4 millimeters. The maximum diameter corresponds to a maximal nominal pressure of 7 atmospheres, which is well below the rated balloon burst pressure of 12 atmospheres. A balloon diameter below 1.2 millimeters is below the diameter of the target vessel, and is inadequate to dilate it; a balloon diameter above 1.4 millimeters may risk overdistension and vessel injury. One hundred sequential measurements of the catheter's balloon diameter were obtained using an animal model. The designing team used a process capability analysis to study the performance of the balloon.

A capability analysis using Minitab© (Minitab Statistical Package, Pennsylvania State University) showed (see Figure 17-4):

1. **An I-mR chart** to assess process stability. The process is stable (all values between the upper and lower control limits). When performing a capability analysis, the current process must be stable and in statistical control in order to be able to predict the process's current and future capability.

2. **A histogram** showing the spread of the data. This is the VOP.

3. **The process data box** showing summary statistics (variation or spread of the data calculated with the mean and the standard deviation), and the **upper** and **lower specification limits**. The distance between the LSL and the USL is the VOC. The LSL and USL are the specifications of the key measurable variables of the process outcome set by the customer that are known, operationally defined, and agreed upon by the customer and the stakeholder. In this case, the specifications are the minimum and maximum catheter balloon diameter. The "within" standard deviation is the short-term variation of the process; the "overall" standard deviation is the long-term variation of the process.

4. **Performance data** that falls outside of the upper and lower specification limits. Data on both sides of the specification limits (defects or defective) is combined to yield the total defectives. The total number of defectives is reported either as **percent defective (PD)** or as **defects per million opportunities (DPMO)**. Observed performance is based on the actual results; expected performance is based on predictions of the proportion that will fail the specification limits.

5. **Capability indexes.** Process capability indexes measure how much natural variation a process has relative to its specification limits, and allow different processes to be compared on the basis of this measure (see next). "Potential capability" is based on the short-term variation; "overall capability" is based on all the variation seen in the data and reflect the true performance of the process.

Using the two graphs in this example, we can conclude

- **The process is stable.** A bell-shaped histogram means data is homogenous. The I-mR chart shows common cause variation and a stable process. (Note: Bell-shaped histogram does not always mean homogenous data and stability; a Control chart is necessary for the diagnosis).

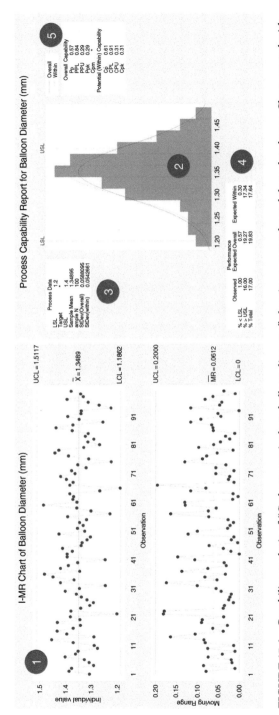

- **The process is not capable.** *The **natural process behavior** or process performance (VOP) varies from 1.18 mm to 1.51 mm (the upper and lower control limits of the I-mR chart). This is above the set specifications of 1.2 mm to 1.4 mm in diameter (VOC): 17% of the observed process performance (balloon catheter diameter measurements) is above the specifications for optimal performance (upper and lower specification limits). The risk of rupture is 16% (percentage of data above the upper specification limit), which is unacceptable in the setting of catheter balloon angioplasty. The designing team should return to the drawing board!*

CAPABILITY INDICES

> **Process capability indices are statistical measures of process capability that assess the extent of variation a process experiences relative to the specifications set by the customer.**

Capability indices are ratios of the variability or spread of the process and the specifications. Because they are unitless values, they are also used to compare the capability of different processes. A process experiences more variation in the long run than in the short term; therefore, the capability of a process, or ability of the process to deliver what the customer needs, also changes when data has been collected over a short or a long period of time. The ratios of the variability or spread of the process, the specifications, and the span of time data is collected determines two types of indices: C and P. Both indices are used to assess the ability of the process to deliver what the customer needs (conformity), and are calculated using a similar equation. The difference is in how the standard deviation is computed.

- **C capability indices** measure the natural variation of the process relative to the specification limits. Because the C indices uses the standard deviation calculated from the subgroups, the C index represents short-term variation, and short-term capability.
- **The P indices** also measure the natural variation of the process relative to the specification limits. Because the P indices use the standard deviation calculated from all the data, they represent long-term variation and long-term capability.

An important consideration is that if the process is not stable, no capability index can be used to assess or predict the performance of the process. Remember, process capability is about using data from the past to try and predict the future. This assumes only common cause variation is present!

The Cp Indices

The Cp metric compares the space available within the specifications (specification tolerance or VOC) with the space required by the process (natural tolerance or VOP), establishing a ratio. To calculate the Cp index, follow these steps:

- Confirm the process is stable (Refer to your histogram and Control chart).
- Identify the USL and LSL.
- Estimate the process (sample) standard deviation (SD) using R(bar)/d2.
- Use the formula Cp = USL – LSL/6SD.

There are three possible outcomes:

1. **Cp < 1.** This defines a process that does not have the ability to operate within the specifications.
2. **Cp = 1.** This process is marginally capable and uses 100% of the tolerance to comply with the specifications of the customer or VOC. This process is operating at the margins.
3. **Cp > 1.** This process is capable. Most experts prefer a Cp > 1.33. A Cp > 2 is excellent, indicating that the VOC is twice the size of the VOP (or vice versa, depending on what we are measuring).

The Cpk Indices

The Cpk index is called the **centered capability ratio**. It measures whether the process is properly centered within the specifications. The Cpk defines the effective space available as twice the distance from the process average to the nearest specification limit, and compares this value with the space required by the process (VOP). The formula is: Cpk = Minimal value when comparing (USL – average/3SD) or (Average – LSL/3SD).
There are three possible outcomes:

1. **Cp = Cpk.** The process is perfectly centered.
2. **Cpk < Cp.** The process is not centered.
3. **–Cpk.** The process average is outside specification limits.

The P Capability Indices (Pp, Ppk)

The P capability indices evaluate the long-term variation and long-term capability of the process. They measure the natural variation of the process relative to the specification limits using the standard deviation calculated from all the data.

Going back to the example in Figure 17-4, we can state:

- Cp <1 (0.57): The process is not operating within the requirements set by the customer.
- Cpk < Cp: The process is not centered.
- The long-term capability of the process (Pp) is <1 (0.57), and the process will continue to not operate within specifications.

PROCESS CAPABILITY FOR DISCRETE DATA

A defect is a product, service, or step that does not meet customer requirement for quality. A primary objective of process improvement projects is to reduce or eliminate defects. Attribute data can be used to assess process capability. There are two options:

1. **Assessment of the number of defective items.** In this case, the units are **% defectives** or **defects per million opportunities** (DPMO) and measures the defect rate (proportion or percentage) of the process. For example, out of a sample of 100 preprepared syringes by pharmacy, 18 had the wrong label. The percent defective would be 18% (number of syringes with the wrong label/ total number of syringes). A **binomial capability analysis** would be used to determine whether the % defective meets customer requirements.
2. **Assessment of the number of defective items per unit.** The unit is **defects per unit** (DPU) and measures the defect rate of the process. A **Poisson capability analysis** would determine the capability of the process.

THE PROCESS SIGMA OR SIGMA METRIC

The sigma metric is a metric derived from the Six Sigma improvement methodology and can be very useful in healthcare as a measure of process capability. Sigma metric is a measure of the variation in a process relative to customer requirements and measures defects on a scale of **defects per million opportunities (DPMO)**. The sigma measurement is the metric that helps us define our current capability in meeting our customer requirements based on their specification.

> **The sigma measurement indicates how many standard deviations or "sigmas" can fit between the process average and the nearest specification limits.**

Sigma can be used to assess how well we are meeting customer requirements, track improvement efforts, and compare performance across fields, as a common metric to make comparisons between different work processes.

Sigma measures

- defects on a scale of defects per million opportunities (DPMO), and
- the variation of the process relative to the customer requirements.

Sigma is more sensitive than percentages as an indicator of process performance. Any instance of failing to meet customer requirements is a defect, so a high number for DPMO is reflective of a suboptimal process performance. Once the defect rate of a process is known (expressed as defects per million opportunities (DPMO) a **process sigma-level conversion table** can be used to determine the process sigma (performance level) for that process (see Table 17-2).

TABLE 17-2   Process Sigma Level Conversion Table

% Yield	DPMO	Sigma	% Yield	DPMO	Sigma
8.0000	920000	0.09	94.5200	54800	3.10
10.0000	900000	0.22	95.5400	44600	3.20
12.0000	880000	0.33	96.4100	35900	3.30
14.0000	860000	0.42	97.1300	28700	3.40
16.0000	840000	0.51	97.7300	22700	3.50
19.0000	810000	0.62	98.2200	17800	3.60
22.0000	780000	0.73	98.6100	13900	3.70
25.0000	750000	0.83	98.9300	10700	3.80
28.0000	720000	0.92	99.1810	8190	3.90
31.0000	690000	1.00	99.3790	6210	4.00
35.0000	650000	1.11	99.5340	4660	4.10
39.0000	610000	1.22	99.6540	3460	4.20
43.0000	570000	1.32	99.7450	2550	4.30
46.0000	540000	1.40	99.8140	1860	4.40
50.0000	500000	1.50	99.8650	1350	4.50
54.0000	460000	1.60	99.9040	960	4.60
58.0000	420000	1.70	99.9320	680	4.70
61.8000	382000	1.80	99.9520	480	4.80
65.6000	344000	1.90	99.9670	330	4.91
69.2000	308000	2.00	99.9770	230	5.00
72.6000	274000	2.10	99.9850	150	5.12
75.8000	242000	2.20	99.9900	100	5.22

(Continued)

TABLE 17.2 (Continued)

% Yield	DPMO	Sigma	% Yield	DPMO	Sigma
78.8000	212000	2.30	99.9930	70	5.31
81.6000	184000	2.40	99.9960	40	5.44
84.2000	158000	2.50	99.9970	30	5.51
86.5000	135000	2.60	99.9980	20	5.61
88.5000	115000	2.70	99.9990	10	5.76
90.3200	96800	2.80	99.9992	8	5.81
91.9200	80800	2.90	99.9995	5	5.92
93.3200	66800	3.00	99.9997	3.4	6.00

> **The goal of any process should be to have a process sigma of 6.0, which is no more than 3.4 defects per million opportunities (DPMO), or a process performance of 99.9997%.**

To calculate the process sigma (sigma level),

- Define the opportunity (output desired by the customer).
- Define the defect (defect is a product, service, or step that does not meet customer requirement for quality).
- Measure the number of opportunities and defects in a given period of time.
- Calculate the **yield**. The process yield is calculated by subtracting the total number of defects from the total number of opportunities, divided by the total number of opportunities, and multiplying the result by 100 (Opportunities – Defects)/Opportunities × 100).
- Then look up process sigma on the process sigma level conversion table.

Example: Improving DVT Prophylaxis

Prevention of deep vein thrombosis (DVT) in hospitalized patients is critical to a safe recovery. The DVT prevention success rate for the neuro ICU, medical ICU, surgical ICU, and the OR is 93.790%, 99.3760%, 99.9767%, and 99.9997%, respectively. The percentage success rate is the % yield. How are the units performing?

Consulting the process sigma level conversion table, we can find their defect rate expressed as DPMO (defects per million opportunities) and the corresponding process sigma capability or sigma level. Sigma level for the neuro ICU, medical ICU, surgical ICU, and the OR is 3, 4, 5, and 6, respectively. For the operating room, there are 3.4 DVTs

TABLE 17-3   DVT Prophylaxis Process Sigma Levels

DVT Prophylaxis Success Rate by Unit			
Hospital Unit	DVT Prevention or % Yield	DPMO	Sigma Level
Neuro ICU	93.3190%	66,800	3
Medical ICU	99.3760%	6,210	4
Surgical ICU	99.9767%	230	5
Operating room	99.9997%	3.4	6

for every million patients. For the neuro ICU, there are 66,800 DVTs per million patients. Sometimes, 99% is not good enough! (See Table 17-3.)

PUTTING IT ALL TOGETHER: IS THE PROCESS STABLE? IS IT CAPABLE?

To understand and assess the performance of a process, we need to answer three basic questions:

1. How is our process behaving? Can we meet the needs of our customer?
2. Are we meeting the needs of our customers?
3. How often are we meeting their requirements?

To answer the first question, we need **two summary statistics** (a measure of central tendency and a measure of dispersion); and **two graphs** (pictures): a snapshot of the process, and a graph of time-ordered data showing performance over time. To answer the second and third questions, we can use a Control chart (graph of time-ordered data) and a capability analysis. See Figure 17-5, an updated version of Figure 14-11 in Chapter 14.

These are the steps:

- Collect data following the three rules of data collection (operational definition, principles of stratification, time-ordered data).
- Answer the **homogeneity question**. Is data homogeneous? Does data come from one process being run under one set of conditions, or does the data reflect different processes or the influence of several conditions? Use a histogram, Run chart, or Control chart.
- Compute **summary statistics.** Use a measure of central tendency (mean, median, mode) and a measure of dispersion (range, variance, standard deviation) to characterize your data and define process performance.

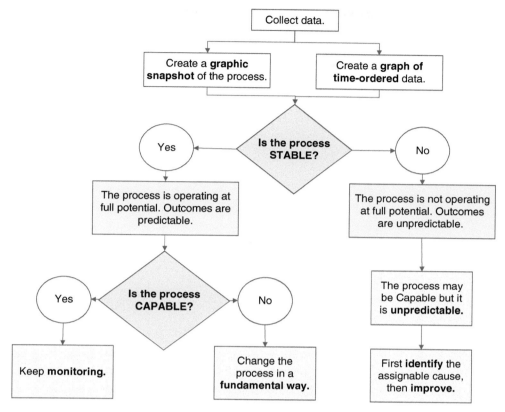

FIGURE 17-5 Assessing a process's performance. Stability and capability guide the improvement strategy.

- Analyze **variation.** Use a histogram. Create a Run chart or a Control chart. Does the process show Common or Special Cause Variation? Is the process stable? How is the process performing over time? Can we predict performance? Can we meet customer requirements?

- Perform a **capability analysis.** Is the process capable? How is the VOP performing compared to the VOC? Are we meeting customer demands i.e. specifications? How often are we meeting these demands?

- Based on the results, apply the appropriate **improvement strategy.** If the process is stable and capable, keep monitoring. If the process is stable but not capable, the process needs to be changed in a fundamental way. If the process is not stable, no matter the results, find the assignable causes of special cause variation and then decide if further improvement is needed.

A properly created histogram and Control chart will tell you all you need to know about process performance.

CHAPTER 18

How to Identify and Prioritize the Most Likely Cause of the Problem

STORIES FROM THE FRONT LINES OF HEALTHCARE: WAIT TIME IN THE ORTHOPEDIC OUTPATIENT CLINIC

Dr. Archivetti was shocked. His clinic's patient satisfaction scores were the worst of any clinic in the outpatient building. Complaints seemed to be focusing on the long waiting times to be seen by a provider. For some patients, wait times had been as long as an hour and a half. Dr. Archivetti considered the possible causes of the clinic's poor performance, and based on his own experience, concluded clinic staffing was inadequate. He scheduled an appointment with the hospital's CEO, and at the meeting, demanded an additional nurse and nurse tech be assigned to his clinic. Wanting to avoid any conflict, the CEO agreed.

Three months after the arrival of additional clinic staff, wait times had not improved. Patients' comments continued to reflect long wait times as the source of their dissatisfaction. Puzzled, Dr. Archivetti enlisted the help of an improvement team. A thorough evaluation of the problem and review of available data revealed an atypical patient scheduling pattern as the main source of the problem. It appeared that while providers were spending an average of 25 minutes with each patient, patients were scheduled to arrive every 15 minutes. This caused a significant back-up starting late morning and throughout the day.

What was the problem? How was it addressed? What were the results?

The Quality Improvement Challenge: A Practical Guide for Physicians, First Edition.
Richard J. Banchs and Michael R. Pop.
© 2021 John Wiley & Sons Ltd. Published 2021 by John Wiley & Sons Ltd.
Companion website: www.wiley.com/go/banchs/quality

THE THINGS WE DO THAT STIFLE OUR ANALYTICAL THINKING

Critical thinking is the objective analysis of information in order to form a judgment. Critical thinking involves **analytical thinking,** a step-by-step approach to thinking that allows the breakdown of complex information. Looking for the cause(s) of a problem requires analytical and critical thinking. We must start with a clear understanding of the problem and a thorough analysis of the available data. Only then can we attempt to make a decision about the true nature of the problem. Unfortunately, we often follow a haphazard approach. We have the tendency to

1. **Rush to judgment.** We are so sure about the cause of the problem that we totally bypass any analytical process. We don't take time to gather additional data to confirm our suspicions; instead we rush to implement a seemingly obvious solution. This often has disastrous consequences with leadership and the frontline stakeholders investing a great deal of time and effort implementing the wrong solution. When additional efforts to resolve the problem are again needed, these are met with skepticism and a significant amount of resistance. Following a step-by-step analytical approach when looking for the cause(s) of a problem is a great investment of time because it increases our chances to come up with the best solution(s). Further, involving the front line in the search for the causes of the problem and finding solutions is a sure way to get their buy-in and acceptance because people support what they help create.

2. **Take information at face value.** We take the first available piece of information and launch into a creative thinking mode without a clear understanding of the problem. There is no effort made to analyze additional data or to confirm the facts. As a result, more time is spent debating the merits of each solution than on finding the true nature of the problem.

3. **Focus on a single issue.** We identify one of the causes of a problem but fail to see other relevant contributing factors. Looking for the cause(s) of a problem requires digging beneath the surface and being open to considering multiple factors. Problems don't happen in a vacuum and "systems thinking" must drive our analytical approach. The results we get are the product of the system that we work in. Systems are the sum of multiple factors: the vision, the mission, culture, leadership, communication channels, policies, procedures, work processes, people, equipment and physical structures. To uncover the cause(s) of complex performance problems, we need to view problems from a broad perspective that includes seeing the system, and all its elements, structures, cycles, and hand-offs as contributors to the final outcome.

4. **Confuse the cause with the effect.** An effect is the problem or the unwanted result(s) we are experiencing. Every effect may have multiple causes, not just one. Cause and effect are on a continuum because a problem (effect) can be

TABLE 18-1 The Cause and Effect Continuum

The Cause and Effect Continuum		
Effect (the outcome or problem)		**Cause**
Infection of a central line site	caused by. . .	Insufficient sterilization
Insufficient sterilization	caused by. . .	Inadequate sterile technique used by the resident
Inadequate sterile technique used by the resident	caused by. . .	Lack of proper supervision or oversight by faculty
Lack of proper supervision or oversight by faculty	caused by. . .	Insufficient faculty for the workload; faculty cannot always supervise residents

the cause of a subsequent problem. A problem can be the cause or the effect, depending on where we look on the **cause-and-effect continuum**. Sometimes people confuse the cause for the effect, finding it difficult to distinguish between both. In the example provided in Table 18-1, "Inadequate sterile technique used by the resident" is both a cause and an effect.

CRUCIAL INTERACTION OF ACTIONS AND CONDITIONS

When looking for the cause(s) of a problem, consider that a problem is generated by the interaction of an **action** and a **condition**. The problem or effect can only exist if the action and the condition both occur at the same time and in the same space:

- **Actions** are usually temporary causes that bring together or enable the condition to produce an effect. They are the **enablers**. However, no action can cause a problem without a contributing or related condition. Actions are created by humans. Humans are responsible for the **human cause(s)** of the problem. Human errors of omission or commission can result in the problem (effect).
- **Conditions** are usually **preexisting**, sometimes unseen, and always present before the action takes place. Conditions can be clearly visible, or dormant and hidden from observation.
  - o **Direct (physical) causes of problems.** This is usually the physical reason why the product, service, or care fails to meet customer expectations. Direct causes often involve the medical and technical explanation of why something fails. For example, a burnt-out light bulb could cause no light to be emitted and the medical equipment to fail.

○ **Hidden causes of problems.** These are the deficiencies in policies, procedures, and systems that allow the human error to go unchecked. Hidden causes can be discovered by tracing them back through the culture of the organization, attitudes of the front line professionals, and assumptions that underpin the decisions taken. We find the hidden causes by going to the gemba and asking the frontline professionals to describe "what was going on when the problem happened." To find the hidden causes of a problem we must understand the **conditions** people are working under when the problem occurred. Then we fix the system and the process to improve the outcome.

> **Problems (effects) happen by the combination of action(s) and conditions; direct (physical) causes are triggered by the actions of humans, but humans are negatively affected by hidden or latent forces (see Figure 18-1).**

The goal of the causal analysis is to find the human causes, the direct causes, and then go beyond them to identify and improve (change) the hidden causes.

Example: Medication Error Before Initiating CPB

During a surgical procedure, a first-year anesthesia resident administered intravenous protamine instead of heparin before initiating cardiopulmonary bypass (CPB). Heparin administration is required at the initiation of CPB to prevent clotting within the CPB circuit. By facilitating the action of antithrombin III, heparin inhibits thrombin and coagulation. Protamine is used after CPB to reverse the anticoagulant effects of heparin and restore coagulation. The error resulted in significant patient harm. A root-cause analysis revealed:

*   **Human cause.** The resident made an error by selecting the wrong syringe and not checking the label on the syringe.*

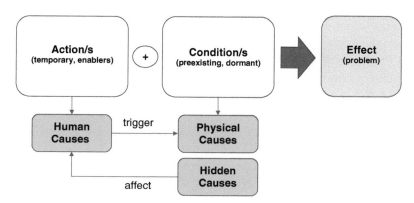

FIGURE 18-1   Problems come from the interaction of actions and conditions.

Conditions: Direct cause. *Drawn-up protamine and heparin syringes were left on the working surface of the anesthesia machine at the time of room setup by a senior resident. Protamine and heparin syringes were appropriately labeled with color-coded labels, but placed on the same working surface, and in proximity to other medications making syringe (label) identification more difficult. Heparin and protamine syringes were labeled using the same white, nonspecific label, with the name of the medication handwritten by the senior resident.*

Conditions: Hidden cause. *Currently, no specific protocols exist as to where each syringe should be placed and the time at which each drug should be drawn. Best practice suggests heparin should be drawn at the beginning of the case and placed on the working surface of the anesthesia machine, and protamine should be drawn after cardiopulmonary bypass (CPB) is initiated and the syringe left on the working surface of the anesthesia cart. The root-cause analysis also found that currently, there is no written policy that requires residents call their supervisor before administering heparin or protamine.*

THE PATH TO THE ANALYSIS OF Y

The outcome y is what the QI project has been launched to improve (also called the primary QI project metric). This outcome may be "long wait times," "defects," "ventilatory-induced pneumonias," or "failed screening tests." Y is the result of the interaction of a number of factors or variables we call x. The relationship between the outcome y and the factors or variables x can be summarized with the equation:

$$y = f(x)\, x_1 x_2 x_3 ... x_n$$

Y is a function of multiple x variables. Once we identify the x factors that interact to produce the undesirable outcome y, we are going to have to filter and prioritize those x variables that have the greatest impact on y. These variables are the vital few, or critical x factors. The goal of our **analytical process** is to identify which input variables or critical x factors are mostly responsible for output y we want to change. Once identified, we can then generate a list of possible solutions, prioritize them, and pilot them. The path to the analysis of y follows these steps (see Figure 18-2):

1. **Identify potential causes of the problem:**
   - **Use your process knowledge** to generate a list of potential causes of the problem. Energize your analytical thinking process (cause-focused analysis) by using tools such as brainstorming techniques, fishbone diagrams, or 5 whys diagrams (see next).
   - **Use a display of data** to find possible causes of the problem. Graph are the preferred tool. Data can be displayed using bar charts (see Chapter 14), pie charts, and Pareto bar charts (see next). These basic tools may be used separately or together to help generate a list of potential causes of the problem.

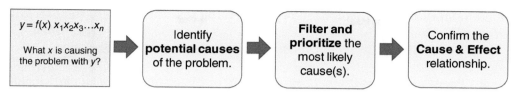

FIGURE 18-2   Path to analysis of *y*.

2. **Filter and prioritize the most likely causes**. Potential causes of the problem need to be filtered and prioritized to focus the team's efforts on the causes with the highest impact on the outcome y we want to change. These are the critical *x* factors. Tools to filter and prioritize the most likely cause(s) are multivoting, cause-and-effect matrix, and bar charts or pie charts of stratified data.

3. **Confirm the C&E relationships**. Confirm the cause-and-effect (C&E) relationships between the outcome y and the critical *x* factors via experimental or quantitative analysis (see next).

TOOLS TO IDENTIFY THE POSSIBLE CAUSE(S) OF THE PROBLEM

To generate a list of the potential causes of the problem we can use our process knowledge, or a display of data. Several tools are available (see Figure 18-3).

Brainstorming Techniques

Brainstorming is a group creativity technique in which efforts are made to generate a large amount of ideas (causes) contributed spontaneously by the QI team and front line stakeholders.

Brainstorming techniques offer a useful way to gather the input of team members. Team members are the front line stakeholders that know the "ins and outs" of the process, experience the process's workflow, and are knowledgeable about barriers to effective and efficient completion of their work. **It is critical that the front line**

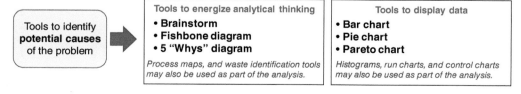

FIGURE 18-3   Tools to identify potential causes of a problem.

stakeholders also be involved in brainstorming sessions because they are the professionals doing the work that is the focus of our improvement efforts. Brainstorming is a technique rooted in two fundamental principles:

1. **Focus on generating a large quantity of ideas.** Encourage all participants to provide a wide array of ideas that might lead to identifying the most likely causes of a problem. All ideas should be recorded and received without criticism or discussion.

2. **Explicitly suppress judgment of ideas**. No judgment regarding the feasibility of ideas should be made during a brainstorming session. Judgment should be reserved for a later stage when prioritization occurs. Brainstorming should be used to generate a thorough list of causes using the teams process knowledge, and "piggybacking" off each other's ideas. Judging the merits of each contribution will stop the flow of ideas.

These principles give rise to the four rules of every brainstorming session, and make the acronym DOVE:

- **D**efer judgment: Withhold any criticism during the brainstorming session so that analytical-thinking is not stifled, and participants feel free to generate a great number of ideas.
- **O**ffbeat ideas are OK: Welcome wild ideas. Participants should be encouraged to express themselves; combine and improve ideas to encourage new ideas.
- **V**ast number of ideas: Participants should generate a large quantity of ideas in order to increase the likelihood of generating a better understanding of the contributing causes of the problem.
- **E**valuate later: Judgment should be reserved for the prioritization phase.

Brainstorming cannot be a random activity. It needs to follow a set of rules that is often best accomplished with the help of a facilitator. With the generation of a large list of possible ideas, the project team can now organize them and get a consensus about the most likely cause of the problem. An easy way to achieve this is with a fishbone diagram.

Fishbone Diagram

> **The fishbone diagram is a basic tool for identifying potential causes of a problem and providing the structure and template on which to arrange and organize all the ideas generated during a brainstorming session.**

The fishbone diagram is also known as an **Ishikawa diagram,** or a **cause-and-effect diagram**. The fishbone diagram relates causes to an effect in an organized and structured manner (see Figure 18-4):

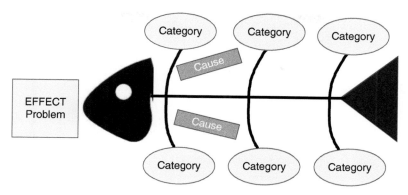

FIGURE 18-4   Fishbone diagram.

- The effect, or problem being investigated, is shown at the end of a horizontal arrow (at the "head" of the diagram).
- The main categories of potential causes are shown as labeled arrows entering the central spine.
- Each arrow may have other arrows entering it to designate the sub-causes of the main category.

Typically, fishbone diagrams have four to six main categories of causes labeling the arrows entering into the central spine. These correspond to general themes of ideas from the brainstorming session. In Six Sigma projects in manufacturing, the main categories are referred to as the six "Ms" for manpower (people), methods (processes), materials (supplies), measurements, machines (equipment), milieu (environment), and "Mother Nature"). Any other categories can be added according to the nature of the project. The fishbone diagram is an excellent tool to help organize thoughts, provide a structure for further investigation of causes, stimulate additional brainstorming, and maintain focus on the issue. A fishbone diagram is a very useful tool when trying to identify possible causes of operational or clinical problems (see example in Figure 18-5).

Steps for creating a fishbone diagram

- Create a detailed, specific, and narrowly defined problem statement.
- With the team, brainstorm a list of possible causes; come up with at least 10 potential causes.
- Write the problem (effect) at the head of the fishbone skeleton.
- Label the main branches; write down the major categories for the arrows entering the "spine."
- Label secondary branches if needed.
- Organize the ideas from the brainstorming session according to the main categories: Place the different causes in their appropriate location (main and

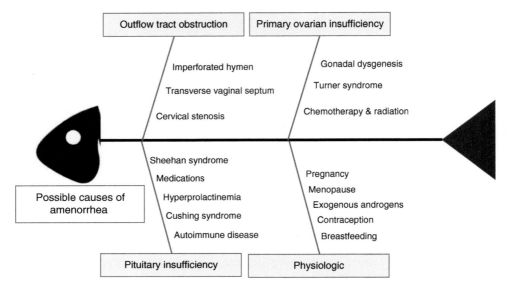

FIGURE 18-5   Fishbone diagram showing the possible causes of Amenorrhea.

secondary branches). Use the words "could **cause**" to make sure you are forced to think in terms of cause-and-effect continuum.

- Do some additional brainstorming as new ideas surface.
- Disregard any cause the team immediately agrees does not apply.
- Brainstorm for more ideas in categories that contain fewer ideas.
- Identify the cause you think are most critical.

Common mistakes when building a fishbone diagram

- assembling a team without an adequate process knowledge (subject-matter expertise);
- brainstorming too few causes;
- not exploring enough ideas, i.e., creating an insufficient number of main branches;
- focusing only on branches that are most familiar;
- mismatching causes or not using "could cause" to make sure each cause is in the appropriate category and relates to the effect; or
- writing down solutions instead of causes.

The 5 "Whys" Diagram

> **The 5 whys diagram is a quick, basic, and focused technique used to explore the potential causes of a problem by asking "why" five times; the 5 whys diagram drills down to the lowest/deepest level of the cause(s).**

When creating a 5 whys diagram, each answer from the preceding question serves as the basis for the following question. By repeatedly asking the question "Why?" an improvement team can drill down into the issues that led to the underlying causes of the problem. The 5 whys diagram is an excellent tool to

- look for the **hidden causes** of a problem;
- practice an **"inch wide and mile deep"** type of investigation; and
- examine a problem without completing a time consuming, resource intensive investigation that requires significant data collection and statistical analysis.

The 5 whys technique helps teams avoid accepting the most obvious explanations of a problem, which are often superficial and do not capture the full essence of the issue. Keep asking "Why?" until

- you have obtained five responses,
- there is insufficient knowledge to continue,
- the cause is not within the control of the team, or
- the cause is too broad and does not specifically address the issue.

Sometimes we may reach a cause that the team can act on after two or three "whys." Take appropriate action and implement countermeasures; however, do not make the mistake of stopping too early, i.e. – stopping at the human causes vs. the hidden causes. Other times the team may have to drill down well past 5 "whys" to find actionable items.

How to create a 5 whys diagram:

- Start with a statement of the problem, or the primary causes identified by the fishbone diagram.
- Ask, "Why did it occur?"
- Turn the answer to the first question into a second question and ask, "Why did that occur?"
- Continue to follow the process until you have asked "why" five times.

With each answer to the 5 whys, you increase the odds of finding the fundamental/systemic causes of the problem. The 5 whys diagram

- can be used as a tool to compliment the fishbone diagram as a way to drill down to the core causes of the problem; or
- can be used to investigate the cause and effect relationship in a **failure event**, building a cause-and-effect tree known as a "why tree" or "fault tree."

When building a 5 "whys" diagram, it is necessary that each "why" question uses the previous answer as the basis for the next question in order to create a clear association

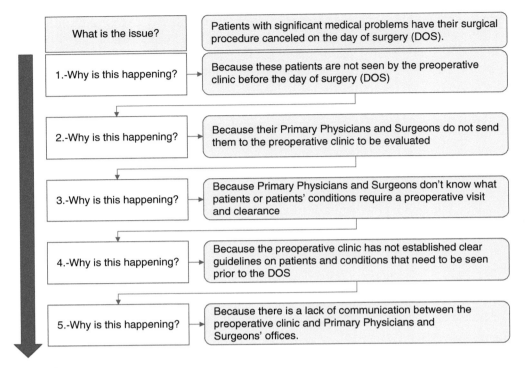

FIGURE 18-6   An example of a The 5 whys diagram.

between them. This link establishes that an effect is due to the stated cause and confirms the failure path from the event to its root. Figure 18-6 is an example of a 5 whys diagram.

The Pie Chart

Pie charts represent data in a circular graph divided into a number of sections, each of which designate a proportion of all the data collected.

Pie charts are used with categorical data to represent percentages of a category or factor, or for giving a quick idea of the proportional distribution of the data (see Figure 18-7).

Pie charts have several limitations when compared to bar charts (see bar charts in Chapter 14):

- Pie charts can only show a small number of categories or segments of data; as the number of segments increase, the size of each segment or slice becomes

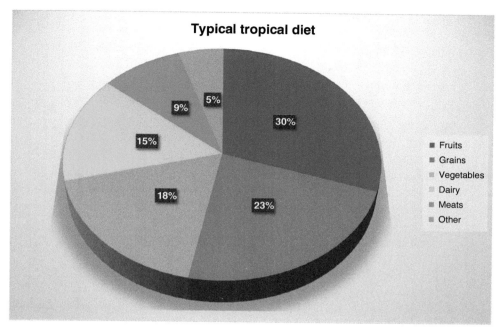

FIGURE 18-7   Pie chart.

smaller, which makes them unsuitable for large amounts of data and lots of segments.

- Pie charts take up more space than some of the other graphic alternatives. This is mainly due to their size and need for extra space for legends.
- Pie charts are not the ideal graph to make accurate comparisons between groups of data. It is harder to distinguish the size of an item by comparing the area of two slices.

The Pareto Bar Chart

> **The Pareto bar chart is a specialized bar chart used with count and attribute data that presents a graphical visualization of the frequency of the individual causes displayed in decreasing order using cumulative percentages. The Pareto bar chart is based on the Pareto principle.**

The Pareto principle (also known as the 80–20 rule, the law of the vital few, and the principle of factor scarcity) states that for many events, roughly 80% of the effects come from 20% of the causes. The Pareto principle was first described by Vilfredo Pareto (1848–1923), an Italian economist who noted that roughly 80% of the wealth in

Italy was concentrated in 20% of the population, and that 80% of the crime was committed by a small percentage of the population.

The Pareto bar chart can be used to

- narrow down your search during your cause-identification efforts,
- focus your efforts on the "vital few" (most important causes of the problem), and
- figure out which categories will yield the biggest gains.

The Pareto chart is one of the most valuable tools to find which inputs or x variables are the greatest contributors to the problem y, and warrant further evaluation. It is the tool of choice to visualize priority opportunities for improvement. *Be aware though that the Pareto bar chart can only be used when the Pareto principle holds* (see Figure 18-8).

Four conditions for the Pareto principle (Pareto effect) to hold:

1. The scale of the vertical axis (y) contains the total number of defects, errors, and causes of the categories represented.
2. Each category (defect, errors, sources, factor, etc.) has the same area of opportunity (AOO), that is, has the same chance of appearing or sample space. For example, February typically has 28 days and March has 31 days. It may not be

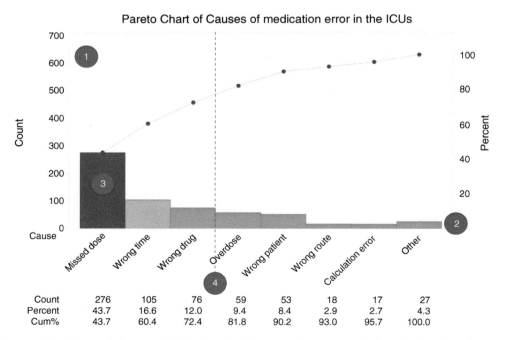

Pareto Chart of Causes of medication error in the ICUs

Cause	Missed dose	Wrong time	Wrong drug	Overdose	Wrong patient	Wrong route	Calculation error	Other
Count	276	105	76	59	53	18	17	27
Percent	43.7	16.6	12.0	9.4	8.4	2.9	2.7	4.3
Cum%	43.7	60.4	72.4	81.8	90.2	93.0	95.7	100.0

FIGURE 18-8 Conditions for the Pareto principle to apply. Chart created with Minitab® Software package. Printed with permission of Minitab, LLC. All rights reserved.

fair to compare the performance of these two months without addressing the three additional days.

3. The first bar is 2–3 times larger than the rest of the bars.

4. The first three bars account for roughly 70–80% of the count or impact (cumulative percentage).

When these four conditions are true, the Pareto principle holds, and we can use the Pareto bar chart to narrow the focus of our efforts to the "vital few." The Pareto bar chart strategy provides a way for the improvement team to focus on the "biggest bang for the buck." If the Pareto principle holds, the target should identify the roughly 20% of causes that are responsible for 70–80% of the problem.

What to do when the Pareto principle does not hold (Pareto effect)?

Sometimes, the Pareto principle does not hold (see Figure 18-9):

1. In Figure 18-9, the first bar is not much larger than the second.

2. The four bars out of a total six account for 82% of the causes. That is almost all the causes!

If the Pareto principle does not hold, data must be stratified to look for additional patterns, or look for another way of analyzing the data. For example, analyze the **impact**

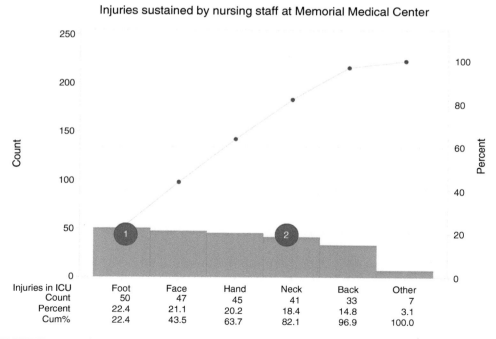

Injuries in ICU	Foot	Face	Hand	Neck	Back	Other
Count	50	47	45	41	33	7
Percent	22.4	21.1	20.2	18.4	14.8	3.1
Cum%	22.4	43.5	63.7	82.1	96.9	100.0

FIGURE 18-9   This Pareto bar chart that does not hold the Pareto Principle. Chart created with Minitab® Software package. Printed with permission of Minitab, LLC. All rights reserved.

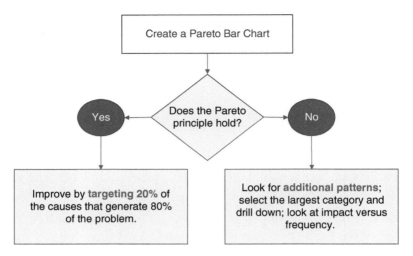

FIGURE 18-10   Pareto bar chart strategy.

of the cause versus frequency of occurrence. Depending on the outcome variable being studied, some of the most frequent causes may not have the biggest impact on the problem. When the Pareto principle does not apply, a Pareto bar chart should be constructed with a different approach to evaluate the contribution of each cause to the problem. A different strategy should be used (see Figure 18-10).

TOOLS YOU CAN USE TO FILTER AND PRIORITIZE THE MOST LIKELY CAUSE

Multivoting

The analytical thinking process to this point has helped us identify potential causes of the problem. They are only potential causes. We must continue to work to filter and prioritize the ones that make most sense to further investigate, i.e. the critical x's. One method of filtering and prioritizing the list is multivoting. *Multivoting takes advantage of the team's process knowledge and facilitates collaborative decision-making.*

> **Multivoting is a simple technique where participants in a group cast multiple votes to identify their priorities and narrow down the possible causes of the problem from a list of ideas generated during an investigative analysis.**

To multivote, follow these steps:

- First brainstorm ideas. After the session, write each idea on a sticky note and place it on a board visible to all participants. Ask each team member to explain the idea in a clear and concise way.
- If two or more ideas have common grounds, place them in close proximity, creating as many groups as needed.
- Set the voting process. Each team member can cast multiple votes equal to 1/3 to 1/4 of the total number of items on the board. Each team member can cast more than one vote per item or choose to place all votes on one item.
- Tally all votes and record the totals.
- Identify the top causes, and keep the top third that scored the highest.
- With the new list, repeat the procedure until the final list is narrowed down to three or fewer options.
- In case of a narrow difference between ideas, perform a second round of multivoting using only the top selections.

The Cause-and-Effect Matrix

> **The cause-and-effect (C&E) matrix is a tool used to assess the effect of multiple inputs on one or more outcomes using ranked priorities and narrows down the focus of your improvement efforts.**

The C&E matrix should not be confused with a C&E diagram (Ishikawa diagram). The C&E matrix establishes a relationship between process inputs x (causes) and outputs y based on ranked priorities. The C&E matrix assigns a **priority score** to each key process output variable and a **correlation assessment** to each input variable. These two numbers determine a total score that can then be used in the identification of the key process input variables (x) that must be addressed to improve the key process output metrics.

There are several ways to create a C&E matrix. Here is one:

- **Create the priority score.**
  - o Use the VOC and CTQ tree to identify the key customer requirements or outputs (y) of the process that are critical for quality; list these outcome(s) across the columns of the matrix.
  - o Assign a priority score to each of the outputs (y) according to the perceived importance by the customer; use a 1- to 10-point scale; you may have to obtain additional data to find this information.

- **Identify process and steps.**
  - ○ Identify all process steps from the process map; for each step find the key inputs (*x*).
  - ○ List all the possible inputs (*x*) on the individual rows of the C&E matrix.
- **Decide on the correlation score.**
  - ○ For each input (*x*), determine its relationship to the output (*y*).
  - ○ At the intersection of the row of the input and the column of the output, place a number that indicates the strength of the relationship as determined by your process knowledge; use 9 for strong relationship, 5 for moderate relationship, 3 for weak relationship, and 0 for no relationship.
- **Compute the results.**
  - ○ For each input *x* (row), multiply the priority score by the correlation score. Add all the products across the row and place result in the "total" column.
  - ○ When all the total scores are entered, calculate the percentage of contribution for each input.
- **Select** the two or three inputs with the greatest % score.

Example: Patient Satisfaction with the ED Visit

A C&E matrix is used in this example to determine which inputs x *(cause) have the greatest impact on the outcome variable* y. *The variable* y *is "patient satisfaction with an ER visit." First, key requirements for patient satisfaction are written on the top of the matrix under outputs. Using the VOC and the CTQs, these are: empathy, effectiveness, efficiency, and comfort. These are the categories found to have the greatest impact on patient satisfaction with a visit to the ED. A priority score is then assigned to each of the requirements, according to patient stated importance. For example, empathy (8), effectiveness (10), efficiency (7), comfort (7). The key steps or inputs during a visit to the ED are then identified: front desk admission, RN intake & placement of IV, RN administration of pain medication, RN execution of treatment plan, provider assessment, provider explanations, provider execution of treatment plan, and discharge process. Each step is placed on individual rows. A correlation score for each desired output is then assigned. Multiply the correlation score by the priority score, calculate the totals, and determine the percentage contribution for each step. Given the results of the C&E matrix in this example, you may conclude that provider explanations (14.2%), getting pain medication (14.2%), and the admission and discharge process are the greatest contributors to patient satisfaction in the ED (see Table 18-2).*

TABLE 18-2   The Cause and Effect Matrix

Cause & Effect Matrix					
Correlation Score 0 = No correlation 3 = low correlation 5 = medium correlation 9 = high correlation	**Desired output for patients** **Priority Score**				Final Rank %
	8	10	7	7	
Key Steps	Empathy	Effectiveness	Efficiency	Comfort	
Front-desk admission	9	5	9	3	13.5
RN intake & placement of IV	5	9	3	7	12.3
RN gives pain medication	5	9	5	9	14.2
RN executes treatment plan	0	9	5	3	8.5
Provider assessment	9	9	5	0	12.25
Provider gives explanations	9	9	5	5	14.2
Provider's execution Rx plan	9	9	3	0	11.38
Discharge process	5	9	9	3	13.58

EXERCISE: IN-TRAINING EXAMINATION AT MASS GENERAL HOSPITAL

The residency program director at Mass General Hospital's Department of Medicine is concerned about the high failure rate of residents in the in-training examination (ITE).

1. Using a **brainstorming session** and a **fishbone diagram**, generate a list of possible causes of the problem. Why do residents perform poorly on the in-training examination (ITE)? What are the possible causes? Generate a list.

2. Using the information gathered up to this point, select the most likely causes of the problem. Filter and prioritize your options with **multivoting**. Once identified, select the cause with the highest score and use a **5 whys diagram** to drill-down to the root cause of the problem; find the "hidden cause."

REVIEW QUIZ

1. A fishbone diagram is a tool to help identify potential causes of a problem.
   A. True
   B. False

2. The 5 whys diagram provides a general, high-level overview of potential causes a problem.
   A. True
   B. False

3. Brainstorming is an effective technique for generating a list of potential causes of a problem. It is based on generating as many ideas as possible given the expertise of participants.
   A. True
   B. False

4. Which of the following is a simple selection technique where participants cast multiple votes to identify priorities and narrow down a list of possible causes of the problem?
   A. Pareto analysis
   B. 5 whys diagram
   C. Fishbone diagram
   D. Multivoting
   E. Cause-and-effect matrix

5. All of the following statements regarding the Pareto principle are true EXCEPT
   A. It can be applied to natural phenomenon.
   B. The Pareto principle is also known as the 80–20 rule.
   C. It cannot be used with normally distributed data
   D. The *law of the vital few* is another name for the Pareto principle.
   E. The Pareto chart is built on the Pareto principle.

6. The Pareto bar chart
   A. can be used with count and attribute data,
   B. shows columns representing the quantity of a value,
   C. columns are usually set in decreasing order,
   D. includes frequency and the percentage of values, or
   E. all of the above

7. The Pareto principle applies to a Pareto chart when
   A. The scale of the vertical axis contains the total number of counts of the categories represented.
   B. The first bar of the Pareto chart is almost two to three times larger than the rest of the bars.
   C. The first three bars account for approximately 80% of the factors.
   D. a, b, and c
   E. a and c only

8. If the Pareto principle does not apply to a Pareto bar chart, look for additional patterns on the data, look for impact versus frequency, or select the largest category and break it down further into another Pareto chart.
   A. True
   B. False

9. Which of the following is true about bar charts and pie charts?
   A. The charts are used with continuous data.
   B. The charts are used to analyze variation.
   C. Both are tools that can be used to focus on the possible causes of a problem.
   D. Bar charts display data with each column representing a range of values.
   E. Pie charts represent data in a circular graph divided into equal sections.

10. Which of the following is NOT TRUE?
    A. The Pareto principle is also known as the 80–20 rule.
    B. The Pareto principle states that for many events, roughly 80% of the effects come from 20% of the causes.
    C. The Pareto bar chart is a specialized bar chart used with continuous data.
    D. The Pareto bar chart shows the frequency of the individual causes displayed in decreasing order using cumulative percentages.
    E. The Pareto principle was first described by an Italian economist who noted that about 80% of the country's wealth was concentrated in 20% of the population.

11. Which of the following is NOT a condition for the Pareto principle (Pareto effect) to hold?
    A. The scale of the vertical axis (y) contains the total number of causes.
    B. Each category has the same area of opportunity.
    C. The first three bars account for at least 70% to 80% of the total.
    D. The first bar is two to three times larger than the rest of the bars.
    E. Causes must come from a brainstorming session.

Key: 1a, 2b, 3a, 4d, 5c, 6e, 7d, 8a, 9c, 10c, 11e

CHAPTER 19

Before Proceeding, Confirm the Cause-and-Effect Relationship

THE CAUSE-AND-EFFECT RELATIONSHIP

Once we have identified and prioritized the most likely causes of the problem, it is time to prove the cause-and-effect (C&E) relationship. Is x the cause of the outcome y? Is there a relationship? To what degree does x contribute to our problem? The stronger the evidence that the critical x is responsible for the outcome y, the easier it will be to find a solution that successfully changes the outcome and resolves our problem. There are two common ways to confirm the C&E relationship (see Figure 19-1):

1. **Experimental analysis**. Experimental analysis is the simplest way to test our assumptions. It involves brainstorming possible causes of the problem; identifying a possible cause; making changes in the process; collecting data; confirming your suspicions that the new "way of doing things" is better.
2. **Quantitative analysis**. Quantitative analysis uses data along with several statistical tools to confirm and quantify the C&E relationship (see Figure 19-2).

Quotable quote: "If your experiment needs statistics, you ought to have done a better experiment." Ernest Rutherford

The Quality Improvement Challenge: A Practical Guide for Physicians, First Edition.
Richard J. Banchs and Michael R. Pop.
© 2021 John Wiley & Sons Ltd. Published 2021 by John Wiley & Sons Ltd.
Companion website: www.wiley.com/go/banchs/quality

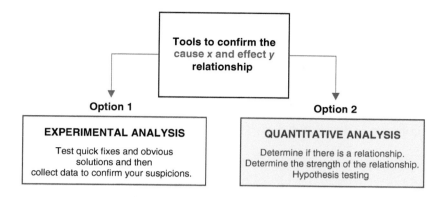

FIGURE 19-1   Options for the analysis of the cause and effect.

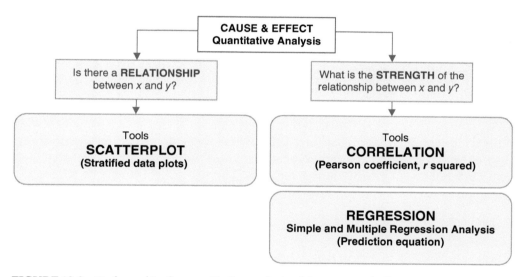

FIGURE 19-2   Tools used in the quantitative analysis of the cause and effect.

THE SCATTERPLOT: IS THERE A RELATIONSHIP?

> A scatterplot (or scatter plot) is a graph consisting of a set of data points plotted on a horizontal and vertical axis used to see patterns that allow us to establish a relation ship or correlation between two variables.

Scatterplots are typically used with **continuous** data. Each point on the scatterplot represents one result with an input (x) and an output (y). The scatterplot helps show the relationship between two factors or variables that can assist with confirming or refuting your hypothesis.

Scatterplots can be used to

- determine the relationship between two variables,
- predict values of one of the variables as the other variable changes,
- help create a hypothesis,
- compare an independent *x* variable to a dependent *y* variable, or
- compare two dependent or two independent variables with one another.

By convention, the independent variable (cause) is placed on the *x*-axis, and the dependent variable (effect) is placed on the *y*-axis. To create a scatterplot, you must have two measurements for each observation, both *x* and the corresponding *y*. When two sets of data are strongly linked, they are said to have a high **correlation**. Correlation is a linear association between two variables. *Statistical evidence of correlation is not evidence of causation.*

Correlation can

- be positive (when the values increase together) (see Figure 19-3),
- be negative (when one value decreases as the other increases), or
- have a complex pattern.

The width, or tightness of scatter, reflects the strength of the relationship (see Figure 19-4). The width or tightness of scatter, however, does not guarantee that there is a C&E relationship between the variables. The two variables may be related to a common cause not included in the analysis.

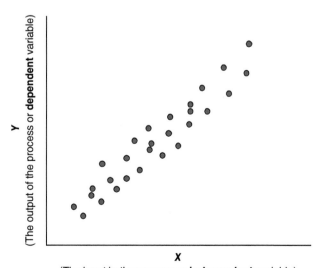

FIGURE 19-3   The scatterplot.

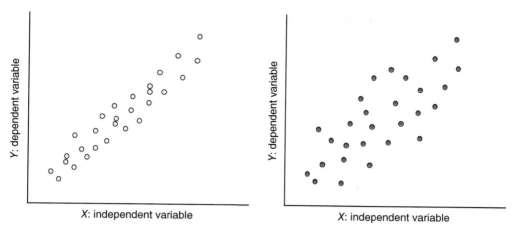

FIGURE 19-4 The scatterplot scatter tightness reflects the strength of the relationship but does not guarantee that there is a cause-and-effect relationship.

THE CORRELATION COEFFICIENT: WHAT IS THE STRENGTH OF THE RELATIONSHIP?

The strength of the relationship is measured by the **correlation coefficient**, using data from the scatterplot.

> **The correlation coefficient is a measure that determines the degree to which two variables are associated.**

While the correlation coefficient measures the degree to which two variables are related, it only measures the linear relationship between the variables. Nonlinear relationships between two variables cannot be expressed by the correlation coefficient.
   The range of values for the correlation coefficient is from –1.0 to 1.0:

- A value of exactly 1.0 means there is a perfect positive relationship between the two variables in which a positive increase in one variable results in a positive increase in the second variable of the same magnitude.
- A value of exactly –1.0 means there is a perfect negative relationship between the two variables in which a positive increase in one variable results in a decrease in the second variable of the same magnitude.
- The strength of the relationship varies, based on the value of the correlation coefficient. A correlation of 0 simply means there is no relationship between the two variables.

The Pearson Correlation Coefficient

> **The Pearson coefficient (r) is a type of correlation coefficient that represents the relationship between two variables that are measured on the same interval or ratio scale. The Pearson coefficient represents the strength and the direction of the relationship.**

The most common correlation coefficient is the **product-moment correlation**, which is also called the **Pearson correlation coefficient**:

- The Pearson coefficient is used to measure the strength of the linear relationship between two variables.
- This coefficient considers both the slope and the clustering of the data on a scatterplot (the graph where a correlation coefficient is plotted).
- The coefficient ranges from –1.0 to +1.0 where –1.0 represents a very strong inverse relationship, +1.0 represents a very strong direct relationship, and 0 represents no relationship (see Figure 19-5).

How is the Pearson coefficient calculated?

- First, calculate the covariance of the two variables in question.
- Next, determine the standard deviations of each variable.
- To find the correlation coefficient, divide the covariance by the product of the two variables' standard deviations.

The statistical significance of the Pearson coefficient must be assessed, as it may have been calculated using insufficient data. The statistical significance of a Pearson

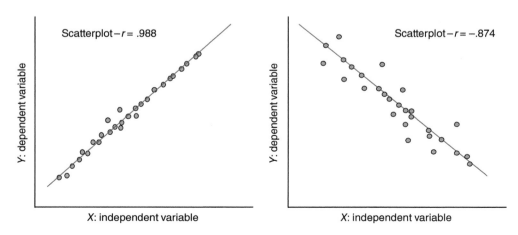

FIGURE 19-5   Positive and negative values for the Pearson coefficient.

coefficient is validated using a *p*-value. *A strong Pearson correlation may have weak statistical strength.* The strength of the correlation is a combination of the angle of the slope and the degree to which the points are tightly clustered, as seen in Figure 19-4.

The Square of the Pearson Correlation Coefficient

> **The squared correlation coefficient (r^2) is the proportion of the variance in *y* that can be accounted for by knowing *x*. Conversely, it is the proportion of variance in *x* that can be accounted for by knowing *y*.**

The squared correlation coefficient is also known as the **coefficient of determination**. It is one of the best means for evaluating the strength of a relationship.

REGRESSION ANALYSIS

> **Regression analysis is a tool that uses data on relevant variables to develop a prediction equation model.**

Regression analysis uses data on relevant variables to develop a prediction equation model that will estimate the changes on a dependent variable by the effects of one or more independent variables. There are differences between correlation and regression analysis:

- In regression, the interest is directional in which one variable is predicted and the other is the predictor; the emphasis is on predicting one variable based on the value of the other variable.
- With correlation, the interest is nondirectional in which the relationship is the critical aspect; the emphasis is on the degree to which a linear model may describe the relationship between two variables.

There are two common types of regression analysis:

1. **In simple linear regression**, a single input variable *x* is used to predict a single output *y*.
2. **In multiple regression**, we are trying to predict the impact of multiple variables *x* on one output *y*.

Correlation and simple linear regression have some similarities and differences. The similarities include

- Pearson's correlation coefficient is the same as the standardized regression coefficient.
- The square of Pearson's correlation coefficient is the same as the r squared in simple linear regression.
- Neither simple linear regression nor correlation answer questions of causality directly.

The main differences are

- Correlation establishes a relationship, while regression makes a prediction. The regression equation can be used to make predictions on the dependent variable y based on the independent variable x.
- Correlation usually suggests a linear relationship, but it can also denote other forms of dependence, such as polynomial or nonlinear relationships.
- While correlation typically refers to Pearson's correlation coefficient, there are other types of correlation, such as Spearman's.

Evaluating Regression Models

There are several methods for evaluating regression models. The most common are

- **Analysis of residuals.** This is the analysis of the sums of squares. Residuals are the difference between the actual data point and the regression model line. Regression models that fit the data have residuals that are random and may be bell shaped. The strength of the correlation between two variables assumes normality and random variation of the residual.
- **R-squared.** This is the amount of the variation of y explained by x, i.e. how much of the variation in the output y is explained by the input factors x in the regression. A high R-squared value indicates a better regression model, since more of the output variation is explained by the input. In Figure 19-6, $a =$ the explained variation (r squared); $b =$ the total variation 19-6.

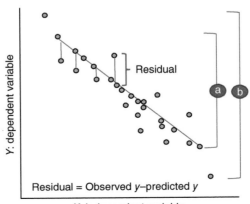

FIGURE 19-6   Analysis of residuals.

HYPOTHESIS TESTING

> **Hypothesis testing is used to make comparisons between two or more groups of data to determine if their differences are due to random variation or if they come from different populations and are actually different.**

Hypothesis testing is an advanced tool due to the number of assumptions that must be made and uses statistical inference to test a theory (hypothesis). The theory is whether there is a statistically significant difference between two or more groups:

- The **null hypothesis** is always that there is no difference between the groups.
- The **alternative hypothesis** is that there is a difference between the groups.

The following assumptions are critical for hypothesis testing:

- When comparing groups of data taken from populations, we assume the samples are random, independent, and unbiased.
- When comparing groups of data taken from processes, we assume the process is stable, only common cause variation is present, the samples are representative and unbiased.

Based on the sample data, *the hypothesis test determines whether to reject the null hypothesis or accept the alternative hypothesis.* The test uses a ***p-value*** to make the determination. The *p*-value represents the probability of obtaining the observed difference between the groups given that the "true" difference is zero (the null hypothesis). If the *p*-value is less than or equal to the level of significance, which is a cut-off point that the team must define, then you reject the null hypothesis and accept the alternative hypothesis. The default significance for most tests is 95%. In other words, if the *p*-value is less than .05, we can conclude there is a statistically significant difference and we must accept the alternative hypothesis and reject the null hypothesis.

The process of distinguishing between the null hypothesis and the alternative hypothesis is aided by identifying two conceptual types of errors, **type 1** and **type 2,** and by specifying parametric limits on how much type 1 error will be permitted. Again, the default is usually .05 for type 1 error, or a 95% significance.

There are several tests available for hypothesis testing (see Figures 19-7 and 19-8).

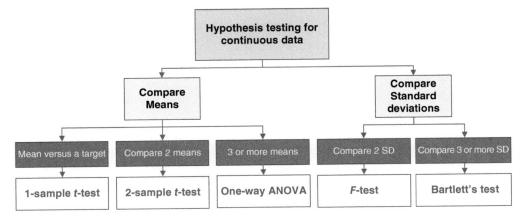

FIGURE 19-7   Hypothesis testing for continuous data.

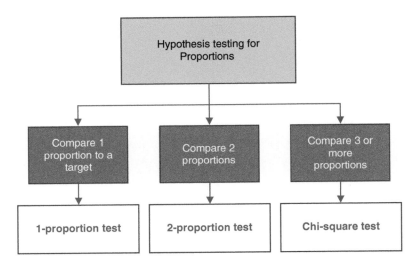

FIGURE 19-8   Hypothesis testing for proportions.

THE THIRD TOLLGATE REVIEW

Periodically, the improvement team needs to confirm that they are on the right track to achieve their project objectives. This is best done through a tollgate review with the Primary Sponsor. A tollgate review is a go/no-go checkpoint where the team leader, team members and the Primary Sponsor meet to: discuss ongoing project activities; review results and deliverables; and assure the project is on track. The third tollgate review should be scheduled with the Primary Sponsor soon after identifying and confirming the most likely cause of the problem, at the end of the fourth "R": the "Right Cause" (see Chapter 25).

REVIEW QUIZ

1. How can you confirm whether a potential cause may contribute to the problem you are trying to improve?
   A. Test quick fixes and obvious solutions and collect data to confirm your suspicions.
   B. Use a scatterplot.
   C. Use a correlation analysis.
   D. Use a regression analysis.
   E. All of the above

2. A cause-and-effect relationship can be confirmed with all of the following tools EXCEPT
   A. scatterplot
   B. pareto bar chart
   C. correlation
   D. simple regression
   E. multiple regression

3. Hypothesis testing can be performed to determine if two or more sets of data are different due to true variation or random variation.
   A. True
   B. False

4. How would you confirm that a variable is a potential cause of the problem?
   A. Test quick fixes and obvious solutions and see the results.
   B. Use a scatterplot.
   C. Use a correlation and determine the r coefficient.
   D. a and b
   E. a, b, and c

Key: 1e, 2b, 3a, 4e

PART VI

THE FIFTH "R": THE RIGHT SOLUTION

CHAPTER 20

Develop and Prioritize Your Improvement Ideas

BARRIERS TO CREATIVE THINKING

Coming up with new ideas is not easy. It is hard to break away from what we know and what we are used to. Because we consider ourselves experts in our field, coming up with a different perspective is hard to do. Most teams experience some difficulties coming up with new ideas in this phase. Barriers to creativity are numerous:

- **Organizational culture.** Organizations with a strong hierarchical structure, traditional views, and inflexible policies make it more difficult for teams to come up with new ideas; there is always the fear new ideas or ways of doing things won't be accepted. These cultures go against the nature of QI and stifle individual creativity.
- **Leadership style.** Leaders that are authoritarian inhibit a team's creativity. Leaders must be open to new ideas, encourage different perspectives, and tap ideas from all ranks.
- **Lack of structure.** The right structure can breed creativity. Team structure and processes to support and channel ideas are important to energize creative thinking.
- **Problem misidentification.** A faulty problem construction and identification, because of assumptions and misconceptions about the issues, often leads individuals to be limited in their capacity to come up with solutions. Creative problem solving first starts with problem identification and construction; then

The Quality Improvement Challenge: A Practical Guide for Physicians, First Edition.
Richard J. Banchs and Michael R. Pop.
© 2021 John Wiley & Sons Ltd. Published 2021 by John Wiley & Sons Ltd.
Companion website: www.wiley.com/go/banchs/quality

idea generation; only at the end do we engage in idea evaluation and selection (Munford 1991). If we don't clearly understand the nature of the problem or focus on the wrong issue, it is difficult to see how we can come up with an appropriate solution.

- **Personal biases**. Biases and preconceptions often stall the flow of new ideas.
- **Fear of change**. We are often averse to creating new solutions because we are uncomfortable embracing uncertainty and change. Entrenched beliefs and old habits cloud our minds, and often make it more difficult to accept change. When we fear change, we can't imagine a new or different way of doing things. It's just human nature.
- **Fear of ridicule or rejection**. Even when we have new ideas, we often don't want to express them for fear of ridicule or rejection.

SETTING THE RIGHT CONDITIONS FOR CREATIVE THINKING

In the right environment and with the right conditions, we can overcome some of the individual and organizational barriers that hinder creativity. Our team's creative thinking can be energized with

- **The right leader**. A leader that is comfortable coaching improvement work; a leader that makes democratizing the source of ideas a priority: great ideas come from all. No idea is dumb and all ideas are welcomed. Ideas can either be shared openly or sent to the leader via email before a brainstorming session. This may help the more reserved members of our team.
- **Clarity of purpose**. A guiding vision and clarity of purpose are key to creation and collaboration. A clearly defined problem is the first step to creative thinking; a well-defined problem is integral to the success of the improvement effort because it ensures all the issues are addressed and change is accepted.
- **Inspiration**. Provide a clear objective and connect the project with the hospital's big picture objectives; the objective is defined in a compelling context that provides motivation and emotional energy.
- **An enabling framework**. Creativity doesn't mean chaos; creativity needs a framework that offers
  - Resources: teams need resources; teams need time to communicate and collaborate. It is difficult to be creative when you have 15 minutes before your next patient!
  - A structure that is consistent with a template where the mind can exercise the creative process.
  - An environment that encourages mistakes. We need to be positive and open-minded. When looking for solutions, we need to be able to generate as many

ideas as we can because improvement is a complicated process that requires our willingness to create, test, and learn from our mistakes. The leader needs to offer positive reinforcement to team members even when their ideas may not work. This enhances the creative thinking process of the team. Just because what has been suggested doesn't work in the current situation does not mean the idea will not work in a similar situation.

○ Visibility for your ideas. Make your ideas and the ideas of others visible. Use boards, diagrams, or build prototypes so everyone can see and share a common understanding.

THE CREATIVE SCAFFOLD

One of the best-known problem-solving and idea generation frameworks is the **Double Diamond. Double Diamond** is the name of a design process model developed by the British Design Council (Design Council 2004). For each "diamond," the Double Diamond model pairs two types of thinking or process, **Divergent** and **Convergent**, where many ideas are created, before refining and narrowing down to the best idea (see Figure 20-1). The Double Diamond applies to both the analytical and creative process:

- **Divergent thinking.** During the divergent thinking phase, a team works to generate as many ideas as possible. In this phase, any filtering or selectivity

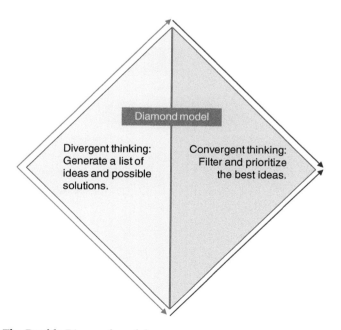

FIGURE 20-1   The Double Diamond model.

is minimized, and the objective is to come up with a great number of possible solutions. Divergent thinking calls for generating ideas, making combinations, changing forms, and identifying connections among different possibilities.

- **Convergent thinking.** Once divergent thinking is complete, information and ideas are structured and organized using convergent thinking. In the convergent thinking phase, a team works towards organizing, prioritizing, and selecting the best solution. Convergent thinking involves refining and narrowing down the best ideas, bringing together different ideas from different sources or fields, and prioritizing the best solutions.

A number of tools can be used to overcome barriers and limitations during the divergent phase (see Figure 20-2); others can be used alone or in combination with the tools of the divergent phase during our convergent phase (see Figure 20-3).

Quotable quotes; "Both tears and sweat are salty, but they render different results. Tears will get you sympathy; sweat will get you change." J Jackson

DIVERGENT THINKING: DEVELOPING IDEAS USING EXISTING SOLUTIONS

Frontline staff and providers who are busy performing their work may not be able to envision completing tasks in a different way. Their workflow has become a habitual pattern and they may have developed a personal attachment to completing their

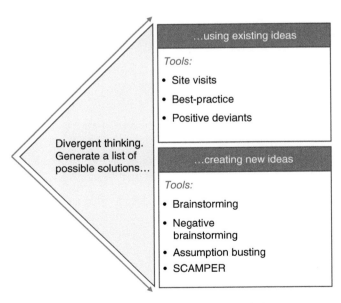

FIGURE 20-2   Tools for the divergent phase to generate a list of ideas.

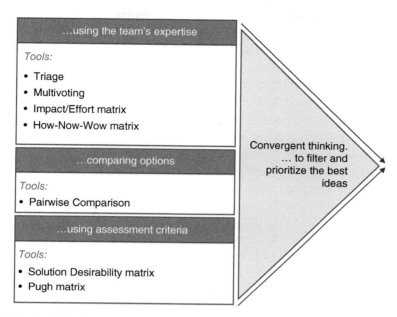

FIGURE 20-3   Tools for the convergent phase to filter and prioritize the best ideas.

job-related responsibilities in a certain way. Attachment to the old ways may be fueled by a fear of the unknown, a sense of loss of control over their work, or a limited knowledge of alternatives and ways of improving the work. Sometimes we can set the stage for productive solutions by facilitating the assimilation of information that demonstrates better ways of doing things. We may also be able to encourage the adoption of different ways of doing things by bringing the experience of teams in other areas, departments, or hospitals that are performing better. There are three general ways of doing this:

1. **Site visits.** Coordinating an opportunity to observe the process being performed at a similar type of hospital (i.e. academic, community, large, small, etc.) during a prearranged site visit may be extremely helpful. In healthcare, many hospitals have identified effective and efficient processes that support best practices inpatient care. Healthcare professionals who are familiar with their counterparts at other hospitals due to their networking activities (professional meetings and conferences) may tap into their colleagues' hospitality to schedule site visits for their teams. It is imperative to confirm that the other hospital demonstrates high performance in accordance with the established best-practices prior to visiting them. Seeing different workflows effectively enacted at other hospitals can be a very powerful motivator. It not only highlights the suboptimal nature of one's current processes, it also emphasizes the improvements that can be realistically attained by modifying one's approach.

Remember: People working in hospitals that are performing well are proud of their accomplishments and are often willing to share their achievements with other healthcare professionals who are struggling in that specific area. When arranging a site visit, make sure not only the formal leaders but a good representation of the front line stakeholders are invited. Opinion leaders and naysayers should also be invited as they may be powerful agents of change.

2. **Best practice.** Compiling benchmarking data or conducting a literature review with a best-practice analysis relative to the issue or process can also be of great value. When it is not feasible to conduct a site visit at another hospital that performs the process according to best practice guidelines, it is a good idea to gather information from a variety of sources and distribute it to team members for review prior to a brainstorming session. Most hospitals have access to industry benchmarking data that compares their performance to other similar hospitals' performance on a multitude of processes and practices and provides recommendations for improvement. A comprehensive review of the literature provides a wealth of information on best practices and evidence-based care in a hospital. Make sure that the potential solutions to the problem they are addressing are supported by **robust data** and can be **implemented locally.**

3. **Positive deviants.** Positive deviants are people within a certain area or department whose uncommon but successful behaviors or strategy enables them to find better solutions to a problem than their peers, despite facing similar challenges and having no extra resources. These professionals may serve as great examples of how to improve one's current processes.

Finding and distributing articles, literature reviews, best-practice recommendations, and other material before a team meeting may facilitate creative thinking and may make the improvement team more open to finding evidence-based solutions to optimize their workflow. These will make it easier to focus on developing a well-designed solution to their problem.

DIVERGENT THINKING: FINDING NEW SOLUTIONS

Brainstorming Sessions

> **A brainstorming session is a team activity aimed at creating ideas and solutions through intensive and freewheeling group discussion.**

Brainstorming is one of the most widely used tools for soliciting a wide variety of creative and relevant ideas from group members. Every participant is encouraged to think aloud and suggest as many ideas as possible, no matter how seemingly outlandish or bizarre they may seem. Brainstorming can be accomplished relatively quickly. With facilitation, brainstorming can also help engage the participants in the tasks at hand by validating their contributions to the process (See Chapter 18 for brainstorming during the analytical process).

A well-designed brainstorming session follows three phases:

1. **Define the objective.** The facilitator clearly explains the aim of the session to all participants. This includes the problem the team is brainstorming, possible or identified causes, and identified solutions, if any. All questions are answered and a time limit for the exercise is set.

2. **Brainstorming phase.** New ideas arise. Participation from everybody is encouraged. No ideas are dismissed or criticized; team members are dissuaded from commenting on other members' ideas until the end of the session.

3. **Decision phase.** The group assesses and evaluates the effects and validity of each idea. Before a brainstorming session, criterion can be developed to prioritize ideas into a more finished list or set of actions or options. The team members must agree on next steps, time frame, and responsibilities to implement ideas.

After the session, team members should be allowed some time to share feedback and get updates. It is important that people feel their effort and contribution are rewarded and have resulted in action and change. If this is done, they will be motivated to help again. Avoid dismissing or rejecting contributions that cannot be used in the current setting by including them in a "second options" list. This will facilitate people's contribution on the next session.

There are a number of techniques to brainstorming. While group brainstorming with the team is most common and preferred, individual brainstorming techniques can be employed when this is not feasible. Regardless of whether group or individual brainstorming techniques are employed, *it is important to solicit the input of all team members and that all team members see the contributions of their peers.*

Group Brainstorming Techniques

These are group creativity techniques where efforts are made to find a solution to a specific problem by gathering a list of ideas spontaneously contributed by its members:

- **Free brainstorming**: Team members brainstorm as a group. The facilitator records every suggestion on a flipchart so it is visible to the whole team. Sticky tape can be used to hang large sheets around the walls and contributions recorded, or ideas can be written on a Post-it note and stuck directly to the wall. At the end of the time limit or when ideas have been exhausted, all contributions are categorized into groups. The team then votes to select and prioritize the best ideas.

- **Guided brainstorming**. Participants are asked to adopt a specific mindset for a period of time and contribute their ideas to a central idea map. Ideas are then ranked for further brainstorming and research. A list is generated with clear and specific actionable items.
- **Electronic brainstorming**. Group members simultaneously and independently enter ideas into a common site. Ideas are collected, organized, and displayed. Software supports categorization of ideas, elimination of duplicates, and prioritization, all of which can be done over extended periods of time and in multiple locations. Electronic brainstorming enhances efficiency by eliminating traveling, and creativity by reducing what Gallupe calls
  - ○ **Production blocking,** or the reduction of idea generation due to turn-taking and forgetting ideas in face-to-face brainstorming.
  - ○ **Evaluation apprehension**, which is a general apprehension experienced by individuals for how others in their presence are evaluating them (Gallupe 1992).

Individual Brainstorming Techniques

These are group creativity techniques where efforts are made to find a solution to a specific problem by gathering a list of ideas contributed by individual members and then shared with the group for review and enhancement.

Idea card. Team members brainstorm individually and then write their ideas on 3×5 index cards. Three options are available:

1. The facilitator collects the ideas, shares them with the team, and the group votes on each idea. The vote can be as simple as a show of hands in favor of a given idea. The top-ranked ideas are selected or they may be sent back to the group for further brainstorming.
2. Ideas are placed onto a large idea map. Each member shares the meanings behind their ideas. If new ideas arise by the association, they are added to the idea map as well. Once all the ideas are captured, the group can vote and take action.
3. Each person's idea is passed to the next person who adds some thoughts. This continues until everybody gets his or her original index card back. Ideas and all the comments are read out loud and the group votes on each group of ideas.

Directed brainstorming. A set of criteria for evaluating a good idea is given to the group to constrain the answers. Each participant is given one sheet of paper and told to write one response only. All the responses are collected and randomly distributed back to the group. Participants are asked to look at the idea they received and create a new idea that improves on the one received based on the initial criteria. The answers are then swapped again. The process is repeated for three or four rounds.

The book technique. An "idea book" is created with a description of the problem on the first page. The "idea book" is circulated with a distribution list included. The first person to receive the book writes his or her ideas and passes the book to the next person on the distribution list who can write new ideas or add to the ideas of the previous person. The process continues until the book has been circulated among all the people on the list. A follow-up meeting is then held to discuss the ideas in the book.

Quotable quote: "Tell me and I forget. Teach me and I remember. Involve me and I learn." Often attributed to Xunzi (Xun Kuang), a Confucian philosopher

Negative Brainstorming Sessions

> **Negative brainstorming is an idea-generation method that, unlike the conventional brainstorming session, focuses on how not to solve the problem.**

Finding the solution to questions such as: "How do we not solve the problem?", "How do we not address the need of our customer?", and "What should we do to completely fail?" will generate much humor and unexpected ideas. This method is often referred to as the brainstorming **tear-down** method. To hold a Negative brainstorming session,

- Identify the problem for which a solution is sought.
- Generate a negative statement such as: "How can we make it fail?", "How can we assure patients are dissatisfied?"
- Brainstorm possible ideas to accomplish the goal.
- Review the ideas and reverse those that have potential.

Assumption Busting

> **Assumption busting is a brainstorming technique that generates a list of potential ideas by doing two things: Identifying and challenging conventional assumptions, and eliminating them if they are obstacles to optimal solutions.**

The problem with creative thinking when a group is made up of people with similar expertise is that team members often come up with the same ideas because they have the same **embedded assumptions**. Assumption busting can be used in most creative situations and is particularly effective when the team is stuck in a current thinking paradigm or has run out of ideas. To do an assumption busting brainstorming session,

- **Collect data.** The first step is to gather data in order to recognize the patterns or thinking paradigms that might be limiting us. Record all the facts that are known about the problem or situation. These are the preliminary assumptions. Defer judgment, and just collect all the information known about the problem. Each statement or data piece is considered an assumption. The basis of assumption busting is the belief that some of the statements that have been made about the problem may not be true.
- **Analyze each assumption.** Review all the assumptions. Choose the assumptions that are too vague or seem constraining and may not be true. Focus on
  - the statements that you believe are true that may not be true,
  - statements that seem to be necessary requirements for something to happen but may not be, and
  - things you believe you don't control but in fact you do.

Deepen your understanding of each statement you want to challenge by making an additional list of assumptions about the assumption.

- **Overturn or "burst" the assumptions.** The easiest assumptions to burst are the things you believe are true but might not be true. Reverse each statement and pretend for a moment the opposite is true. Challenge your preconception: Does the reverse statement make sense? You may gain a new perspective by asking this question. Ask yourself "what if. . .?" to help make the reverse statement seem more possible. What other reverse statements might be true? Sometimes this line of questioning leads to a breakthrough. Many reverse statements will not make sense and you can discard them. Some reverse statements will give you a different perspective, and others, new wisdom about the problem at hand.

The process of assumption busting is a very useful way to break the patterns in our brain and the barriers that limit creative thinking.

SCAMPER

SCAMPER is an acronym for an idea-generating method that is based on the notion that everything new is a modification of something that already exists.

SCAMPER is a structured approach to creating new solutions. SCAMPER stands for: S = Substitute, C = Combine, A = Adapt, M = Magnify, P = Put to other uses, E = Eliminate or modify, R = Rearrange or reverse. Every new idea is a substitution, combination, adaptation, magnification, new use, modification or rearrangement of something that already exists.

SCAMPER starts with an idea-generating list that aims at sparking a team's creativity. SCAMPER represents the different ways one can adapt the characteristics of the problem to trigger new ideas. SCAMPER works best with a facilitator. To use SCAMPER,

- **Generate a list of ideas.** Ask: Can we substitute something from elsewhere? Are there functions, elements, features, or processes that we can successfully combine? Can we adapt ideas from other processes to our needs? Can we modify a feature or function by increasing it, decreasing it, or changing its shape or attributes? Can we use a solution, idea, product, or process and put it to other uses? Can we eliminate or remove an element or a step in the process? What would happen if we rearrange the order, or reverse the sequence turning it inside out or upside down?
- **Organize the ideas.** After generating as many possible ideas as you can, organize them according to their commonalities using an affinity diagram. Affinity diagrams sort and categorize ideas into groupings based on the general themes that emerge from the team.
- **Narrow down and focus.** After using the affinity diagram, narrow down the options; add focus to certain areas; further investigate the areas with potential. Finally, filter and prioritize the potential solution(s); test your ideas.

SCAMPER is the basic framework for creating a solution in the popular 1995 movie: *Apollo 13*!

CONVERGENT THINKING: USING THE TEAM'S KNOWLEDGE TO PRIORITIZE IDEAS

These **idea selection tools** can be used on their own or to filter and prioritize ideas from the divergent thinking phase.

Triage

While we may have come up with many great ideas and ways to resolve our problem, only a few solutions can be selected for trial in a time and resource-constrained environment such as healthcare. Triage can help us narrow down the list of possible ideas to the ones that best meet the specific needs of the project.

> **Triage is a simple approach for selecting improvement ideas that involves removing the ideas that are unsuitable for implementation because they negatively affect other outcomes, conflict with organizational strategy, or do not address the entirety of the problem.**

How to use triage:

- Review each idea individually; evaluate them against exclusionary criteria.
- Discard any idea that does not meet the specific criteria.
- Any disagreements between team members are resolved according to a preestablished process.
- Purge the list of incompatible solutions.

A team can quickly narrow down a long list of potential solutions into a smaller list that can be used to focus on discovering the optimal solution to a problem.

Multivoting

As discussed in Chapter 18, Multivoting provides another option for filtering and prioritizing possible solutions in QI improvement efforts. Refer to Chapter 18 (possible causes) for the specific details.

The Impact/Effort Matrix

> **The Impact/Effort matrix provides a quick way to prioritize possible solutions according to their impact on the problem and the amount of effort required for implementation.**

The Impact/Effort matrix allows teams to quickly visualize the optimal solutions to the problem and eliminate those that are not expected to make the desired impact (see Figure 20-4).

How to create an Impact/Effort matrix:

- List each possible solution on a sticky note.
- Evaluate where each option falls on the Impact/Effort diagram; this decision is made based on team members, experience, subject-matter expertise, and previous experiences. The Impact/Effort matrix provides the structure to an otherwise subjective assessment.
- Place the sticky note with its name or identifying number in the designated area of the grid.
- When the Impact/Effort designations of all possible solutions have been made, filter potential solutions according to their placement on the matrix.

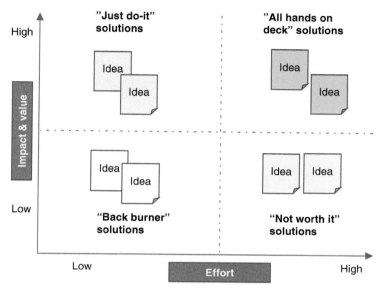

FIGURE 20-4   The Impact Effort matrix.

Filtering strategy

- **High-impact, low-effort solutions.** Implement these "just-do-it" solutions expeditiously as they are projected to significantly impact the resolution of the problem without expending considerable effort.
- **High-impact, high-effort solutions.** Plan to invest time and effort into the implementation of these solutions. These solutions are typically part of a long-term strategic improvement agenda. These solutions take substantial energy to implement, but will have a visible impact when completed.
- **Low-impact, low-effort solutions.** Place these options on the back burner, as they are not expected to provide the impact needed to resolve the issue, even though they do not require much effort.
- **Low-impact, high-effort solutions.** Avoid these solutions. They are not anticipated to yield the desired results and will consume a great deal of effort to execute them.

The How-Now-Wow Matrix

When developing new solutions, people can be creative, think "out of the box," and come up with all sorts of ideas. However when it comes to the convergent phase, people often end up picking ideas that are most familiar to them. This is called the

creative paradox. This paradox states that even when people are trying to be creative and support creativity as a desired goal, they reject creative ideas. This implicit bias against the acceptance of creative ideas exists for two reasons:

1. People want to avoid uncertainty and the associated risk, real or imagined of the unknown.
2. People are not able to identify what creativity is and when confronted with a new idea, reject it (Mueller 2010).

> **The How-Now-Wow matrix is an idea selection tool that forces people to categorize ideas based on their originality and the ease of implementation counteracting the tendency to select only ideas that are the most familiar.**

The How-Now-Wow matrix organizes ideas around three different categories (see Figure 20-5):

1. **How** – represents ideas that are innovative but difficult to implement. These ideas are worth keeping and implementing when possible.
2. **Now** – represents unoriginal ideas that are familiar, easy to implement, and can work well.
3. **Wow** – represents innovative ideas that are easy to implement. These ideas should be planed for and implemented.

The How-Now-Wow matrix is straightforward and easy to use. It encourages team creativity and allows ideas to flow to create groundbreaking innovation.

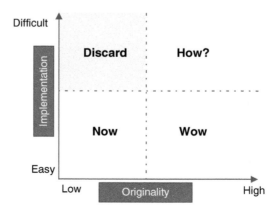

FIGURE 20-5   The How-Now-Wow matrix.

CONVERGENT THINKING: PRIORITIZE IDEAS BY COMPARING OPTIONS

Pairwise Comparison

The Pairwise Comparison or Paired Comparison Analysis is a selection technique for weighing potential ideas against each other.

When choosing between many different options, it is difficult to decide on the best option if they all are very different, seem acceptable, and the decision criteria are subjective. Paired Comparison Analysis helps establish the relative value of each of the options and set priorities when there are limited resources.

The project team considers each pair of ideas in turns and decides which of the two is "better" against each other. The ideas are then ranked against each other based on how often the team voted for them. To create a Paired Comparison Analysis table, follow these steps:

- Make a list of all of the options to be compared and assign each option a letter.
- Write the options on both the row and column of the table.
- Block out the cells where the different options are compared to themselves and the duplicates.
- Decide on the score you want to use when comparing options; for example, 0 = no difference or same importance, 3 = difference with one more important than the other, 5 = substantial difference with one much more important than the other.
- On each blank cell, compare the option in the row to the option in the column. Decide which of the two options is most important, write down the letter of the most important option and the score (see Table 20-1).
- Add the values for each of the options; convert them to a percentage of the total score (see Table 20-2).

TABLE 20-1   Paired Comparison Analysis

Paired Comparison Analysis table				
Options	**A**	**B**	**C**	**D**
A		B, 0	A,3	A,5
B			B,5	C,3
C				D,3
D				

TABLE 20-2   Paired Comparison Analysis Results

Paired Comparison Analysis Results			
Option	Total	Percent	Rank
A	8 (3 + 5)	42%	1
B	5 (5)	26%	2
C	3 (3)	16%	3
D	3 (3)	16%	4

Paired Comparison Analysis can also be used to weigh assessment criteria against each other. The number of votes that each assessment criteria receives drives the weighing score that is assigned.

CONVERGENT THINKING: PRIORITIZE IDEAS USING ASSESSMENT CRITERIA

Assessment criteria provide a basis for developing and selecting the best improvement idea(s). Typical assessment criteria focus on factors such as

- Will the idea work? (probability of success)
- How easy is it to implement?
- How long will it take?
- What personnel are needed?
- What level of risk is involved?
- How much does it cost?

Not all assessment criteria are equal. It's important to weigh assessment criteria against each other in order that the most important criteria are more influential in our decision-making process. Assessment criteria can be weighted using a Paired Comparison Analysis or Multivoting with the team. When using the Multivoting approach for weighing assessment criteria, each team member can be given 100 "points" to distribute across the assessment criteria.

Solution Desirability Matrix

A Solution Desirability matrix is a team-based decision tool for evaluating various improvement proposals against weighted criteria established by either the organization or the team according to the goals of the project.

The Solution Desirability matrix is an evaluation method that allows the project team to determine the necessary components of an optimal solution, which are then used as a basis for comparing the alternative options. The comparisons of possible solutions result in the calculation of a numerical score for each proposal based on criteria selected by the team. The highest score is for the improvement option that best matches the project's goals.

To create a Solution Desirability matrix:

- **Create assessment criteria.** Start by creating assessment criteria based on the needs of the customer (patient, staff, or provider), available resources, organizational mandates, or regulatory and safety requirements:
  - Questions such as "What will the best solution look like?", "What are the most important issues to be addressed?", "What is more cost-effective?", or "What are barriers to implementation?" can help generate a list of assessment criteria and provide a standardized way to compare solutions.
  - When creating assessment criteria, include pertinent project-specific criteria such as, "The solution needs to resolve the problem completely," "The solution cannot conflict with organizational values," or "The solution needs to meet strategic objectives."
  - Other pertinent criteria can be, "will receive leadership support and commitment", "will adapt to organizational culture", "can be implemented quickly", "is cost-effective", "will not negatively impact frontline professionals", or "does not pose regulatory risk or safety concerns for the patient."
- **Prioritize the assessment criteria.** Using a Paired Comparison Analysis or a Multivoting technique, determine the relative value of each assessment criterion. When using a Multivoting technique, you can assign each team member 100 points to apportion across the potential criteria. Calculate the relative contribution of each criterion.
- **Complete the table.** Code each solution with the letters A, B, C, D, and so on, and place them on the columns of the Solution Desirability matrix; place the assessment criteria on the rows of the matrix. For each solution, assign a value of 1 to 10 for each of the assessment criteria.
- **Calculate the scores and select the option.** For each option, multiply the assigned value by the weighted score. Add all the scores and determine the total weighted score. Select the best ideas according to the highest score.

Pugh Matrix

A Pugh matrix is an idea selection technique that can be used to develop and refine potential ideas. The first step is to compare each criterion for each idea against a standard idea and assess it as being better (+), the same (s), or worse (−). Second, the scores for each idea are weighted and totaled. Each positive is multiplied by the weighting to give a weighted sum of positives. Similarly, negatives are added to create a weighted

TABLE 20-3   A Pugh Matrix

Pugh Matrix				
Assessment Criteria	Solutions			Weighting
	A	B	C	
>Addresses the problem completely	+	−	Standard	1
>Will get leadership support	+	+	Standard	3
>Can be quickly implemented	−	+	Standard	5
>Is economic and >cost-effective	S	S	Standard	2
>Will not affect other measures	−	+	Standard	3
>Provides a great healthcare experience for parents	+	−	Standard	3
>Weighted sum of positives	7 (1 + 3 + 3)	11 (3 + 5 + 3)		
>Number of "same"	1	1		
>Weighted sum of negatives	−8 − (5 + 3)	−4 − (1 + 3)		
>TOTAL	-1	+ 7		

sum of negatives. Each solution is compared according to their weighted sum of positives and negatives. Using the Solution Desirability matrix example (see next), if we considered option C the standard, the Pugh matrix reveals option B to be superior to option A (see Table 20-3).

CASE STUDY: DECREASING UNPLANNED READMISSIONS AFTER TONSILLECTOMY

John, Mary, Peter, and Sofia are part of an improvement team. They have been tasked with finding a way to decrease the number of unplanned readmissions after tonsillectomy. Unplanned readmissions after tonsillectomy are frequently caused by dehydration, pain, and postoperative bleeding. Parental awareness, adequate treatment, and early recognition can decrease the risk of hospital readmission in the convalescent child.

Three possible options are being evaluated by the QI team to increase parental awareness and early recognition of possible complications: Provide parents with written instruction upon discharge (A), provide parents with an instructional video (CD) upon discharge (B), or provide parents with instructions and an access key to an instructional website (C).

*Peter suggested the team use a **Solution Desirability matrix** to select the best option. After developing assessment criteria, the team Multivoted and assigned each* *criterion a relative value, each member apportioning 100 points among the criteria (see Table 20-4).*

Assessment criteria and their weighted values were then placed in the rows of the Solution Desirability matrix. For each solution, the team members assigned a score of 1–10 points corresponding to how each solution performed against the assessment criterion. The final score was calculated by multiplying the assigned score by the weight of each assessment criterion. The total weighted score was placed at the bottom of the matrix. Option C was selected as the highest ranked solution (see Table 20-5).

TABLE 20-4 Solution Desirability Matrix Assessment Criteria

Solution Desirability Matrix Assessment Criteria						
	John	Mary	Peter	Sofia	Total	Weight
Addresses the problem completely	>20	>25	>20	>15	>80	>0.2
Will get leadership support	>15	>10	>10	>15	>50	>0.125
Can be quickly implemented	>20	>25	>15	>20	>80	>0.2
Is economic and cost-effective	>15	>5	>15	>15	>50	>0.125
Will not affect other ongoing efforts	>10	>15	>15	>10	>50	>0.12
Provides a great healthcare experience for parents	>20	>20	>25	>25	>90	>0.225
Total	>100	>100	>100	>100	>400	>1

TABLE 20-5 Solution Desirability Matrix Rank Results

Solution Desirability Matrix Ranked Results				
Assessment Criteria	Weight	Solutions		
		A	B	C
>Addresses the problem completely	0.2	8	7	9
>Will get leadership support	0.125	6	8	6
>Can be quickly implemented	0.2	7	4	7
>Is economic and >cost-effective	0.125	5	6	3
>Will not affect other ongoing efforts	0.125	4	7	5
>Provides a great healthcare experience for parents	0.225	8	6	9
>Total weighted score	1	6.675	6.175	6.975
>Rank		2	3	1

ASSESSING RISK: FAILURE MODE AND EFFECTS ANALYSIS (FMEA)

When designing and implementing a possible solution, it is important to anticipate potential problems so that you can take measures to reduce or eliminate the risk. This is especially important in the deployment of solutions that may incur patient harm. Failure Mode and Effects Analysis (FMEA) is a tool designed for this purpose, i.e. to address problems and correct weaknesses before the solution is implemented.

> **Failure Mode and Effects Analysis (FMEA) is a highly structured, systematic technique for failure analysis. It is used to proactively evaluate a process to identify where and how it might fail, the possible causes of failure, their relative impact, the steps or parts of the process involved, and the strategies to mitigate or eliminate that risk.**

Risk analysis has the fundamental purpose of answering four questions:

1. What can go wrong?
2. If something does go wrong, what is the probability of it happening?
3. What are the consequences?
4. How can I avoid or mitigate that risk?

FMEA can be used to analyze potential problems in systems (Systems FMEA), designs (Design FMEA), processes (Process FMEA), or the implementation of solutions. From a perspective of Systems and System's steps, the FMEA assesses the manner in which the item, product, service, or step can potentially fail, the way in which it can occur, the consequences of the failure, and the methods or actions that are currently in place to reduce or eliminate the risks. FMEA considers

1. three elements of the failure: Mode, Effect and Cause;
2. three assessment scales: Severity (SEV), Occurrence (OCC), Detection (DET);
3. one index: Risk Priority Number (RPN); and
4. a list of recommended actions

The FMEA is set up as a table with 11 columns (see Figure 20-6):

1. **Item or step.** This is the focus of the FMEA: a component, step of the process, or solution that we need to evaluate.
2. **Function.** This is what the item, process, or step is intended to do.

Failure Mode and Effects Analysis										
1	2	3	4	5	6	7	8	9	10	11
Step	Function	Failure			Controls	SEV	OCC	DET	RPN	Actions
		Mode	Effect	Cause						

FIGURE 20-6   The FMEA tool.

3. **Failure mode.** The manner in which the item, product, or step can potentially fail to perform or function and the way in which it can occur. A Failure mode may generally have five potential possibilities: complete failure, partial failure, intermittent failure, failure of time (functions too soon or too slow), or over-performance of function.

4. **Failure effect.** The consequences of the failure in the process or the consequences to the patient, staff, or providers.

5. **Failure cause.** This is the specific reason for the failure mode found by asking: "Why does this happen?" A team can use different techniques, such as brainstorming and cause-and-effect analysis, to generate a list of possible causes of failure.

6. **Controls.** The methods or actions that are *currently in place* to reduce or eliminate the risk associated with each potential cause.

7. **Severity.** This is a ranking number associated with the impact of the effect of the failure mode on the patient or customer. It is usually based on a scale from 1–10, determined without considering the likelihood of occurrence or detection.

8. **Occurrence.** This is a ranking number, usually on a scale of 1–10, associated with the likelihood that the failure mode and its associated causes will be present in the item or step in question.

9. **Detection.** This is a ranking number, usually on a scale of 1–10, associated with the ability of current controls to detect the failure mode and cause, determined without accounting for the severity or the likelihood of the occurrence.

10. **Risk Priority Number (RPN).** A numerical ranking of the risk of each potential failure and its cause calculated from the arithmetic product of the Severity number, Occurrence number, and Detection number.

11. **Actions.** Refer to the recommended actions and tasks to reduce or eliminate the risk associated with the potential causes of failure. These actions should reduce the risk of failure (RPN) to an acceptable predetermined level.

The Problem with the Risk Priority Number (RPN)

> **The RPN is a numerical ranking of the risk of each potential failure and its cause, calculated from the arithmetic product of the Severity number, Occurrence number, and Detection number.**

A number on a scale of 1–10 is assigned for each failure mode and on each scale. The Risk Priority Number (RPN) is computed for each failure mode (see Figure 20-7). The failure mode with the largest RPN value is prioritized. There are 10 levels of severity, 10 levels of occurrence, and 10 levels of difficulty of detection.

There are several concerns or problems with the Risk Priority Numbers:

- **Ranking.** While the RPN ranges from 1 to 1000, there are only 120 possible values for the RPN and these values are not uniformly spread out between 1 and 1000. Some RPN values will group up to 24 problem descriptions together, while other RPN values will correspond to only one problem description. So, values sort the 1000 problem descriptions into 120 artificial groupings of different sizes. A ranking of problems is not possible.
- **Scale.** Rankings are on an **ordinal scale**. When we place a series of categories in order in some continuum such as Severity, Occurrence, or Detectability, we may represent this ordering with numbers such as 1–10. The value of 1 is the lowest-ranked category in the continuum, which is below 2, and below 3, and so on. Values with this property of order are called ordinal-scale data. Before you can add or subtract numbers you must have **interval scale data,** which possess both ordering and distance—not only is 1 less than 2, and 2 is less than 3, but also the distance from 1 to 2 is exactly the same as the distance from 2 to 3. Equal distance gives meaning to addition and subtraction. Before you can multiply and divide, you need to have **ratio-scale data**, which

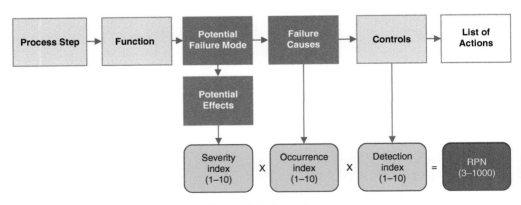

FIGURE 20-7   Calculating the FMEA's Risk Priority Index.

possess ordering, distance, and an absolute zero point. With ratio-scale data we can add, subtract, multiply, and divide numbers to get meaningful results. With interval-scale data we can only add and subtract numbers. With ordinal-scale data addition, subtraction, multiplication and division are all nonsense operations. The product of three ordinal-scale values on any RPN value is not meaningful. As Donald Wheeler states ". . .the lack of a distance function, and the lack of an absolute zero will combine to result in inconsistencies where both serious and trivial problems have the same RPN value and where some trivial problems end up with larger RPN values than other, more serious, problems. This is why any attempt to use RPN values is an exercise in absurdity" (Wheeler 2011).

- **Threshold.** Using a threshold for RPN assumes RPNs are a measure of relative risk and that below the threshold, continuous improvement is not required. It is not recommended to use a threshold with the FMEA.

USING THE FMEA WITHOUT THE RISK PRIORITY NUMBER (RPN)

Rather than focusing on the RPN, determine the severity, occurrence, and detection scores for each Item or function of the process and then proceed as follows:

- Give the severity score of an item or step the first priority. Focus your efforts on redesigning the step with the highest SEV score. (It should be noted that many believe that the only way to change a severity value is via a design change and even then, it may not absolutely affect the severity.)
- Give the occurrence score of an item or step the second priority. Focus your efforts on removing or controlling one or more of the causes through assessment. Analyze the variation in the step that can reduce the occurrence.
- Give the detection score the third priority. Focus your efforts on identifying and understanding the special causes or circumstances that can be targeted for detection and implement error-proofing.

REVIEW QUIZ

1. Which of the following statements is TRUE?
   A. Site visits are good opportunities to come up with a list of improvement ideas.
   B. Benchmark data and literature reviews cannot be used to create solutions.
   C. Positive deviants are people that tend to see problems in a positive light.
   D. Focusing on a single good idea is better than trying to generate a list of possible ideas.
   E. Team members that support the QI project are the only ones that should go on to a site visit.

2. All of the following are rules for brainstorming EXCEPT
   A. No judgment or criticism allowed.
   B. Generate the maximum number of ideas.
   C. Brainstorming can be achieved by developing or combining ideas.
   D. All ideas should be feasible at first sight.
   E. Participation from everybody is encouraged.

3. All of the following are brainstorming techniques EXCEPT
   A. free brainstorming as a group,
   B. brainstorming ideas and then emailing the ideas to the brainstorming organizer who will judge their merit,
   C. guided brainstorming where participants adopt a specific mindset for a period of time,
   D. free individual brainstorming using ideas placed onto a large idea map, or
   E. brainstorming using an "idea book".

4. All of the following statements regarding solution ideation are true EXCEPT
   A. A useful way to filter and prioritize ideas is through triage.
   B. Negative brainstorming is an idea-generating method that focuses on how not to solve a problem.
   C. Assumption busting identifies and challenges paradigms that are obstacles to new ideas.
   D. Negative brainstorming is also called the tear-down method.
   E. SCAMPER is an idea-generating method that is based on the notion that solutions can be created by teams using ideas that have been shown to be best-practice.

5. All of the following are true of the Impact/Effort matrix EXCEPT
   A. The Impact/Effort matrix provides a quick way to prioritize possible solutions according to their impact on resolving the problem and the amount of effort required.
   B. High-impact, low-effort solutions will require a complex strategy to be deployed.
   C. High-impact, high-effort solutions need an investment in time and effort by a QI team.
   D. Low-impact, low-effort solutions should be placed on the back burner.
   E. Low-impact, high-effort solutions should be avoided.

6. A Solution Desirability matrix
    A. is a team-based decision tool for evaluating various improvement proposals against weighted criteria,
    B. uses a calculation of a numerical score for each proposal based on criteria selected by the team,
    C. ensures that the solution chosen by the team provides the best chance for achieving the project's goals,
    D. uses weighted criteria that are established by either the organization or the team according to the goals of the project, or
    E. all of the above.

7. Which of the following is TRUE about the Failure Mode and Effects Analysis (FMEA)?
    A. It is a highly structured, systematic technique for failure analysis.
    B. It is used to proactively identify where and how a process might fail.
    C. FMEA is used to evaluate possible causes of failure and their relative impact.
    D. FMEA helps the team brainstorm strategies to mitigate or eliminate that risk.
    E. All of the above

8. Which of the following is NOT TRUE of the FMEA?
    A. FMEA has three elements of the failure: mode, effect and cause.
    B. FMEA has two scales: severity (SEV) and occurrence (OCC).
    C. There is one risk number: Risk Priority Number (RPN).
    D. FMEA tables include a list of recommended actions.
    E. There are usually 10 levels of severity, 10 levels of occurrence, and 10 levels of detection.

Key: 1a, 2d, 3b, 4e, 5b, 6e, 7e, 8b

REFERENCES

1. Design Council. The Double Diamond. 2004.
2. Gallupe B. Electronic Brainstorming and group size. *Academy of Management Journal*, 1992.
3. Mueller JS. The bias against creativity: Why people desire but reject creative ideas. *Psychological Science*, 2010.
4. Mumford MD. Process Analytic Models of Creative Capacities. *Creat. Res. J.* 1991. 4: 91–122.
5. Wheeler D. Problems with the Risk Priority Numbers. Avoiding more numerical jabberwocky. *Quality Digest Daily*, 2011.

CHAPTER 21

Test the Effectiveness of Your Ideas with a Pilot

THE PILOT STUDY

What Is a Pilot?

> A pilot study is a localized, small-scale, controlled trial of a possible solution conducted to test its feasibility and effectiveness, understand its limitations, and find any adverse effects before full implementation.

A pilot study allows us to

- Evaluate ideas.
- Validate and measure the effectiveness of our ideas.
- Understand potential limitations: learn what works and what doesn't before attempting full-scale implementation.
- Fine-tune ideas, allowing for adjustments on a small scale.
- Decrease disruption, time, money, and risk by making small-scale changes.
- Get buy-in: Pilot studies facilitate change management and decrease barriers to change by focusing on stakeholders who are supportive and engaged in the process improvement initiative and invested in problem solving challenges that arise during the small-scale trial.

The Quality Improvement Challenge: A Practical Guide for Physicians, First Edition.
Richard J. Banchs and Michael R. Pop.
© 2021 John Wiley & Sons Ltd. Published 2021 by John Wiley & Sons Ltd.
Companion website: www.wiley.com/go/banchs/quality

For best results with a pilot study,

- **Test on a relatively small scale.** For example, start with one patient or one clinician at one clinic. Increase the numbers as you refine the ideas.
- **Test the proposed change initially with people who believe in the improvement.** Don't try to convert people into accepting the change at this stage. Start with supporters. People who do not support the change may inadvertently or willingly sabotage the results.
- **Complete testing before the full-scale roll-out.** Only implement the idea when you're confident you have considered and tested all the possible ways of achieving the change.

Quotable quote: "Everyone gets the experience; some get the lesson." TS Eliot

How Do We Conduct a Pilot?

A pilot study must be conducted in an organized manner. Consider what to do before, during, and after the pilot.

Before the go-live date:

- **Get approval for the pilot from the Project Sponsor/s and senior leadership.** If the Primary Sponsor and leadership team have not been involved in selecting the solutions to pilot, it is critical you meet with them and present the pilot proposal for their approval. They will be instrumental in monitoring stakeholder compliance with the pilot solutions and using their influence to engage the front line in adopting the new processes. Their feedback regarding the details of the pilot plan will support its success as they will need to oversee and participate in various parts of the pilot.
- **Develop a detailed pilot plan.** The pilot plan provides the specificity needed to ensure all stakeholders understand what changes are occurring and what their roles will be during the pilot. It contains the pilot logistics of *who, what, when, where, and how.* You will need a starting date; clear scope; a defined area, patient care unit, or department in which to conduct the pilot; a mutually-agreed upon duration for the pilot – usually 2–4 weeks; and any other logistic preparation that is appropriate.
- **Prepare the data collection plan.** Be clear on what will be measured. Define the process metrics and data collection plan. You will need a plan prepared in advance of the go-live date that outlines the process objectives that will be measured during the pilot and the logistics behind the data collection, analysis, reporting, and dissemination procedures.
- **Make sure all stakeholders have been informed.** Develop a communication plan. Think of other groups you may want to involve. It is often helpful

to pull in additional supportive stakeholders, or champions, to assist with the pilot education, data collection, and monitoring.

- **Educating all frontline stakeholders on the standard work involved in the processes that will be piloted.** Depending on the extent of the changes, one to two weeks will be needed to train the stakeholders on the pilot processes using the standard work that was developed. During the education sessions, the project team and champions solicit the feedback of the front line and address their concerns in order to decrease their resistance to the changes. The education can be presented in a 1:1 session, during staff meetings, and at morning huddles and should have a sign-off to ensure that all stakeholders have been trained prior to the pilot go-live. Hand-out materials and email notification can reinforce the information provided during the education.
- **Set a go-live date.**

During the pilot,

- **Ensure "all hands-on deck" for the pilot go-live with frequent leadership rounding.** Remember a pilot is a change. The presence of the leadership team on the pilot go-live date and with follow-up rounding during the course of the pilot demonstrates their commitment to the successful implementation of the solutions. It also provides an opportunity for the front line to share their input on the changes, which facilitates buy-in and real-time problem-solving. Frequent feedback from the frontline professionals may help modify the piloted solution if unforeseen issues arise.
- **Communicate ongoing results.** Instituting frequent data collection and reporting of process metrics to the stakeholders is key during the pilot. Frequent data collection and reporting provides valuable information on the effectiveness of the piloted solutions and encouragement to the front lines. It will also give you the ability to correct any problems as soon as possible. When the resistance to the new processes is significant, it is optimal to provide the data on a daily basis initially with follow-up action plans as needed. This can be accomplished by convening daily debriefings that last less than 10 minutes and implementing structured leadership rounding with checklists. The frontline professionals will become aware that their behaviors are being recorded and usually conform to the expectations. It also provides a venue for addressing and resolving any issues as soon as possible.

At the conclusion of the pilot,

- **Meet with the Primary Sponsor.** The meeting serves to objectively determine whether the piloted solutions are effective in improving the outcome metrics as well as whether the stakeholders have been compliant in performing the processes according to the agreed upon best practice. If the sponsor and leadership team support the ongoing implementation of the new processes, a sustainability plan is developed.

- **Meet with the key frontline stakeholders.** Pilot studies can foster stakeholders' acceptance of new processes when they have input into evaluating the effectiveness of the changes. Often, the pilot showcases the improvements in the stakeholders' workflow, which encourages stakeholders to adopt the new processes.

THE BEST-KNOWN PILOT IS THE PDSA CYCLE

What Is a PDSA Cycle?

The PDSA cycle is one of the best-known approaches to conducting pilot studies. PDSA is an acronym for Plan-Do-Study-Act (see Figure 21-1). The PDSA cycle is used to test an idea by temporarily trialing a change on a small scale to assess its impact.

> **A PDSA is an iterative four-step problem-solving model used for improving a process or carrying out change.**

The PDCA (Plan-Do-Check-Act) cycle was first made popular by **Walter Shewhart** in 1939 based on the scientific method developed by Francis Bacon. The scientific method states that all advances are based on a cycle of "hypothesis-

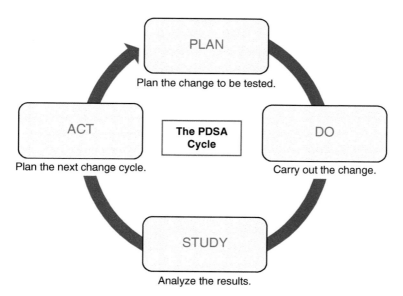

FIGURE 21-1   The PDSA is an acronym for Plan-Do-Study-Act.

experiment-evaluation." In 1951, W. **Edwards Deming** modified the original PDCA cycle (Plan-Do-Check-Act) from Walter Shewhart calling it the Shewhart Cycle for learning and improvement or the PDSA (Plan-Do-Study-Act) cycle. He modified again in 1986 and 1993 describing it as a flow diagram for learning and improvement of a process through small tests of change. In 1991, **Moen, Nolan and Provost** in 1991 added a required prediction and associated theory to the planning step of the improvement cycle. The process of comparing the observed results to the prediction is the basis for learning (Moen 1991). In 1994, **Langley, Nolan, and Nolan** added three basic questions to supplement the PDSA cycle: "What are we trying to accomplish?", "How will we know that a change is an improvement?", and "What changes can we make that will result in an improvement?" (Langley 1994). These became the basis for the **Model for Improvement** (Langley 1996).

Each step of the PDSA cycle requires specific actions to allow the transition from idea to full implementation (see Figure 21-2). When using the PDSA cycle, it's important to include the customer and the frontline stakeholders because they can provide feedback about what works and what doesn't. Involving them in the process will increase acceptance of the end result.

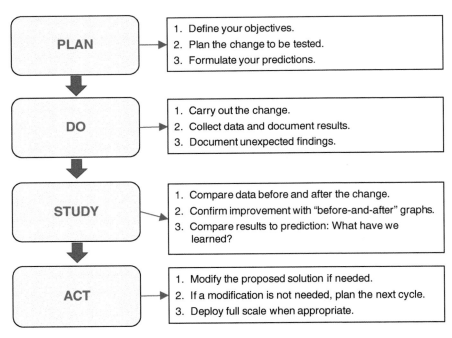

FIGURE 21-2   The PDSA cycle steps and actions.

ADVANTAGES OF THE PDSA CYCLE

Similarly to what was said for the pilot study, the PDSA cycle

- **Decreases disruption** by testing ideas on a small scale before wholescale implementation; it involves less time, money and risk.
- **Allows us to gain knowledge** about the proposed changes from the structured test cycles that support the implementation of new ideas and processes with greater success; the PDSA cycle is a powerful tool for learning from both ideas that work and those that don't work (sometimes learning what does not work is most important).
- **Facilitates change management** by giving stakeholders the opportunity to see if the proposed change will work. As with any change, ownership is key to implementing the improvement successfully. If you involve a range of colleagues in trying something out on a small scale before it is fully operational, you will reduce the barriers to the change when it is rolled out on a larger scale.

Quotable quote: "Failure is only the opportunity to begin again more intelligently." Henry Ford

THE PDSA CYCLE IS A "LEARNING RAMP"

The PDSA cycle is a systematic series of steps to gain valuable learning and knowledge for the continual improvement of healthcare services and clinical care. It's like a **learning ramp** (Langley 2009). To gain process knowledge and encourage buy-in, we

- Perform small scale tests with small groups of patients (or frontline stakeholders).
- Repeat testing with the required modifications to the original proposed changes.
- Increase the scale and scope of the PDSAs and perform additional **tests,** changing the conditions to gain any additional process knowledge.
- Modify the proposed solution according to the results of each pilot. With each cycle, we are going to increase our knowledge and buy-in from the professionals involved in piloting the solutions.
- When ready, deploy the full-scale change that will result in an improvement of the service or care you want to provide (see Figure 21-3).

Conducting a PDSA cycle can be made easier using a PDSA template (see Table 21-1).

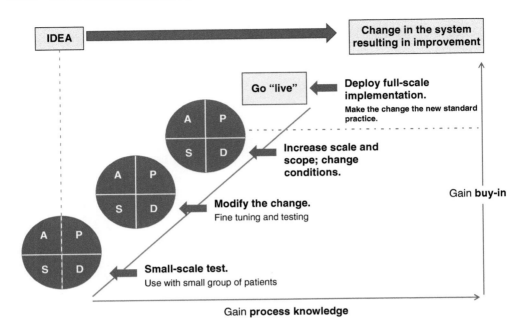

FIGURE 21-3   The PDSA cycle is a systematic series of steps to gain valuable knowledge and buy-in.

TABLE 21-1   The PDSA Cycle Template

The PDSA Cycle Template	
Plan	What change are we testing?
	Where are we testing it?
	What question(s) do we want to answer?
	How are we going to collect data?
	What is our prediction?
Do	What did we observe?
	Were there any unexpected findings?
	Did anything go wrong?
Study	What did "before-and-after" data show?
	Was there an improvement?
	Do results agree with the prediction?
	How are we going to address the problems and unexpected findings?
Act	Based on the results: • A number of modifications need to be made before proceeding to next phase. • The change resulted in an improvement, and we can move to next phase. • The change resulted in an improvement and can be implemented to all shifts, all conditions.

REVIEW QUIZ

1. Regarding pilots, which of the following is NOT TRUE?
   A. Pilots are full-scale deployments of new solutions.
   B. Require less time and resources than a full deployment of a solution.
   C. Are localized controlled trials of a possible solution in order to test its effectiveness and understand its limitations before implementation.
   D. Produce less significant disruption for the front lines.
   E. Are tools for testing solutions and learning.

2. All of the following are best practice for a pilot EXCEPT
   A. Communicate with the front lines about the nature and expected results of the pilot.
   B. Test the proposed changes initially with people that believe in the improvement.
   C. Complete the testing before the full-scale change.
   D. Test on a relatively small scale.
   E. During a pilot, leadership support is not required because a pilot is a small test of change.

3. Regarding a PDSA,
   A. PDSA requires an initial prediction of the expected results.
   B. PDSA stands for Plan-Do-Study-Act.
   C. It was originally described by Walter Shewhart.
   D. It is a cycle for learning and improvement.
   E. All of the above.

   Key: 1a, 2e, 3e

REFERENCES

1. Langley GL. The foundation of improvement. *Quality Progress*, 1994; 81.
2. Langley GL. *The improvement guide: A practical approach to enhancing organizational performance.* Jossey Bass Publisher, 2009.
3. Moen R. *Improving quality through planned experimentation.* McGraw-Hill, 1991.

CHAPTER 22

Improve "Flow" and Work Conditions

PROCESS FLOW

What Is "Flow"?

Along every care pathway, there are many moving parts that need to be coordinated to provide quality care and enhance the patient's experience. For example, a patient visit requires a number of steps: efficient scheduling, verifying insurance, providing patient instructions, checking and obtaining necessary equipment and supplies for care, checking provider availability, and ensuring the patient's comfort, privacy, and understanding of the process. When one of these steps is performed inefficiently or incorrectly or a long time elapses in between steps, patient care may be impacted, experience negatively affected, and the staff and providers may have to work harder to correct the situation. Faster is usually better!

> **Flow is how work progresses through a process. When a process is working well, steps and actions are executed in synchrony and the people, information, services, equipment, supplies, and patients in that process move through it steadily and predictably.**

The Quality Improvement Challenge: A Practical Guide for Physicians, First Edition.
Richard J. Banchs and Michael R. Pop.
© 2021 John Wiley & Sons Ltd. Published 2021 by John Wiley & Sons Ltd.
Companion website: www.wiley.com/go/banchs/quality

Why Is Flow Important?

Think of flow as all the starts and stops of our work. Patients will want steady flow, not having to constantly wait in between work activities. Flow creates speed; speed creates efficiency; efficiency creates quality for patients, staff, and providers. A well-designed process is a process that has optimal flow through the care value stream within an optimized work environment.

> **For patients, optimal flow means the right care (effective), at the right time, in the right place, on the first attempt, and in the right manner. For staff and providers, optimal flow means that they get what they need, when they need it, in the right quantity, on time every time.**

A well-designed process benefits the frontline stakeholders who perform the work, the local sponsors who oversee the work, the leaders who monitor the results of the work, and most importantly in healthcare organizations, the patient who receives the care from the professionals that do the work. Failing to achieve optimal flow puts patients at risk for suboptimal care and increases the burden and frustration of staff and providers that must deal with a poorly designed process and suboptimal work environment and conditions. It is generally accepted that healthcare has seven flows:

1. patients,
2. families,
3. staff and providers,
4. medications,
5. supplies,
6. equipment, and
7. information.

Remember in Chapter 10 we learned the Value Steam Map considers three flows: the flows of information, work, and time.

STRATEGY FOR CREATING PROCESS FLOW

A process is defined as the collection of related steps, actions, decisions, and handoffs that are used to transform inputs into outputs. From the perspective of the customer (the patient, staff, or provider) steps can be divided in three types (see Figure 22-1):

- **Non-value-added steps** (NVA): These steps do not add value from the customer's perspective; they do not transform or change a product, service, or

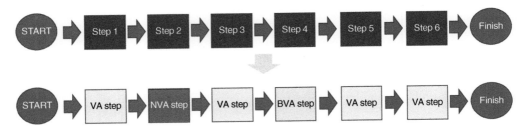

FIGURE 22-1   The three types of process steps.

the course of the disease; they are not welcomed and contribute to waste and delays.

- **Business value-added steps** (BVA): These steps do not specifically add value to the customer but must be done to fulfill the requirements of the "business of medicine" or to comply with regulatory agency mandates.

- **Value-added steps** (VA): From the perspective of the customer, these steps are essential in producing the service the patient or customer desires or needs. These steps change information, provide a service, modify the course of the disease toward health, or provide an outcome the end-user is willing to pay for (see chapter 11). These steps must be done right the first time.

Flow creates speed between value-added (VA) steps; speed creates efficiency; efficiency creates quality for patients, staff and providers. There is a clear relationship between the elapsed time between value-added activities and flow.

> **The goal of creating flow is to move patients from one value-added activity to the next with minimum delay while maintaining the highest quality of care.**

The goal of creating flow is also to move items, supplies, equipment, and information to a value-added activity with the minimum delay. A time delay between successive value-added activities or steps occurs because of these three possibilities (see Figure 22-2):

- **Non-value-added steps (NVA).** Staff and providers spend time doing something that does not add value; they spend time "doing something that shouldn't be done"; examples of NVA steps are: transporting patients to distant locations, moving excess inventory, making more items than what is needed to create value, looking for supplies, etc. Remember the seven wastes (TIM WOOD) we saw in Chapter 11: Transport, Inventory, Motion, Waiting, Overproduction, Overprocessing, and Defects.

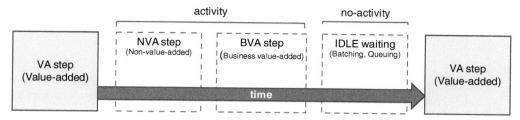

FIGURE 22-2 Causes of time delay between value-added (VA) steps.

- **Business value-added steps (BVA).** Staff and providers spend time doing something that does not specifically add value to the customer but must be done to fulfill the requirements of the "business of medicine" or to comply with regulatory agency mandates; a typical example is getting patients' insurance information so the hospital can bill the insurance company; a hospital must bill patients and their insurance companies or it will go out of business. However, many times because there is a fear of not meeting a requirement or mandate, multiple checks and double checks/approvals are added that can hinder flow significantly. While we may not be able to remove these steps, many times they may be minimized.
- **Idle waiting.** The patient (customer) is just waiting for a service or the staff and providers are not performing any activity; Idle waiting occurs for a number of reasons. The three most common reasons for idle waiting are (Crane 2011)
  - Lack of a visual management system such as a signal indicating the next activity can proceed; for example, we delay discharging a patient because we are waiting for a consult without realizing the consult is already in the chart; there was no way for us to know the consult had already been done unless we periodically check in the EMR.
  - Batching; we wait to provide a service, perform a task, or process an item for a number of requests to accumulate before we process them. A typical example is the lab not processing a sample, waiting for more samples to arrive, and then processing them at the same time.
  - Queuing is the most common cause for idle waiting for patients (customers). This is when we are busy providing a service or performing a task for an earlier request, and an arriving request for a service or task must wait until we can address it.

STEPS AND SEQUENCE TO CREATE FLOW

The strategy to create flow and move patients from one value-added activity to the next with minimum delay involves removing non-value-added (NVA) steps, minimizing the time spent doing Business value-added (BVA) steps, and eliminating idle waiting time (see Figure 22-3). Following the steps in order creates a pathway or **sequence to flow** (see Figure 22-4):

- **Map the process.** Functions performed as part of our professional duties are processes. All processes can be broken down into a series of steps and actions. These steps and actions are used to transform inputs into outputs and can be graphically depicted with a map.
- **Critically evaluate the process steps**. Identify the process steps:
  a. Non-value-added steps (NVA): These steps do not add value.
  b. Business value-added steps (BVA): These steps must be done to fulfill requirements.
  c. Value-added steps (VA): These steps are essential in producing the service the patient or customer desires.
- **Remove NVA steps.** A well-designed process creates flow, adds value, and has minimum waste. Waste is a step that does not create value for the customer (patient, staff, or provider) and should be removed. A NVA step is a step that "spends time doing something that shouldn't be done," or using anything other than the minimum amount of equipment, material, technology, space, staff, and time that are essential to add value. Waste results in increased time needed for performing key activities as well as the increased staff frustration.
- **Minimize the time spent doing BVA steps**. Whenever possible, eliminate or minimize the Business value-added steps;
- **Eliminate idle waiting time.** Idle waiting time can be eliminated by: improving signaling with a robust visual management system; eliminating batching; improving the performance of a queue; reducing the number of queues (Crane 2011).
- **Optimize value-added (VA) steps by creating Standard Work**. Optimize the timing and decrease the variability in the performance of the value-added (VA) steps by consistently performing VA steps in a predetermined sequence according to best practice and a specific time frame as determined by patients

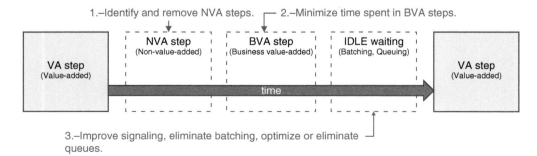

FIGURE 22-3   Strategy to create and improve process flow.

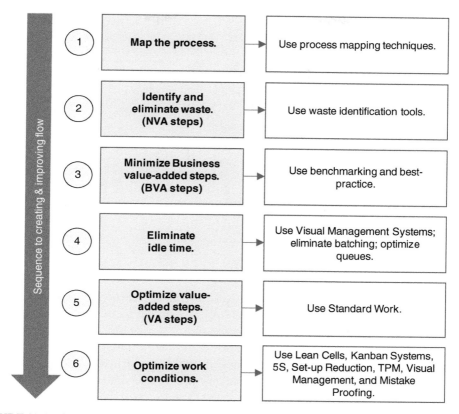

FIGURE 22-4   Sequence to creating and improving flow.

demands or **takt time**. Takt time is the rate at which you need to complete a product or service in order to meet customer demand.

- **Optimize work conditions.** Once the VA steps are standardized, NVA steps removed, BVA steps simplified, and idle time eliminated or minimized, focus on optimizing work conditions. A well-designed process cannot perform optimally (optimal flow) if we cannot provide what is needed, when it is needed, where it is needed, in the quantity needed, on time, every time (Zidel 2006). Delays and variability in the performance of the value-added activities (Standard Work) are often caused by poor layouts, lack of supplies, and faulty or unreliable equipment.

A queue can be improved (decrease or eliminate queuing time) by reducing the demand for service or care (not always possible), increasing the capacity and rate of service (increasing the number of people performing the service or decreasing the time it takes to provide the service), reducing the variation in the rate of demand (better predicted), or reducing the variation in the service (see Figure 22-5).

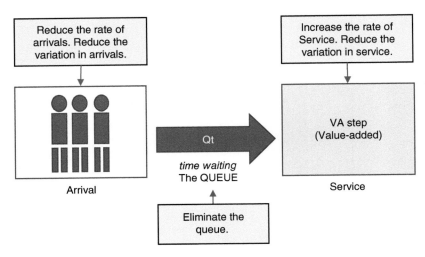

FIGURE 22-5   Approach to improving a queue.

The process for creating flow follows the principles of **Lean improvement methodology**. Lean aims to eliminate non-value-added steps (NVA), minimize the number and time spent on Business value-added steps (BVA) and standardize the value-added steps (VA). High quality work is delivered when it is needed, without error, efficiently, and safely. While the traditional improvement strategy focuses on increasing flow by working harder, *Lean improvement strategy focuses on improving flow by eliminating NVA activities first in order to work smarter.*

WHAT IS STANDARD WORK?

A standard is a description of how a work process should be done:

- Standards allow for a comparison between what is actually happening and what we want to happen.
- Standards allow us to create work outputs that are effective, repeatable, efficient, and reproducible.
- Standards allow us to create high quality outputs on a reliable and consistent basis.
- Key elements of a process are performed with the best method, in the same way every time no matter who, when, or where the work process is performed.

Without a standard, people do whatever they think is best, often whatever is easiest, leading to an enormous variation and therefore delays in the completion of the value-added steps.

The standard must be understood and practiced by all who do the work. *The standard is our best collective knowledge.*

Standardization is the practice of defining and communicating a standard.

> **Standard Work is an agreed-upon set of work practices that establishes the best and most reliable method and sequence of tasks for each clinician and support staff member to follow.**

Standard Work is a Lean tool for maintaining high levels of safety, quality, and productivity. It allows for a consistent service that meets patients' expectations regardless of who the provider is. Standard Work reduces process steps to a series of individual tasks, executed in a specific predetermined sequence and devoid of NVA activity. Standard Work is practiced in the same way every time no matter who, when, or where the service or care is delivered. Once Standard Work is set, performance can be measured and constant improvement can be initiated on the basis of the standard. In other words, without a standard there can be no real improvement.

Standard Work

- maximizes performance while minimizing waste in each person's operation and workload,
- serves as the basis for retaining and sharing knowledge,
- provides a map or compass for tracing problems (difficult if everybody does things differently),
- serves as the basis for initiating process improvement,
- serves as a basis for providing training to new professionals, and
- can be revised as best-practice recommendations for clinical care change.

Optimizing value-added steps with Standard Work allows for the creation of flow (of people, information, material, patients) through the value stream. The patient can move from one value-added activity to the next with minimum delay; flow creates efficiency; efficiency results in increased quality of the care we provide to the patients. With Standard Work completed, it will be necessary to ensure all staff and providers are familiar and have been properly trained in the new work process. Training should be evaluated to ensure customer requirements and standards are being consistently met.

Many times, processes are performed in certain ways because healthcare professionals have always done them that way. Habits become ingrained in the fabric of the workflow and provide a sense of stability and competence. As a result, staff and providers often perceive the current processes to be very reliable and often cannot understand why they would ever change it, even when the evidence shows the process to be clearly outdated or plagued with dysfunctional work-arounds. Change is often dismissed and seen as contrary to the individualization of patient care. This highlights the importance of acknowledging the change dynamics involved in implementing new processes and the necessity of including the frontline stakeholders from the beginning of the QI project. When the frontline stakeholders participate in the transformation of a process and creation of Standard Work, they are able to identify the areas of opportunity that exist in their current workflow and become engaged in developing future-state processes that are more effective and more efficient that the current processes. *Standard Work takes best-practice born out of our collective knowledge and creates a well-defined process embedding it within the unit's workflow, ensuring its consistently performed by all healthcare professionals.*

THE CRITICAL ROLE OF WORK CONDITIONS

Standard Work, or the agreed-upon set of work practices that establishes the best and most reliable method and sequence of tasks for each clinician, cannot be carried out if the environment does not support it. How can we work safely, effectively, and efficiently if we do not have what we need?

> **Optimal work conditions provide what is needed, when it is needed, in the quantity needed, on time, every time, so that the agreed-upon set of work practices that establish the best and most reliable methods and sequences of work can be carried out.**

In order for a process to function as intended and achieve the expected results, the environment in which the work is done must also be optimized. Standard work and unobstructed throughput are the hallmarks of a process that is effective, repeatable, efficient and reproducible. Quality care can only be delivered when

- The patient is available and ready.
- The process is clearly defined and standardized.
- Work is done in the right location with the right infrastructure and optimal layout.
- There is adequate staffing.
- Equipment is available, capable, and in good working condition.
- Supplies are readily available.
- Medications are at our reach, clearly identified, in the right dosages, and in the right quantities.

With the proper work conditions, we can perform our clinical duties effectively; provide a safe environment for our patients; support standard work and unobstructed throughput; and create efficiency and increased quality. An optimal work environment

- Has optimal workflow. This may be achieved using a **Lean cell,** as applicable.
- Has the right supplies. It is easy to find what we need in the quantities needed, on time, every time. This can be achieved using a **Kanban System** and **5S.**
- What is needed is ready to go. Supplies are organized and ready to be used. This can be achieved using **Set-up reduction/make ready.**
- Has the right equipment. Equipment is located in the right place, is reliable, and is always in good working condition. This can be achieved with **Total Productive Maintenance.**
- It is easy to understand how to do the right thing. Achieved with a **Visual Management System.**
- It is hard to do the wrong thing. Achieved with a **Mistake-Proofing System.**

Lean Cells, Kanban Systems, Set-up Reduction, and Total Productive Maintenance are tools from the Lean methodology toolbox. We will discuss 5S, Visual Management, and Mistake Proofing.

5S TO OPTIMIZE YOUR WORKSPACE

What Is 5S?

5S stands for Sort, Set in Order, Shine, Standardize, and Sustain.

> **5S is a systematic way to organize a workspace that allows work to flow in a safe, efficient, intuitive, and sustainable manner.**

5S is integral to improvement efforts; by using 5S in our work areas, staff and physicians find what they need, when they need it, in the quantities needed, on time, every time. The **5S** approach empowers professionals to work efficiently, improve their work space, and remove the frustration that comes with wasting time looking for the items we need to deliver care. **5S** should be standard in our healthcare environment. Instead of **5S**, healthcare professionals often have to

- search for what they need,
- scramble to find needed items,
- swear that somebody must have taken the needed items,
- steal to get what they need from other areas, and
- stash what they could find so they can have it next time they need it.

The Significance of **5S**

- **5S is reliability.** Because every item is in a specific, well-labeled location, **5S** allows the frontline professionals to quickly confirm the availability of the needed equipment and supplies, which saves time and improves the reliability of the process.
- **5S is safety. 5S** establishes a standard and sustained way to clean and organize our environment that facilitates the inspection and rapid detection of missing or damaged items. This prevents errors, making **5S** an effective safety tool.
- **5S is communication. 5S** is frequently viewed as an element of a broader construct known as Visual Control. The **5S** approach allows the environment to "communicate" with professionals, allowing them to see and find what they need when they need it.
- **5S is a cost-reduction strategy. 5S** increases space efficiency by reducing clutter and decreases costs associated with overstock and expired inventory.

The First Pillar of 5S: Sort or S1

The problem. Every working environment accumulates items that are not needed. The workspace is cluttered and forces us to constantly search for items that we need.

The solution. The "Sort" pillar of a **5S**. Follow the sort process to take charge of the work environment. We should be left with only the essentials to complete our work. To do that, we can use the **Red tag** technique, which is a basic method that allows us to identify the unneeded material, supplies, and equipment in the work area, evaluate their usefulness, and deal with them appropriately. First, identify the items that are not needed. Then place red tags on the unneeded supplies and equipment and move them to an area outside of the storage. Send out a notice to the department for feedback. Unless you receive a legitimate rationale for reinstating the removed equipment or supplies, decide for the relocation or disposal of the items (see Figure 22-6). The simple act of identifying and removing unneeded items is the

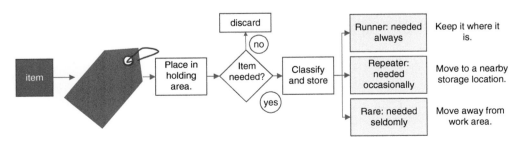

FIGURE 22-6   The red tag technique used for Sort in 5S.

first acknowledgment of our commitment to the safety of our patients. 5S requires dialogue and collaborative decision-making about the workflow, location of items, and priorities. This dialogue about how to best achieve success is a valuable tool that builds understanding among the healthcare professionals. **5S** clearly communicates that the frontline healthcare provider and supporting staff have the ownership of their environment and they are driving the change!

The Second Pillar of 5S: Set in Order or S2

The problem. Items are placed in locations that make it difficult to find them, hidden among the clutter or on shelves away from our workflow. We scramble to find them and when we do, we scrounge and stash them to make sure we will have them when needed.

The solution. The "Set in order" pillar of a **5S**. With set in order, every item has a place and every place can be clearly identified. Set in order is a systematic planning technique for the placement of all equipment, items, and medications. Items are organized so that they are easy for anyone to find and use. This pillar helps eliminate or reduce various kinds of waste such as wasted motion and excess inventory. All locations and storage areas are easy to find, clearly marked, color coded, and arranged according to workflow. Locate items according to the frequency of use and store items together if they are to be used together. This step requires open discussion among the frontline stakeholders to ensure the equipment and supplies are placed in the optimal location and following workflow. Once this decision is made, diagrams may be posted and distributed to all the frontline stakeholders to communicate the changes. Use location indicators, item indicators, and amount indicators to standardize the new order.

The Third Pillar of 5S: Shine or S3

The problem. Overstocking and clutter causes us to overlook broken items and malfunctioning equipment, making them unavailable for use when we need them most.

The solution. The "Shine" pillar of a **5S**. Shine is not only about having a clean work area, but also about having a work area that allows us to inspect, detect, and prevent mishaps. An uncluttered, clean space allows us to see cracks and leaks, detect missing items, and anticipate future equipment failures. When broken items and malfunctioning equipment are uncovered, the front line follows the established protocols to fix or replace them so they are available when needed. Shine applies to our space, medications, monitors, video equipment, etc. "Sorting," "setting," and "cleaning" entail checking, which is the first step in preventive maintenance for safety. Workspace cleanliness is the responsibility of everyone who works in the area. To implement Shine, we can create assignment maps that show the area to be cleaned, who is responsible for them, and the schedule of activities.

The Fourth Pillar of 5S: Standardize or S4

The problem. We often organize our workspaces according to our own preferences and methods. Others might not understand our system of organization and find the work environment incompatible with their own workflow. The work environment soon reverts to the old ways, piles of unneeded items are left everywhere, material storage becomes disorganized and excess supplies take up space and money.

The solution. The "Standardize" pillar of a **5S**. Standardization assures that our new workspace arrangement can be reproduced and communicated visually to all frontline professionals. By standardizing, we reduce variation, identify the roles for maintaining the area as we have designed, and assure that visual management signs and cues will be in place to help us achieve our goal. Standardize is implemented by deciding who is responsible for which activity regarding sorting, straightening, and sustaining. Everyone must know exactly what they are responsible for doing and exactly when, where, and how to do it.

The Fifth Pillar of 5S: Sustain or S5

The problem. We do the best to clean and organize our workspace, but it becomes disorganized again within a short period of time.

The solution. The "Sustain" pillar of a **5S**. Sustain helps us set up routines and schedules for cleaning and maintenance. We commit to a course of action because the rewards for keeping the course of action are greater than the rewards for departing from it. With sustain, we make sure that everyone keeps up the daily 5S in the same sequence and that the 5S becomes an intricate part of our daily work. This is often accomplished with the use of checklists, photos, storyboards, maps, or pocket manuals.

5S has five steps; each step has specific actions that are carried out to fulfill a specific aim (see Table 22-1).

A 5S Audit Checklist

A **5S** checklist is a tool to evaluate work conditions relative to 5S best-practices. It can and should be used regularly to make sure 5S is fully implemented and has been integrated into the workflow and culture of the organization (See Table 22-2).

VISUAL MANAGEMENT

What Is Visual Management?

Visual Management is the ability to quickly convey the current status or needed and important information to anyone that stands and observes within seconds. Visual

TABLE 22-1 The Aim of the 5S Steps

5S to Improve Work Conditions	
Step	Aim
Sort	Aim: Make a decision. When in doubt, move it out using the Red Tag technique.
Set in Order	Aim: Label and locate. A place for everything and everything in its place.
Shine and Inspect	Aim: Prevent. Clean so we can diagnose; diagnose so we can prevent. Inspect through cleaning.
Standardize	Aim: Reduce variation. Make rules, follow and enforce them to make sure the best way to organize the work environment is kept.
Sustain	Aim: Make it "stick." Make the process repeatable and reproducible, a part of our daily work that has become a habit.

TABLE 22-2 5S Audit Checklist

The 5S Audit Checklist			
SORT Remove all items from the workplace that are not needed to eliminate waste.	Poor = 1 Not followed	Good = 3 Applied in most cases	Excellent = 5 Applied in all cases
All items on surfaces have been sorted, are necessary, and there are no unneeded items.			
All items on shelves have been sorted, are necessary, and there are no unneeded items.			
All items in drawers have been sorted, are necessary, and there are no unneeded items.			
All items on floors have been sorted, are necessary, and there are no unneeded items.			
Needed items have been placed in the nearest location according to workflow.			

(Continued)

TABLE 22-2   (Continued)

SET IN ORDER Organize the needed items so that they are easy for anyone to find and use.	Poor = 1 Not followed	Good = 3 Applied in most cases	Excellent = 5 Applied in all cases

Locations of needed items are clearly marked and allow for easy identification of all contents.

All items have been stored in their correct locations.

All drawers and cupboards have a labeling system to indicate their contents.

Minimum and maximum pars are clearly indicated where appropriate.

Locations for equipment and movable items is clearly indicated.

All equipment and movable items has been stored in the correct locations.

SHINE Ensure the work area is maintained in a state of cleanliness to allow for inspection and prevention.	Poor = 1 Not followed	Good = 3 Applied in most cases	Excellent = 5 Applied in all cases

Floors and walls are clean and shiny; surfaces are clean and have been cleared of all dust or debris.

Equipment has been wiped clean; surfaces have been disinfected where appropriate.

All equipment has been inspected and properly maintained; maintenance records are up to date.

There is a checklist to identify ongoing Shine duties and the status of the list has been updated.

STANDARDIZE Assure that our new workspace can be reproduced and communicated visually to all.	Poor = 1 Not followed	Good = 3 Applied in most cases	Excellent = 5 Applied in all cases

Documents are available to review approved location for each item.

Graphic documentation is available for each storage location.

(Continued)

TABLE 22-2   (Continued)

STANDARDIZE Assure that our new workspace can be reproduced and communicated visually to all.	Poor = 1 Not followed	Good = 3 Applied in most cases	Excellent = 5 Applied in all cases
Information displays, signs, color coding, and other markings are clearly displayed and in good condition.			
Standard operating procedures (SOP) are available and are up to date.			

SUSTAIN Assure 5S becomes an intricate part of our daily work.	Poor = 1 Not followed	Good = 3 Applied in most cases	Excellent = 5 Applied in all cases
There is a supervisor responsible to maintain 5S; the supervisor's signature is up to date.			
Results of the previous 5S Audit have been posted and are clearly visible.			
5S is routinely reviewed for best practice and was updated less than 6 months ago.			

Management system is a system of tools used to share work standards, information, and highlight problems so that they can be either stopped or prevented.

> **Visual Management is a system of visual cues that provides information so that instructions, workflow, steps, limits, and performance metrics are easily understood and the correct work is performed.**

Visual Management creates a visual workplace that makes it easier to "do the right thing." Visual Management centralizes the available information and can cut down the time it takes to understand and process the information. Visual Management allows teams to

- Share information and standards about how work should be completed; this decreases variability, eliminates waste, and allows processes to be effective, repeatable, efficient, and reproducible.
- Share information about the day to day operations, flow of work, and metrics. It is able to convey the information quickly so that everybody can get on the same page.

- Make the right decisions on how to proceed with just one glance.
- Reduce opportunities for errors and variation in the process.
- Avoid problems as unusual circumstances occur and deviations from the standards are noticed; where the outliers are immediately obvious, health professionals can easily correct them to make care safer and/or to keep the process flowing.
- Resolve problems as they arise; visual management provides the necessary time-ordered data for analytical and creative thinking.
- Improve both individual accountability and team performance.

With Visual Management, anyone that enters the area within a few seconds can determine what is the status of the work, if there are abnormal conditions that require action, and what the performance of the area is.

Visual Management helps with two types of communication:

- **Vertical.** This is the top-down communication within the organization between management and frontline professionals. A Visual Management System helps people because they can figure out what to do without asking management; it gives them a sense of independence.
- **Horizontal.** This is communication between professionals in the front line along the process flow. Visual Management Systems allow communication between steps and at hand-off points helping with safety, effectiveness and efficiency.

Types of Visual Management Systems

Based on the information they provide, Visual Management Systems can be classified into two different groups:

1. **Visual measurements.** Display data to tell us how each area is performing and the current performance of a process against the expected performance standard or goal. An important point is that Visual Measurements must drive action. For action to be possible, Visual Measurements need to be displayed in a timely fashion and clearly so that everyone in the area understand the current status.

2. **Visual controls.** They cover more broadly how work is done. Visual Controls increase the chance of "doing the right thing" and decrease the chance of "doing the wrong thing." They must be unambiguous, quick to register in the mind, and created in such a way that they transcend languages. There are different types of Visual Controls (Abad 2020):

    a. **Visual signals**, used to give information about the process, the area, the equipment, and safety-related signs. Common visual signals include the marks on the floor used to define certain spaces, color-coded lines on the floor helping us to identify different areas, markings on equipment defining the status of machines (on-off), or signs indicating the location of fire extinguishers and emergency exits.

b. **Visual instructions**, which aim to easily show us what to do. This ranges from job instructions, Standard Work instructions, or traffic light systems telling us what to do based on the light color. A Kanban signal is used as a visual cue to manage inventory levels and tells us it is time to reorder.

c. **Visual representations**, which convey information about processes or concrete activities, including process maps, Gantt charts for project timelines, project status boards, to preventive maintenance boards for a cell.

To create a Visual Management System, the first step is to define the standard. Once the standard has been agreed upon, make the standard visual, incorporate it into the workplace, communicate to all, and implement Mistake Proofing to prevent doing the wrong thing (see next), and constantly improve it.

MISTAKE-PROOFING SYSTEMS

What Is It?

To "err is human." Healthcare organizations are high-stress, high-stakes environments. When errors occur, they can have devastating, if not fatal, consequences for patients and life-changing corollaries for the staff and providers involved in the events. Multiple competing priorities are commonplace for healthcare providers which result in significant stress and overload. These conditions must be mitigated whenever possible to protect patients' safety and provide a supportive environment in which providers can practice.

There are two ways to avoid mistakes:

- **Demand that people be extra vigilant.** This is the traditional approach. Exhorting staff and providers to be more careful does not usually work. We are all plagued by the "human condition."
- **Error-proofing the system.** Instead of depending on people's performance, eliminate the chance of making mistakes. This is a better way where a system generates a signal and people can take action to avoid the mistake.

> **Mistake-Proofing is a Visual Management System that uses any device or method that either makes it impossible for an error to occur or makes the error immediately obvious once it has occurred.**

Mistake-Proofing Systems make it difficult to **do the wrong thing.** Mistake-Proofing prevents or detects mistakes before they occur and is a great way of assuring ownership of an improved process when designed with the input of the front line Defects are caused by individual cultural factors, variability, complexity of the tasks, or mistakes. Minimizing or eliminating mistakes is one of the ways to achieve zero defects.

The Mistake-Proofing Strategy

When designing a Mistake-Proofing System, there are two strategies:

1. **Prevention.** Design a system that eliminates the **mistake**, targeting the cause of error at the source; it eliminates the possibility of a mistake.
2. **Detection.** A system that signals when the mistake has been made.
   a.   The system detects the **mistake** as it is being made and allows the healthcare professional to take action.
   b.   The system detects the defect soon after it has been made but before it reaches the next step in the process.

Where Can We Use the Mistake-Proofing System?

A Mistake-Proofing System should be used

- when a process step has been identified in which human error can cause mistakes or defects to occur, especially in processes that rely on the frontline professional's attention, skill, or experience;
- in a process where the customer can make an error that affects the output;
- at a hand-off step in a process when there is a transfer of service or care of the patient to another staff member or healthcare professional;
- when the occurrence of a minor error early in the process causes major problems later in the process; and
- when the consequences of an error are expensive or dangerous for the patient or end-user.

Characteristics of a Good Mistake-Proofing System

A well designed Mistake-Proofing System should be simple, part of the process, placed close to where the error can occur, give immediate feedback and utilize prevention rather than detection. The optimal design is one that eliminates the mistake and the cause of the defect. There are three types of Mistake-Proofing Techniques: Warning, Shutdown, and Control (see Table 22-3). A garage door not closing when an object

TABLE 22-3   Mistake-Proofing Techniques

Mistake-Proofing System (MPS) Techniques		
Technique	Prediction strategy	Detection strategy
Warning	The MPS signals that something is about to go wrong.	The MPS signals immediately when something does go wrong.
Control	The MPS makes errors impossible.	The MPS prevents defective items from moving to the next step.
Shutdown	The MPS shuts down the process or equipment when a mistake is about to be made.	The MPS shuts down the process or equipment when a mistake has been made.

or being is detected is an example of a Shutdown technique; a saw stopping when it detects human flesh is an example of a Control technique; the sound made by a car when keys are left in the ignition and the driver's door is opened is an example of a Warning technique.

Approach to Mistake Proofing

To create a Mistake-Proofing System

- Obtain or create a flowchart of the process.
- Review each step, thinking about where and when human errors are likely to occur.
- For each potential error, work back through the process to find its source.
- For each error, think of potential ways to make it impossible for the error to occur.
- Consider ERF – Elimination, Replacement, and Facilitation – for each step that contributes to a potential error.
  - **Elimination.** Eliminate the step that causes the error.
  - **Replacement.** Replace the step with an error-proof one.
  - **Facilitation.** Make the correct action far easier than the error.
- If you cannot make it impossible for the error to occur, think of ways to detect the error and minimize its effects.
- Choose the best Mistake-Proofing method or device for each error.
- Test it and then implement it.

For more information on Mistake-Proofing Systems, check "Mistake Proofing the Design of Healthcare Processes" by John Grout on the AHRQ website.

REVIEW QUIZ

1. All of the following steps should be considered in the overall strategy to create flow EXCEPT
   A. Observe, map, and reduce the entire process to a series of individual tasks.
   B. Minimize the business value-added (BVA) steps.
   C. Focus on the value-added (VA) steps and train the team so that these steps can be performed faster.
   D. Optimize the work environment so that it provides what is needed when it is needed.
   E. Eliminate non-value-added (NVA) steps.

2. What type of step in your process should be targeted for elimination?
   A. Value-added (VA) steps
   B. Sequential steps
   C. Business value-added (BVA) steps
   D. Non-value-added (NVA) steps
   E. Standardized steps

3. The purpose of evaluating work conditions is to determine if the environment provides what is needed, when it is needed, in the quantity needed, on time, every time to support Standard Work.
   A. True
   B. False

4. An agreed-upon set of work practices that establish the best and most reliable way to do things is called
   A. best practice,
   B. standard work,
   C. a clinical pathway,
   D. optimum performance, or
   E. an optimized process.

5. Regarding Standard Work:
   A. Standardization is not making the standard visual.
   B. Standard Work often increases the number of steps required in a process.
   C. Standard Work is an agreed-upon set of work practices that establish the best and most reliable method and sequence of work.
   D. Standard Work improves effectiveness but decreases flow.
   E. The best way to retain knowledge and provide a basis for training is to allow the creativity, independence, and personal choice of the frontline professional in performing work.

6. Tools for optimizing work conditions include all of the following EXCEPT
   A. Set-up escalation
   B. 5S
   C. Visual Management Systems

D. Mistake-Proofing Systems
E. Visual Controls

7. One of the drawbacks of using a Visual Management System is the need to refer to a complex instruction manual when trying to ascertain the correct steps of a process.
   A. True
   B. False

8. Mistake Proofing is commonly used in all of the following scenarios EXCEPT when
   A. A process step is repetitive.
   B. A process step has been identified in which human error can cause significant mistakes or defects to occur.
   C. A process step is part of a long sequence.
   D. A process step involves a handoff or transfer of care to another healthcare professional.
   E. A process step is part of a work-around.

9. All of the following statements regarding 5S are true EXCEPT
   A. 5S is frequently viewed as an element of a broader construct called Visual Control that allows us to inspect, detect problems, and prevent errors.
   B. 5S empowers the front line.
   C. 5S is only a way to organize a workspace and keep it clean.
   D. 5S requires a "sustaining" phase.
   E. The best way to "sort" is to use the "Red Tag" technique.

10. All of the following are advantages of Standard Work EXCEPT
    A. Standard Work creates a stable and predictable work process.
    B. Standard Work creates a baseline to monitor and improve performance.
    C. Standard Work eliminates the practice of medicine based on clinical expertise.
    D. Standard Work provides a basis for training.
    E. Standard Work retains the organizational knowledge.

11. All of the following are true about 5S EXCEPT
    A. 5S is a systematic way to organize the workspace.
    B. 5S should only be done in complex work areas.
    C. 5S is safety because it allows us to inspect and prevent errors.
    D. 5S creates flow.
    E. 5S empowers healthcare professionals.

Key: 1c, 2d, 3a, 4b, 5c, 6a, 7b, 8e, 9c, 10c, 11b

REFERENCES

1. Abad S. Understanding lean visual management tools. Lean Coach, Instituto Lean Management, Barcelona. In Planet Lean. Accessed May 2020.
2. Crane J. *The Definitive Guide to Emergency Department Operational Improvement.* CRC Press 2011
3. Zidel T. *A Lean Guide to Transforming Healthcare.* ASQ 2006.

CHAPTER 23

Now Roll-Out Your Improvement Ideas and Make Them "Stick"

STORIES FROM THE FRONT LINES OF HEALTHCARE: THE EARLY DISCHARGE QI PROJECT AT MEMORIAL HOSPITAL

The Early Discharge QI Project at Memorial Hospital had been a huge success. It had been coordinated by Linda James, the director of med-surgical nursing, and Dr. Sampson, the CMO. The multidisciplinary team of nurses, physicians, care managers, nurse techs, unit secretaries, and transport staff had worked for months to define the current state, identify the root causes of late discharges, and select and pilot the best solutions. The new process resulted in a decrease in the average time to discharge of 3.5 hours, and as a result, a significant improvement in patient flow in the Emergency Department (ED). Nurse James and Dr. Sampson quickly became absorbed in resolving other priority issues. Three months after the project's completion, a sharp rise in ED boarders prompted Carol, the ED nursing director, to contact Linda about the status of the Early Discharge QI Project. Linda compiled data on the average patient discharge times and was alarmed by what she saw. The average patient discharge times had reverted to the pre-project level of performance.

What happened? Why did the discharge times revert back to pre-project performance? What should have been done differently?

The Quality Improvement Challenge: A Practical Guide for Physicians, First Edition.
Richard J. Banchs and Michael R. Pop.
© 2021 John Wiley & Sons Ltd. Published 2021 by John Wiley & Sons Ltd.
Companion website: www.wiley.com/go/banchs/quality

BEFORE YOU ROLL-OUT, YOU NEED AN IMPLEMENTATION PLAN

Preparation for a full-scale implementation is frequently overlooked by QI teams, and is often done in an ad-hoc manner. Preparation and proper planning are critical as it yields deliverables that support the long-term success of a project. When preparation is disregarded, full-scale implementation often fails and the gains made as a result of the project work are difficult to sustain. A proper implementation plan should provide a structure for *creating and detailing the steps, actions, timing, and people responsible for the full-scale implementation of the new process or process changes.*

First Decide on the Scale-Up Approach

After completing the pilots, the first thing we need to consider is how to scale up the new process or process changes. There are three main approaches to scaling up (Blackburn 2011):

1. **Linear.** The roll-out of the new process or process changes is done sequentially, one area (unit or department) after another. This is the preferred choice when changes are complex, substantial support from the QI team will be needed, or there is a strong resistance to the proposed changes.
2. **Exponential.** The roll-out of the new process or process changes is done in different areas at the same time, with each wave of implementation bigger than the last one. This is the best approach when there is a time constraint, areas share common features that make joint implementation better, or buy-in will be relatively easy.
3. **Global.** The roll-out of the new process or process changes is done in all the areas at once. This approach is best suited for changes that cannot be deployed in stages (for example, a new Electronic Medical Record throughout the hospital), there is a time-sensitive issue, the solution is straightforward, or there is ample support for the change.

Put the Right Team in Place

During the scale-up, QI team members and leaders from the pilots should be actively involved in supporting the changes, coaching and teaching the front line, and solving problems as they arise. The success of any full-scale implementation depends on having the right team in place. Select the leader, an appropriate roll-out team, and make sure there is a clear understanding of the changes, the goals, and the timelines. All areas should also have clear and defined leadership and leadership roles.

Make Sure the Process Is Standardized and Documentation Updated

The new process or process changes should be clearly defined. Imbedding the new process or process changes in the area's workflow should not be left up to individuals, and should not be performed differently depending on the particular area or unit.

- **Standard Work should be in place, assuring an** agreed-upon set of work practices that establishes the best and most reliable method and sequence of tasks for each clinician and support staff member to follow. Standardization (Standard Work) allows the front line to know what the new process steps are, who is responsible for performing them, when they are to be performed, and how to imbed them in the current workflow.
- Detailed information on the changes should be widely disseminated, new roles and responsibilities clearly defined, and job descriptions modified and updated as needed. Make sure all documents have been updated to reflect the changes and clear standard operating procedures (SOPs) are available for all to follow. Orientation manuals and procedural checklists should also be updated as needed.
- Make sure mechanisms exist for the front line to ask for help, and how to find help and who to talk to is well known by all staff and providers.

Make Sure the Work Environment Supports the New Way of Doing Things

Before rolling out the new process or process changes, make sure the work environment has been modified, if needed, to accept the change. If you make it more difficult for people to do things the new way, people will quickly revert to doing things the old way rather than to adopt the change. Remember, change requires a willingness to endure a temporary sense of loss: loss of identity and loss of ability. Make it easy by having all needed machines / equipment / manuals / information and resources available as required. Check that proper **visual controls** (job aides) have been deployed to ensure optimal performance. **Mistake-proofing** aids should be in place to reduce errors and avoid mistakes.

Choose the Right Training Method, Time, and Location

Training programs, coaching, and mentoring should be provided on a wide scale before rolling out any full-scale change. Remember that when we lead an improvement effort, we often experience a **projection bias**, or tendency to assume others have the same information and see things the same way we do. How to proceed or perform a certain task may be clear to the leader and QI team members may not have been easily understood at the front line. **Training** and **coaching** of the "new way" are essential. Training activities require significant preparation and ensuring that it is successful is crucial when you are investing time, money, and the efforts of other team members to coach and train. Keep in mind the content, location, specific learner's needs, and the timing. In healthcare, timing is particularly important since training activities often have to compete with patient care responsibilities.

Monitor, Monitor, Monitor

During the scale-up,

- Use the **metrics** tested in the pilots as part of the performance assessment.
- Track all areas and make sure the new process or process changes are being implemented effectively and according to the agreed-upon plan and schedule.
- Monitor and record the ease of use, effectiveness of each change, and the response of the frontline stakeholders.

An Improvement Plan checklist can help with all aspects of the roll-out of the full-scale change (see Table 23-1).

TABLE 23-1   The Implementation Plan Checklist

Implementation Plan Checklist	
The start	<ul><li>A go-live date for full-scale implementation has been set and communicated.</li><li>Agreement with all mid-level managers and senior leaders has been obtained.</li><li>A local sponsor analysis and stakeholder analysis has been completed.</li><li>A strategy for leveraging and maximizing the support and influence of the local sponsors has been developed.</li></ul>
The team	<ul><li>An implementation team and team leader have been identified.</li><li>The team has a clear understanding of the implementation process and goals.</li><li>The team and team leader have agreed to the timelines.</li></ul>
Process & documents	<ul><li>Changes have been identified; detailed information on the changes has been widely disseminated.</li><li>Standard work has been defined, implemented, and communicated to all.</li><li>New roles and responsibilities have been clearly defined.</li><li>Job descriptions updated as needed.</li><li>Guidelines, policies & procedures, and reference manuals have been updated.</li><li>All changes have been discussed and accepted by key stakeholders.</li><li>Detailed information has been widely disseminated.</li></ul>

(Continued)

TABLE 23-1   (Continued)

Implementation Plan Checklist	
Work environment	• All needed machines and equipment are available as required. • Manuals and guides are available and their location know by all. • The proper visual controls (job aides) have been deployed to ensure optimal performance. • Mistake-proofing aides have been put in place to reduce errors and avoid mistakes.
Training	• An effective education and training program are in place. • Staff and physicians have received the appropriate training or have been scheduled to attend training as needed. • A schedule for coaching and mentoring has been created; superusers will be in place to assist the front line with the roll-out. • Additional mechanisms to seek help are available and have been discussed with all key stakeholders.
Monitoring	• Metrics have been selected to follow the roll-out of full-scale changes • All personnel involved in data collection have been properly trained. • Clearly defined procedures / methods for recording data are available. • Location of data collection has been identified, and a data collection sheet has been prepared.

ASSESS THE POTENTIAL IMPACT OF YOUR IMPROVEMENT IDEAS

Before you roll out a full-scale change, you may want to have an idea of the potential impact the change may have at the front line. This assessment can help you gauge the potential for pushback, assess the adequacy of resources, and create an appropriate implementation strategy. There is no easy way to do this. Each area may be different and react to change in a different way. In addition, change may impact individuals and teams differently at different times in the life of the organizations. Nevertheless, what remains clear is that success when rolling out a change at the front line is generally influenced by a number of factors that can be grouped in five categories:

1. the leader (type of leader, presence of the leader, actions of the leader);
2. the team (composition, resources, experience of team rolling out the change);
3. the change (type and magnitude of the proposed change);
4. the organization (type, culture of the organization); and
5. the experience, beliefs, and attitudes of the people working in the area affected by the change.

Our **Impact Assessment tool** can be used to provide a subjective assessment of the impact of the change and the response to change at the front line to inform your roll-out strategy (see Table 23-2). The Impact Assessment tool considers a list of criteria in the five categories of factors influencing the impact of a change. For each criterion, a score of 1, 3, 5, 7, or 10 is assigned according to whether the answer to the statement is yes (1), probably (3), maybe (5), probably not (7), or no (10). Each score is multiplied by an assigned weight. Criteria with a high impact on change have double the weight. All scores are added to generate a total score. The total score is compared to a reference key that assigns a change impact and risk for each range of scores. The higher the score, the greater impact the change will have at the front line, and the greater pushback and resistance you will find. The Impact Assessment tool assumes all five categories have the same impact, which is not always the case. Nevertheless, the tool is helpful to create a buy-in strategy, assess resources, and get an idea of the time and effort you will need to roll out the full-scale change.

TABLE 23-2   The Impact Assessment Tool

Impact Assessment Tool		
Leader & leadership structure		
Evaluation criteria	Weight	Score
Changes are supported by the Primary Sponsor.	1	
Changes are supported by the Local Sponsors.	2	
Local Sponsors are going to be engaged in actively supporting the changes.	2	
Local Sponsors have the required knowledge and experience with change.	1	
There are clear lines of communication between leaders and the front line.	1	
The roll-out team		
Evaluation criteria	Weight	Score
A team has been selected to facilitate the roll-out process.	1	
The team has experience and has been successful with prior projects.	2	
The team has been given adequate time to prepare the roll-out.	1	
The team has been given resources and funding to support communication, coaching, and training.	2	
The type and magnitude of the change		
Evaluation criteria	Weight	Score
The proposed changes are aligned with current improvement initiatives.	1	

(Continued)

TABLE 23-2   (Continued)

Impact Assessment Tool		
The proposed changes will affect a small number of people or teams.	1	
The proposed changes will affect all stakeholder groups the same.	1	
The likelihood changes will impact job descriptions or workflow is low.	2	
The likelihood changes will impact work schedules is low.	2	
The likelihood changes will impact salaries is low.	2	
The frontline professionals		
Evaluation criteria	Weight	Score
The area is innovative and supports changes to the way of doing things.	1	
Change initiatives in the area are frequent and usually successful.	1	
Staff and providers have had a significant role in creating the changes.	2	
Are motivated and support a change to the current way of doing things.	2	
Are willing to accept a temporary discomfort to improve quality care.	2	

TOTAL SCORE

Instructions: For each criterion, assign a score of 1, 3, 5, 7, or 10 if the answer to the statement is yes (1), probably (3), maybe (5), probably not (7), or no (10). Multiply the score by the weight and place the result in the score column.
Reference Key: 30–120 points = low-impact change; some pushback; low risk; 121–210 points = medium impact; pushback will be significant; medium risk; 211–300 points = high impact; generalized pushback; pockets of resistance may try to derail the project; high risk.

ASSESS THE POTENTIAL FOR PUSHBACK: THE STAKEHOLDER ANALYSIS

The Crucial Role of the Stakeholders

While front line stakeholders have valuable insights into their processes and the barriers they face in delivering high-quality patient care, they often have minimal opportunity to share that proficiency in modifying their workflows. As we have said in previous chapters, it is important to make a concerted effort to solicit the stakeholders' input and engage them in the improvement efforts. Change management is most successful when the frontline stakeholders are included in all the phases of the project. Their involvement should not be postponed until a solution has been fully worked out. This is especially important when the frontline stakeholders are the subject-matter experts (SMEs). A proactive approach to engage the front line is always better than a reactive approach where we have to work against resistance. *Proactive planning results in change management. Reactive planning results in resistance management.* The latter is much more difficult. Many improvement teams address change only when faced with pushback from the frontline professionals. This is a tactical and costly mistake.

The stakeholders are the frontline experts – the healthcare professionals who do the work and bring relevant experience and expertise to a particular process. These frontline healthcare professionals are the ones who are going to experience the pain or the gain if the new process is either not functioning properly or doing well. They also hold a position from which they can influence the success of the improvement initiative. To get their support and buy-in, we have to know and understand their interests and engage them early in the improvement initiative.

A robust strategy is a key component of a successful QI project that functions to plan communication, gain support, uncover resistance, and identify competing priorities among the stakeholder groups. It starts with the assessment of who the key stakeholders are, their influence on the project, and the impact they may have on the expected outcome. Properly done, this evaluation leads to the development of a stakeholder engagement strategy that focuses the QI team's efforts on meeting the needs of the different groups of stakeholders to maintain their engagement and support of the project. An important component of stakeholder engagement is to get their agreement and support early on in the project regarding the scope, metrics, and goals of the project.

To create a strategy

- First identify all stakeholders; create a stakeholder list.
- Complete a **Stakeholder Analysis** to determine the level of impact each stakeholder or stakeholder group may have based on their power, influence, and involvement in the project; and to document their attitude toward the project and its expected outcomes in order to plan the best management approach for each stakeholder or stakeholder group.
- Create a **Power & Influence (P&I) diagram**. The P&I diagram provides a graphic depiction of each stakeholder's potential impact on the project that is easy to visualize, and helps you guide your overall engagement and communication strategy.
- Create a list of actions; use the information gathered by the team to create the best approach to engage and get buy-in from each stakeholder and stakeholder group.

The Stakeholder List

To identify the stakeholders,

- Brainstorm with the team to identify the internal and external stakeholders.
- Identify every stakeholder group, including smaller groups and individuals who may influence the project's success. This will minimize the risk of "surprises" from overlooked stakeholders who may oppose the project changes and create roadblocks as the project progresses.
- Stratify the key stakeholders in groups. Identify the subset of stakeholders who potentially have the most influence over the project, are most affected by the project, or will offer the greatest resistance.
- Code the list. Assign a code letter by which to refer to each stakeholder or stakeholder group (A, B, C, D, etc.); document their role in the organization.

The Stakeholder Analysis

The Stakeholder Analysis is a process of analyzing the impact different stakeholders or stakeholder groups may have on the project based on their power, influence, involvement, and attitude toward the project in order to plan the management approach that is best suited to get their support and buy-in.

> **The Stakeholder Analysis identifies the key stakeholders and groups them according to their levels of participation, interest, and influence in the project to determine how best to engage and communicate with them.**

The Stakeholder Analysis helps the project team understand and address the needs of the front line stakeholders, defining how the project impacts them, and how they can impact the project. This evaluation helps with the development of a stakeholder strategy focusing the QI team's efforts on meeting their needs and maintain their engagement and support. The Stakeholder Analysis is crucial in managing change and mitigating resistance; it is a systematic way to assess each stakeholder group in order to understand their interests, positions, alliances, and their potential impact on the project.

The goals of the Stakeholder Analysis are to

- identify the key stakeholders;
- understand their interests, position, and alliances;
- assess the impact of the project on their work;
- assess their influence on the project and the changes being rolled out;
- help develop a communication and action plan; and
- help create the best strategy to get their engagement and project buy-in.

To complete a Stakeholder Analysis,

- **Collect all available information** for every stakeholder group, gathering and reviewing data from all sources; speak to the Primary Sponsor as he/she may have additional information from previous improvement efforts.
- **Interview stakeholders directly.** This will give you an accurate picture of their positions, interests, and potential impact on the project. It is better to ask them than assume you know what they think; a formal discussion or interview process may be the best approach.
- **Record all information** into a concise and standardized format. The purpose is to make systematic comparisons, highlight significant information, and ensure stakeholder identity anonymity if required.
- **Organize** all the available information in a **Stakeholder Analysis template** (see Table 23-3).

How to complete the Stakeholder Analysis template

- **Code.** Assign each stakeholder a letter and place letters on the left-hand column.
- **Complete the Impact column.** Complete the impact column by answering the question "How will the project affect this stakeholder?" Score this column as high (H), medium (M), or low (L).
- **Complete the Power column.** Complete the power column by answering the question "How will this stakeholder affect the project?" Score this column on a scale of 1–5, with 1 being low and 5 being high.
- **Complete the Influence column.** Complete this column by answering the question "What is the influence of this stakeholder over the success of the project?" Score this column on a scale of 1–5, with 1 being low and 5 being high.

TABLE 23-3   A Stakeholder Analysis Template

Stakeholder Analysis									
Stakeholder Key	Impact (High, medium, low)	Power (1 to 5)	Influence (1 to 5)	Attitude					Pxl zone
				SO	O	N	S	SS	
A									
B									
C									
D									

Reasons

- **Complete the attitude column.** Attitude refers to whether the stakeholder supports or opposes the project. This column is scored using SO = strongly opposes, O = opposes, N = neutral, S = supports, SS = strongly supports. Document the reasons for the specific score in the space below the columns.
- Complete the Power and Influence diagram (see next) to fill the PxI zone column.

A stakeholder analysis can be done at the beginning of a project and repeated several times throughout the project lifecycle to monitor changes in the stakeholders' attitudes toward the project or proposed changes that warrant adjustments to the change management strategy.

The Power and Influence diagram

> **The Power and Influence (P&I) diagram is a tool used to categorize and graphically depict each stakeholder group according to their power and influence on the project.**

The P&I diagram defines four distinct zones that correspond to four different needs for communication and change management (see Figure 23-1):

- **Zone I.** Key players; focus efforts on this group; these stakeholders should be involved in all levels of the project planning, decisions, and full-scale roll-out; engage and consult regularly.
- **Zone 2.** These stakeholders require frequent communication on project status and progress; engage and consult on key areas; try and bring to zone 1.

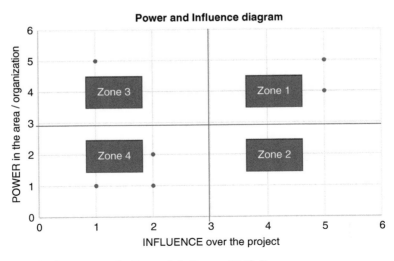

FIGURE 23-1   The four zones of a Power & Influence (PxI) diagram.

- **Zone 3.** Keep informed on a regular basis and consult on interest areas; these stakeholders need communication to address questions and concerns.
- **Zone 4.** These stakeholders can be informed via general communication. They require a less intense level of communication and management.

To create a P&I diagram, plot the numeric values from the stakeholder analysis' power column and influence column on the Power and Influence diagram. Use the diagram to identify the optimal stakeholder strategy for each stakeholder group.

Here is an example of a P&I diagram for seven stakeholder groups coded A to G (see Figure 23-2). The numeric values from the stakeholder analysis' power and influence column are shown in Table 23-4. Based on the P&I diagram presented, stakeholders A, C, and D, in the lower left quadrant, require minimal management effort as they have low power in the organization and low influence over the project; stakeholder F, in the upper-left quadrant, must be kept satisfied by frequent sharing of information and ensuring concerns and questions are addressed adequately; stakeholder G, in the lower right quadrant, has a low power base but exerts significant influence over the success of the project so must be kept informed through frequent communication on the project's status and progress; stakeholders B and E, in the upper-right quadrant, are key players since they wield significant power in the organization and have substantial influence over the project; they must be involved in all levels of project planning and change management.

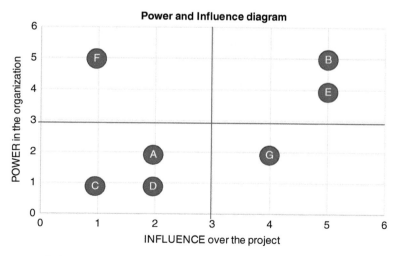

FIGURE 23-2 Stakeholder analysis using a Power & Influence diagram for stakeholder groups A to G.

TABLE 23-4   Power & Influence Scores for Stakeholder Groups A to G

Scores for Stakeholder Groups A to G		
Stakeholder Key	Power (Y-values)	Influence (X-values)
A	2	2
B	5	5
C	1	1
D	1	2
E	4	5
F	5	1
G	2	4

The Stakeholder Analysis Bar Graph

A Stakeholder Analysis Bar Graph is another way information about the stakeholders can be organized to graphically depict each stakeholder's attitude towards the project (see Figure 23-3).

YOUR STAKEHOLDER ENGAGEMENT STRATEGY

The Stakeholder Engagement Strategy integrates the information gathered in the stakeholder analysis and the Power and Influence (P&I) diagram to create a plan for managing the expectations of the stakeholders and engaging them throughout the QI project and full-scale roll-out. It prioritizes the needs of the stakeholders who are most powerful within the organization and have the most influence over the project. In this manner, the QI team is able to expend their energies in the most productive way.

Regardless of the zone in which the stakeholder group falls on the P&I diagram, the most important component of the stakeholder strategy is **communication**. The QI team must communicate with stakeholder groups early and often to ensure project success. Effective communication allows the QI team to gain support and input for the project and solution roll-out. When stakeholders are not aware of the project or the changes, they may develop misperceptions about the project that will negatively influence their adoption of the improvement initiative. Early and frequent communication is crucial. Frontline professionals (stakeholders) may have interests that are impacted by the project and can be leveraged with early and frequent communication to enlist their engagement and support. Thorough communication with key stakeholders is crucial to make sure their concerns are addressed and the resources they control are available for the project.

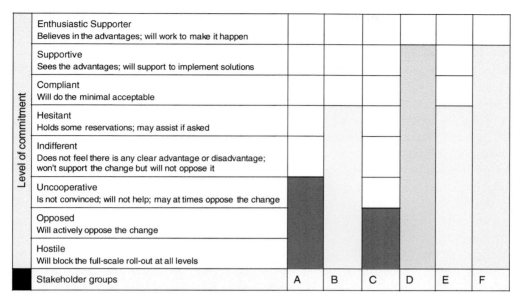

FIGURE 23-3   Stakeholder Analysis using a Stakeholder Bar Graph.

ASSESS THE LEVEL OF SUPPORT: THE LOCAL SPONSOR ANALYSIS

The Role of the Local Sponsors

Within the organizational leadership hierarchy are individuals who are in key positions to impact the project's success – the Local Sponsors.

> **The Local Sponsors are the supervisors (mid-level managers, division chiefs, department heads) who are responsible for and oversee the work being done.**

The Local Sponsors are the middle managers, division chiefs, and department heads in the hospital who are responsible for the effective and efficient performance of the work and the quality of care delivered. They typically have an intimate understanding of the workflow, work patterns, and workforce in their area and leverage that information to support their own agenda, which may or may not correspond to that of the QI team and the goals of the project. It is easy to see how the Local Sponsors have been identified as the group of stakeholders who often demonstrate the most resistance to the roll-out of the improvement initiatives. Similarly, it is clear that the Local Sponsors' perceptions of the changes the QI projects are about to bring warrants significant attention to ensure they are engaged in supporting the project work and outcomes.

The Local Sponsors are the people who are "needed to advocate for, and are in a position to authorize the improvement project and the subsequent changes" (Hiatt 2012). The Local Sponsor has been defined as the individual or group who has the power to sanction or legitimize a change. The Local Sponsors play a critical role in any change effort. They have the ability, through the use of their local power, to make change happen and ensure that the change is sustainable. The Local Sponsors have usually developed a strong network of colleagues that band together in their support of or opposition to the improvement initiatives. When we are able to secure their backing, the Local Sponsors prove to be resilient partners. They collaborate to cascade the change throughout their area of responsibility, serving as role models for the actions and behaviors required by the change. Moreover, they are often instrumental in mitigating the barriers that threaten the implementation of the full-scale roll-out. Hence, the Local Sponsors have the greatest role in promoting the acceptance of the change and the success of the project. *The greatest resistance to change is usually not at the top or the bottom of the organizational hierarchy but in the middle* (Nonaka 1995).

Change sponsorship needs to happen at every level. The best way to identify the Local Sponsors, their reporting structures, and to understand the Local Sponsors' perceptions of the project and upcoming changes is by performing a **Sponsor Analysis**.

The Sponsor Analysis

An organizational chart provides a good way to identify the key Local Sponsors and to organize the information that is compiled about their attitudes and opinions about the project. This information can later be used to develop a Sponsor Strategy aimed at achieving a strong **Sponsor Network** that supports the project changes.

> **A Sponsor Analysis is a structured approach for identifying and assessing the sponsors and their willingness to support and positively impact the outcome of the project.**

The process for completing a Sponsor Analysis is straightforward:

- Identify all groups who will be impacted by the changes.
- For each group, determine who is responsible or in charge of the area.
- Using an organizational chart, create a leadership diagram with the areas involved.
- Follow the formal reporting structures. Add any senior leaders between the Local Sponsors (managers) and the primary sponsor. Make sure to include only the key leaders necessary for the project to succeed.

- For each of the sponsors, determine if they openly support the project, oppose the project, or are neutral; you can interview them or use common knowledge to support your assessment. For the sponsors that fall in the unknown category, get additional information and the opinion of the Primary Sponsor.
- With this information, highlight each sponsor in green if the sponsor will support the project, in red if the sponsor will probably oppose the project, or in yellow if the sponsor is neutral or ambivalent about the project.
- Create an action plan for each sponsor.

This Sponsor Analysis helps the QI team recognize the Local Sponsors who may be resistant to the QI project so they can intervene promptly to mitigate potential issues that would impact the change efforts (see Figure 23-4).

THE LOCAL SPONSOR STRATEGY

To create a strong sponsor network of support,

- **Meet with Local Sponsors individually**. Ensure your Sponsors understand what is required of them, including the responsibilities related to their role and the expected level of commitment. Make sure they are aligned with the change and they are willing to support their frontline staff during the change initiative.
- **Get feedback**. Local Sponsors may not immediately endorse the change. Make sure they have the information they need and a clear process of two-way communication is in place to work through their concerns. Allow them the time to evaluate and affirm the change before requesting of them to role model adoption of the change.
- **Meet with all the Local Sponsors.** Bring together all the Local Sponsors in a cross-departmental meeting. Make sure you discuss the nature of the change, what is in it for them, how the change will affect the units /departments, and how each Local Sponsor is expected to support the front line. Share ideas for addressing the problems encountered. Sponsors will probably face a similar degree of opposition independent of the unit they supervise.
- **Provide feedback**. Provide ongoing feedback about the change, the rate of change, and the success of the area in implementing the new process or change.

The Local Sponsors have an established network of colleagues who are influential in supporting the adoption of change efforts or thwarting them. It is critical that you observe their actions and engage them in the project to leverage that influence in accomplishing the project's objectives.

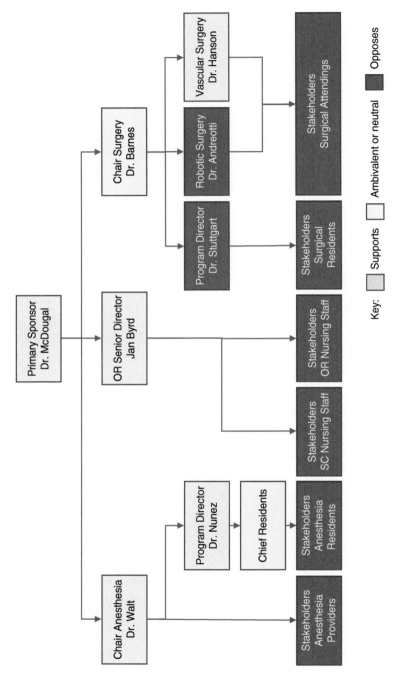

FIGURE 23-4   Sponsor Analysis using an organizational chart.

THE MONITORING AND CONTROL PLAN

A detailed Monitoring & Control plan is essential to monitor the performance of the process and ensure that staff and clinicians do not discard the new processes and revert to their former ways of working. It is critical to monitor the processes with ongoing data analysis and reporting techniques, such as process control charts, debriefings, and daily checklists. The Monitoring & Control plan helps detect changes when they occur and assures that improvements continue to hold moving forward.

A Monitoring and Control plan covers:

- What metrics will be monitored moving forward?
- How is data going to be collected; how often and by whom?
- How are results going to be analyzed and reported?
- What to do if data shows a deviation from the expected performance; what actions should be taken and by whom?

A method used to monitor a process is **Statistical Process Control** (SPC). SPC is a set of methods for ongoing improvement and monitoring of processes and outcomes based on the analysis of variation. SPC has been widely used in the healthcare environment to manage change and monitor improvements (Thor 2007). One of the most important tools in SPC is the Control chart (see Chapter 16). As described, the Control chart computes upper and lower control limits (UCL & LCL) as a threshold to monitor the behavior of a process.

The Monitoring & Control plan checklist should include these items:

- Metrics have been selected to track the performance of the new process.
- A well-planned and clearly defined data collection system is in place.
- Responsible stakeholders have been selected to collect and analyze the data.
- Reports have been designated for tracking and dissemination at known intervals.
- Selected metrics have been included as part of stakeholders' annual performance evaluations as required.

THE FOURTH TOLLGATE REVIEW

The improvement team meets with the Primary Sponsor to discuss ongoing project activities; review results and deliverables; assure the project is coming to a successful conclusion. The fourth tollgate review should be scheduled with the Primary Sponsor:

- before rolling out the changes; and
- soon after completing the full-scale change to discuss results, monitoring plan and project closure.

This is usually best accomplished during and at the end of the fifth "R": the "Right Cause" (see Chapter 25).

PROJECT CLOSURE

Complete the Project Review

The final project review provides a summary of the work performed during the project and the outcomes achieved as a result of that work. This summary allows the Primary Sponsor, QI team, and process owners to determine whether the results obtained substantiate the ongoing implementation of the project's components.

Gather the Lessons Learned

Gather the lessons learned during the project and acknowledge the achievements. The compilation of the positive and negative lessons learned during the course of the project supports a culture of continuous and constant improvement. These lessons become organizational assets that promote the adoption of best practices and the avoidance of mistakes made during previous projects. The final project review meeting serves to solidify the team-building efforts that were realized during the project as the stakeholders reflect on their accomplishments and identify future goals. It also offers the opportunity to celebrate their success and distribute the incentives that had previously been negotiated.

Essentially, the closing phase provides a time to evaluate the value of the project and its impact on our work processes, workflow, and work environment to provide effective and efficient care to our patients.

Transfer the Ownership of the Processes and Deliverables to the Process Owners

Throughout the project life cycle, the project team has facilitated the completion of the project work. As the project ends, the team empowers the process owners and frontline stakeholders to continue the work that has resulted in the successful accomplishment of their goals. This is achieved by maintaining clear communication of the project accountabilities and structuring the standardization of the work to ease the transition process. For example, if the project team has been primarily responsible for performing data analytics during the project, they must ensure that the persons designated by the process owner to assume this function are adequately trained and have access to any programs or templates required to complete this task.

The Project Closure checklist should include these items:

- All the project documentation has been compiled, recorded, and completed by the QI team and final preparations have been made for distribution.

- All the lessons learned have been captured and communicated to all stakeholders.
- Acknowledgments **by executive management** and celebrations have been planned.

REFERENCES

1. Blackburn S. *How to implement complex change at scale? Organization Practice.* McKinsey & Company. 2011

2. Hiatt J. Change Management. The People Side of Change. Prosci Learning Center Publications 2012.

3. Nonaka I. *The Knowledge Creating Company. How Japanese Companies Create the Dynamics of Innovation.* Oxford University Press 1995.

4. Thor J. Application of Statistical Process Control in healthcare improvement: systematic review. *Qual Saf Health Care* 2006. 16(5):387–399.

PART VII

ADDITIONAL THINGS YOU MAY NEED TO KNOW

CHAPTER 24

How to Prepare and Conduct a Tollgate Review

THE TOLLGATE REVIEWS

What Is a Tollgate Review and Why Do We Need One?

Periodically, the improvement team needs to confirm they are on the right track with the work they are doing to achieve their project goals. This is best done by conducting a tollgate review.

> **A tollgate review is a checkpoint at the end of a phase where project activities and deliverables are reviewed with the Primary Sponsor to assure the project is on track and the goals of the phase are being met.**

A tollgate review is a sort of go/no-go decision point. A project should not proceed without a "go" decision by the appropriate senior sponsors for a specific stage tollgate.

The intent of the tollgate review is to actively engage both the project team and the Primary Sponsor in the decisions to be made to either:

- move forward to the next stage of the project, or
- complete needed work in the current stage before proceeding.

The Quality Improvement Challenge: A Practical Guide for Physicians, First Edition.
Richard J. Banchs and Michael R. Pop.
© 2021 John Wiley & Sons Ltd. Published 2021 by John Wiley & Sons Ltd.
Companion website: www.wiley.com/go/banchs/quality

The tollgate review has three purposes:

1. meet,
2. communicate, and
3. m**ake a decision**.

The tollgate review gives the Primary Sponsor the ability to evaluate the completed deliverables and either approve them or request revisions, if needed, to ensure that the project remains on track and achieves the established objectives. An additional purpose of the tollgate review is to **improve communication** between all parties. Clear communication ensures the Primary Sponsor is aware of the issues and the QI team has the support it needs to succeed.

How to Conduct a Tollgate Review

A tollgate review with the Primary Sponsor should have a target time of about **30 minutes.** The idea is to get "in and out." To maximize the efficiency and effectiveness of the meeting,

- Schedule the meeting directly with the administrative staff of the Primary Sponsor.
- Prior to meeting, send an updated presentation detailing the status of the project. You should send all materials a couple of days before so that the Primary Sponsor has the time to review it and prepare possible questions.
- Review all the information collected in the previous steps. Use a **tollgate review checklist** for each phase to make sure all deliverables have been addressed.
- If team members will be presenting, make sure each team member is aware of their role and is comfortable presenting their own work.
- Set the agenda for 30 minutes. For each item, make a brief presentation and get feedback.
- At the end of the meeting, make a joint decision to advance to the next phase or review current steps.

Quotable quote: "Obstacles are those frightful things you see when you take your eyes off your goals." Henry Ford

FOUR TOLLGATE REVIEWS OF A FIVE "R" PROJECT PHASE

The First Tollgate Review

The first tollgate review should be scheduled with the Primary Sponsor soon after organizing your team. This will be at the end of the second "R": the "Right People."

The goal is to discuss with the Primary Sponsor the project feasibility, to make sure the project is focused and well defined, and has clear objectives and the right metrics. The goal is also to make sure the team has the appropriate knowledge and mix of skills. There are three deliverables for this tollgate:

1. **Problem Statement,**
2. **Project Charter, and**
3. **QI team roster.**

You can use a tollgate checklist to prepare your meeting with the Primary Sponsor (see Table 24-1).

Second Tollgate Review

The second tollgate review should be scheduled with the Primary Sponsor at the end of the third "R": the "Right Problem." The goal of this tollgate is for the team to agree with the Primary Sponsor on the project scope and boundaries, to give an update

TABLE 24-1   First Tollgate Review Checklist

First Tollgate Review Checklist
Assign red (no, probably not), yellow (maybe, probably) or green (yes, completed) to each of the statements:
The QI project has support from Senior leadership.
A Primary Sponsor has been selected and will be able to actively and visibly participate through the life cycle of the project.
Resources (time, personnel, and money) have been set aside for the improvement project.
A focused Problem Statement has been written.
A Project Charter has been completed; the charter includes specific metrics and clearly defined goals and targets.
The goals of the project are ambitious but realistic.
The project has a clearly defined timeline, with key milestones and project deliverables.
A QI team has been selected; team members have the appropriate knowledge and mix of skills.
A leader has been selected to lead the team, manage project resources, and help complete the project tasks.
The team leader has clearly identified the purpose, goals, and work strategy for the team members; members of the team have identified "what's in it for me" (WIIFM).

on the Voice of the Customer, and the issues that challenge the stakeholders in the performance of their work. There are three deliverables for this tollgate:

1. **SIPOC diagram;**
2. **Critical-to-Quality (CTQ) tree,** showing the attributes and requirements for customer satisfaction; and
3. **Critical Needs (CN) tree,** so we can understand the drivers of stakeholder performance.

Before this tollgate, the team should update and complete the Problem Statement and Project Charter. You can use a tollgate checklist to prepare for the second tollgate meeting with the Primary Sponsor (see Table 24-2).

Third Tollgate Review

The third tollgate review should be scheduled with the Primary Sponsor at the end of the fourth "R": the "Right Cause." The goal of this tollgate is to discuss process behavior and the causes of poor performance. There are three deliverables for this tollgate:

1. **Process Map,**

TABLE 24-2   Second Tollgate Review Checklist

Second Tollgate Review Checklist
Assign red (no, probably not), yellow (maybe, probably) or green (yes, completed) to each of the statements:
The start and end of the process to be improved has been clearly identified; a completed SIPOC diagram shows the critical activities and elements of the process.
The scope and boundaries of the project are well defined and have been clearly communicated to all stakeholders.
The customer has been identified (patients, staff, physicians); the Voice of the Customer (VOC) has been collected.
Critical-to-Quality (CTQs) attributes and requirements for customer satisfaction have been identified and validated with data.
The Voice of the Stakeholder (VOS) has been obtained, and the Critical Needs of the frontline stakeholders identified and recorded.
A detailed, focused Problem Statement has been completed; the Project Charter has been updated as needed.
A Communication Planner has been prepared; information has been shared with each stakeholder group multiple times and through multiple channels.

2. **Graphic Summary** of the process performance, and
3. Analysis showing **most likely cause/s** of the problem.

Use the third tollgate checklist to prepare your meeting with the Primary Sponsor (see Table 24-3).

Fourth Tollgate Review

The fourth tollgate review should be scheduled with the Primary Sponsor. We often do it in two sessions:

1. Before rolling-out the improvement ideas full-scale. The goal of the meeting is to share with the Primary Sponsor the results of pilots and get feedback and support for the Implementation plan.

TABLE 24-3 THIRD TOLLGATE REVIEW CHECKLIST

Third Tollgate Review Checklist
Assign red (no, probably not), yellow (maybe, probably) or green (yes, completed) to each of the statements:
The team created a detailed process map; the process map has been validated with key stakeholders.
Potential bottlenecks, disconnects, redundancies, and other waste have been identified and targeted for improvement.
Project Metrics have been selected; project metrics include metrics of effectiveness and metrics of efficiency.
Data has been collected and analyzed; power and sample size calculations have been applied as needed.
The type of variation has been properly identified; graphs have been created to reflect current process behavior; based on the results, an action plan has been identified.
A process capability study has been performed; process sigma calculated when applicable.
The potential causes of the problem have been identified; the team filtered and prioritized the most likely cause(s).
The hypothesis has been thoroughly investigated and tested to confirm the cause-and-effect relationship.
Information has been shared with each stakeholder group multiple times and through multiple channels.
All documents have been reviewed and updated to reflect the learning from the previous phase.

2. After rolling-out the improvement ideas full-scale to review results and discuss the monitoring plans and project closure.

There are four deliverables for this tollgate:

1. the **list of ideas** and results of **pilots,**
2. the **Implementation** plan,
3. results of the roll-out and **Project Summary, and**
4. **Monitoring Plan.**

Use the fourth tollgate checklist to prepare your meeting with the Primary Sponsor (see Table 24-4).

TABLE 24-4   Fourth Tollgate Review Checklist

Fourth Tollgate Review Checklist
Assign red (no, probably not), yellow (maybe, probably) or green (yes, completed) to each of the statements:
A list of ideas has been proposed; improvement ideas have been filtered and prioritized, and the best ideas selected. Ideas have been assessed for risk and potential constraints.
Pilot studies (PDSA cycles) have been conducted and lessons-learned applied. Modifications to the initial proposed ideas have been made as required.
A full implementation plan has been developed and worked through by the team and key local sponsors.
Standard Work, 5S, Visual Controls, and Mistake-Proofing have been implemented.
All documents and job descriptions have been reviewed and updated to reflect the new change; the team has planned for all needed equipment as required.
The upcoming changes have been thoroughly communicated to all stakeholders up and down the process. A strategy for leveraging and maximizing the support and influence of the key stakeholders has been developed.
Coaching and training plans have been made to address the needs of the front line.
Appropriate metrics (CTQs) have been identified for tracking the progress of the change and monitoring future process performance.
All lessons learned have been captured, properly documented, and communicated to the stakeholders.
All project documentation has been compiled and recorded. Final copies have been distributed as needed.
The Standardized process has been completely transferred to the process owners.
The goals and targets in the Project Charter have been achieved; The QI team has been properly recognized and rewarded.

CHAPTER 25

How to Communicate Effectively to Engage the Front Line

STORIES FROM THE FRONT LINES OF HEALTHCARE: THE NICU TEAM AT ST. AGNES HOSPITAL

Cathy, the assistant nurse manager for the Neonatal Intensive Care Unit at St. Agnes Hospital, decided to assemble a QI team to organize their unit's supply room. The problem was evident: critical items were difficult to find, poorly organized, or stored in insufficient numbers. Cathy recruited Alex, the day shift charge RN; Derek, the evening shift charge RN; Yolanda, the night shift RN; and Jolene, the NICU fellow to participate on the project team. Together, they evaluated the current inventory and organization of the supplies, removed items never used, and thoroughly cleaned the area. They then reorganized the remaining supplies according to their function using color-coded labels for easier identification. Satisfied with their achievement, the project team sent out an email to all NICU providers and staff that described the goals of the project, the work they had completed, and the new location of the supplies as depicted on a map of the room. Two days later, Cathy was stopped in the hallway by Dr. Finks, one of the NICU Attendings. He was visibly upset with the new layout and the fact that he had been unable to find critical items during a crisis. He claimed he had not been informed, was never consulted, and he did not know anything about the supply room reorganization.

What just happened? What failed?

The Quality Improvement Challenge: A Practical Guide for Physicians, First Edition.
Richard J. Banchs and Michael R. Pop.
© 2021 John Wiley & Sons Ltd. Published 2021 by John Wiley & Sons Ltd.
Companion website: www.wiley.com/go/banchs/quality

THE IMPORTANCE OF COMMUNICATION

> **Effective communication is a critical aspect of any quality improvement project and is recognized as a key component for stakeholder's behavior change in any change management effort.**

Improvement is always a change. All QI projects are in essence change initiatives. Communication provides the information people need to make their personal decision about engaging in an improvement initiative and adopting a change. Studies have shown that effective communication is critical in the spread of small (Nolan 2005) and large (Cooper 2015) improvement efforts (changes) in healthcare.

When improvement teams come up with a great solution, they will fail and their improvements will be short-lived if frontline professionals don't support them or understand what they are trying to achieve. Frontline stakeholders need to be informed; they need to understand the problem, the challenges in solving these problems, and the reasons for change. Change is threatening. When we don't have information about why a change is happening and we are uncertain about how it is going to affect us, we **feel anxious.** Anxiety comes from our inability to predict what is going to happen; we feel lost. Uncertainty creates anxiety, and anxiety triggers a conscious or subconscious fight or flight response (Scarlett 2019). When we don't have information, we create our own stories to fill the void; our stories are a distortion of reality and usually present a picture of the change that is much worse than the actual reality. When we don't have information about an upcoming change, we tend to create a negative view of what's coming; our reaction is to reject the change, even when the change might be an improvement to the current situation.

Communication helps the front line gain an understanding of the problem, the project, the options for improvement, and the possible changes. Communication helps people understand how change is going to affect them. Communication is knowledge, and knowledge is control. We need a sense of control even when the change will negatively impact us. While uncertainty creates anxiety, knowledge generates a certain sense of well-being; we feel better when we know, even if the change will negatively impact us. Communication allows us to create awareness of the problem at the front lines key stakeholders can discuss ideas, share views, and co-create solutions. By communicating with the front line, we create an environment that fosters engagement in the improvement initiative and builds support and buy-in for the change. Communication reduces the misunderstandings that lead to conflicts, and instead builds trusting relationships and teamwork. There is a second reason why all QI project teams need to focus their efforts on effective communication: communication is as much to fill the need for information of the professionals at the front line as it is for the QI team to get feedback on the issues affecting the people at the front line.

WHY PROJECTS OFTEN FAIL

...Because We Don't Communicate

Team members are too busy looking for the solution. All the focus is on creating the right solution to achieve the goals of the project. A good solution does not guarantee the desire to change and the adoption of the solution at the front lines. Buy-in does not stem from the characteristics or appropriateness of the solution, but from the successful transition of people through their own change line. Communication helps achieve this transition.

Team members don't want to say anything to the front line until they know more about the final solution. Improvement teams and their sponsors often feel uncomfortable with communicating too early because much about the project and the changes to come are unknown. But when information is given too late, the lack of participation in the decision-making process results in resistance and opposition to the needs of the project. Communicating early sets the right expectations.

Team members assume everybody knows the issues so they don't engage in communication. This is called **projection bias**. People in the know tend to assume others have the same information and see things the same way they do. When communication is insufficient or inexistent, it creates a knowledge gap resulting in pushback from the frontline professionals who feel uninformed, uncomfortable, and anxious about the change.

...Because We Don't Have a Good Communication Strategy

The team just "checks the box." Team members underestimate the importance of communication and communicate just to check the box. Communication is done haphazardly and with little preparation. The message is delivered as an email or brief statement at a meeting with no time for the fron tline to discuss it or get feedback. With no engagement and the inability to get feedback, the front line feels uncertain about the nature of the change, and cynicism or pushback ensues.

PEOPLE'S BRAINS OFTEN CREATE BARRIERS TO EFFECTIVE COMMUNICATION

People's brains create barriers that challenge even the best attempts to communicate effectively:

Internalization. Different people interpret the same message in different ways. We all filter what we hear and then internalize the message, creating our own personal meaning. Differences in past experiences affect the way we process information.

Positive experiences of similar events shape the interpretation of a message in a different way than if the experience was negative. Reality can be highly subjective. The internalization process is also affected by our beliefs, personal choices, and professional circumstances. While we cannot know what people have experienced and how they are going to interpret what we say, we can rely on getting feedback during the communication process to make sure we understand how people receive our message. We need to know what our audience has understood and then respond accordingly if we are to engage them in our improvement initiative.

Confirmation bias. Confirmation bias is the tendency to interpret or recall information in a way that confirms one's preexisting beliefs. People want to keep connected to the ideas they already have. Confirmation bias is especially strong in emotionally charged issues and for deeply entrenched beliefs.

Sometimes we communicate with people to create an understanding of the problem and the need to change, but communication fails because people cling to their views and only recall the information that confirms their preexisting opinions.

Cognitive dissonance. The cognitive dissonance theory suggests that we have an inner drive to hold our actions and beliefs in harmony to avoid "dissonance" (Festinger 1957). If our actions and beliefs don't match, we experience a state of anxiety. This state of anxiety propels us to do three things:

1. Act differently.
2. Reject the ideas that cause dissonance, allowing the beliefs that do not cause dissonance to prevail.
3. Create a new view of the situation that justifies our actions and avoids the internal conflict.

Dissonance generates a painful feeling in our brain. When people are presented with a problem and are told they need to change, people reject the evidence and cling to their opinions (their beliefs match their current behavior) in order not to create a state of dissonance. Cognitive dissonance can be evidenced by observing neural activity in the anterior cingulate cortex on an MRI (Van Veen 2009).

WHAT SHOULD YOU DO TO COMMUNICATE EFFECTIVELY?

Effective communication does not only depend on what is said but when it is said, the person delivering the message, the delivery method, and the strategies to enhance communication.

...Start Early

- **Communication should start at the beginning of the project, even if only partial information is available.** We need information and the sooner we get it, the better. The objective is to build frontline stakeholder engagement at the beginning of the QI project. Communication should start early, be frequent, and consistent (Hiatt 2012).

- **Communicating early sets the right expectations.** If we communicate with people early, then they have a chance to digest the issues and prepare for the coming changes. Frequent updates should be made to inform sponsors and front line stakeholders about the progress of the project, findings, significant dates in the project lifecycle, and next steps.

...Begin with the Leader

- **Improvement is change, and change brings uncertainty.** Improvement and change generate uncertainty and uncertainty creates a state of anxiety in people. People need the presence of a leader to understand the QI project, the changes, and how it all fits in the scheme of things. Leaders help convey clarity, inspire trust, and provide hope in times of difficult changes. Leaders need to be accessible and spend as much time as possible connecting with the frontline professionals.
- **Leaders need to explain why.** The leader must explain why the change is needed and what will happen if we do not change. The benefits of improvement need to be clearly stated. Knowing the "why" provides certainty, legitimizes the improvement project, and gives credibility to the improvement team. Details of what we are going to do, and how we are going to change, i.e. the details, can come from the QI team and mid-level managers with direct contact with the front lines. Different project stakeholders have different roles in the communication strategy (see Table 25-1).

...Communicate Face-to-Face

Choose face-to-face communication when possible. We all know the preferred method of communication is face-to-face. In an era of internet, social media, and 24 / 7 connectivity, face-to-face communication is still the most effective way to communicate with the frontline stakeholders. Face-to-face communication is advantageous because it is more personal and provides a better platform for feedback with questions and answers from the target audience.

...Create a Compelling Argument

- **Start with the aim.** The primary aim of the communications strategy is to promote awareness and understanding of the QI project and to engage the hearts and minds of front line staff and providers in achieving the goals of the project.
- **Explain the what and the why.** Share the hospital's (unit, area, department) vision and commitment to excellence. Share the role of the frontline staff and providers in facilitating the hospital's commitment to excellence. Highlight the

TABLE 25-1   The Different Roles for Communication

Roles in the Communication Strategy		
Key player	What is their role?	Why?
The Primary Sponsor	• Help identify the problem; explain the importance of addressing the problem now. • Clarify and define the project; explain the "why" behind the project; explain why the project is important. • Place the project in the context of the organizational mission and vision.	The leaders legitimize the project and the QI team.
The QI team members	• Update leaders and key stakeholders on the status of the project. • Share findings; share data; interpret findings. • Explain the changes.	The QI team delivers the information needed for engagement and ownership of the improvement initiative.
The mid-level frontline managers	• Explain and embrace the changes. • Explain the why behind the changes. • Explain what is going to change and what is not going to change. • Help the front line understand how we are going to operationalize the changes.	The mid-level managers deliver the information needed to operationalize the changes.

excellent work the unit (area, department) is doing; address the problem and how it affects the customer (patient, staff, provider). Share the performance gaps and why we are addressing the problem now. What will happen if a change is not made?

...Use Stories

- **Bring the power of stories to your communication.** Stories can be powerful triggers of emotions which are powerful influencers of change. Formal presentations, such a PowerPoint slides, activate our analytical brains and result in the analysis and scrutinization of the information we receive. As a result, when faced with a formal presentation, rather than build buy-in, we look for weaknesses in the arguments to dismiss the need for change. Stories on the other hand activate brain centers involved in feelings and emotions. This creates a much more powerful, engaging, and less-threatening message. The more engaged we feel with the story, the more likely we are to relate to it. As a result, stories tap into our emotions and help us accept the need for change.

- **Use images.** Images are easier for the brain to comprehend and create a better understanding of the issues. When delivering a compelling message, a picture is worth a thousand words.

...Leverage Early Adopters

Involve the frontline staff. Involve the early adopters and frontline staff in communication activities so that they can share their experience and promote engagement and ownership of the QI project (Copper 2015).

...Create Certainty

Uncertainty creates anxiety; anxiety creates a fight or flight response. While we cannot create certainty about every aspect of a change, we can create certainty about the need for change and the communication process we are going to follow to inform people about the change.

- **Create certainty about why the improvement and the change are needed.** The leader must explain why the change is needed and what will happen if we do not change. Use **myth-busting sessions** where rumors and speculations about a change are addressed and issues are clarified to avoid uncertainty and the natural state of threat that comes with it (Scarlet 2016). Make sure communication is clear about what needs to be improved, what doesn't, what is going to change, what is not. It is often said that people prefer to receive bad news and know what the future holds rather than no news. In the latter, people often imagine the worst.
- **Create certainty about the frequency of communication.** Make sure people know they are going to be informed at regular intervals and they also know who to contact for information and how information can be obtained.
- **The three questions.** All communication with the front line or the local sponsors should end with an answer to these three questions:
  o Who is going to answer questions if I have a doubt?
  o Where can I get feedback and an update about the project?
  o How often will you inform me of changes?

...Give Hope

- **Issues can be resolved.** Communication should give a certain measure of hope. A good way of doing this is to give examples of similar problems that have been resolved by other teams or examples of other hospitals that had the same problem and have successfully resolved the issue.

- **The early adopters.** Share the experience of early adopters to encourage others to accept the change.

Quotable quote. "Everything looks like a failure in the middle of a QI project." Rosabeth Moss-Kanter, Six Keys to Positive Change

...Repeat the Message Often

- **Communication should not be a single event**. Communication is a process. To understand the problems and create awareness for the need to change, people require the message to be repeated and digested. The acceptance and buy-in for the change evolve over time. Individuals and groups adapt to the change at their own pace.
- **Internalization, confirmation bias, and cognitive dissonance sometimes makes it difficult for people to accept the project and the need for change**. Give them time; communicate often; make sure people understand the issues and how change will affect them.
- **Messages should be repeated at least four times through multiple channels.** We chose four times as a starting number. The more you communicate, the better the message flows through the different stakeholder groups. Use the available communication channels in the hospital: email, bulletin boards, desktops on computer screens, departmental staff, and provider meetings, etc. Communication should be appropriate and relevant for each audience and for each phase of the project.

... Listen and Get Feedback

- **Understand their issues.** Make sure you understand the issues of the front line. Allow for time and a mechanism for feedback; clarify your understanding of their issues and express to the listener that you are on the same team and focused on the same goals by using the words "we," "our," and "us."
- **Understand the effectiveness of your message.** Communication without feedback often fails because it doesn't provide the communicator a way to assess the effectiveness of the message. Communication must always be evaluated according to the goal and desired outcome to make sure people heard what was intended. With feedback, misunderstandings can be properly addressed. Listen more often than you speak; observe the verbal and nonverbal messages delivered with an awareness of the situational context. Nonverbal communication influences the interpretation of the message significantly when expressing feelings and personal information, as it accounts for over 55% of the message

during in-person communication (Mehrabian 1967). Nonverbal communication includes eye contact, posture, facial expression, tone of voice, and physical proximity, and requires an awareness of the situational context to fully understand what is being conveyed by the sender and how the message is being perceived by the listener.

- **Empathy creates trust.** Conveying empathy by acknowledging and showing an understanding of the barriers and challenges faced by the listener helps pave the way for engagement and buy-in. Before people consider the problem, they need to know leaders understand their issues and care about them. This can only happen when project leaders listen. If people feel understood, they can progress to trusting us and seeing the facts that are presented more clearly.

Quotable quote: "Courage is what it takes to stand up and speak; courage is also what it takes to sit down and listen." Winston Churchill

TIPS FOR ONE-ON-ONE COMMUNICATION

Similar to the ways in which healthcare professionals communicate during high-stakes patient care situations, it is critical to embrace effective communication strategies when communicating one-on-one during a QI project. Often, QI team members and frontline stakeholders will have different opinions about the problem and the ways to resolve it. To avoid misunderstandings that may negatively affect the project's progress, here are some useful communication tactics:

Speaking

- **Manage yourself first.** Managing your stress and negative emotions tends to reduce the likelihood of conflicts.
- **Practice.** Think what you are going to say; practice assertive communication in which you convey your message in an open, honest, and respectful way while avoiding aggressive communication in which you convey your message in a hostile, forceful, or demanding way.
- **Be clear.** Practice speaking clearly and concisely in an even tone of voice.
- **It's not personal.** Avoid criticism, judgment, or blame of the other person's position. Remember, the stakeholder is the expert in the front line.

Listening

- Listen more often than you speak.
- Take it all in; listen to what the other person says. Observe verbal and non-verbal communication. Nonverbal communication It requires an awareness

of the situational context to fully understand what is being conveyed by the sender and how the message is being perceived by the listener.

- Make sure you understand what people say. Ask for feedback; paraphrase and clarify your understanding of their message.
- Express to the listener that you are on the same team and focused on the same goals by using the words "we," "our," and "us."
- Convey empathy by acknowledging an understanding of the barriers and challenges faced by the listener.

USE A COMMUNICATION PLANNER TO MAKE IT EASIER

While effective communication is a critical aspect of any quality improvement project, a systematic and structured communication strategy is often not formally incorporated into QI projects. This is a mistake. A communication strategy that provides a roadmap for how information relating to the project and the changes will be communicated to the frontline staff and providers is critical. Cooper and colleagues talk about the need for a **communication bundle** to enhance communication and achieve a more successful outcome. They define their communication bundle as "a small, specific collection of communication components that enhances engagement with a program, and promotes awareness, understanding, and adoption of change" (Copper 2015). Their communication bundle incorporates six components:

1. The aim (What do you want to achieve?)
2. The audience (Whom do you need to engage?)
3. The message (What do you need to say?)
4. The channel (How will you reach your audience?)
5. The story (How will you engage your audience?)
6. The review (What was the impact, and what will you learn for next time?)

For any strategy, communication should start at the beginning of the project and continue throughout the life cycle of the project. Initially, the objective is to build awareness of the problem and the project; later, the goal is to provide knowledge to get buy-in and support for the change.

In the authors experience, any communication strategy should address seven factors:

1. the goal,
2. the timing,
3. the audience,
4. the messenger,

5. the message,
6. the channel, and
7. feedback.

Based on these seven factors, a **Communication Planner** to deploy the QI team's communication strategy should be created (see Table 25-2).

TABLE 25-2 The Communication Planner

The Communication Planner: Phase I	
The goal	What's the problem? What's our project? Create awareness of the problem. Explain the project; get support and buy-in.
Timing	At the beginning of the project, set a time and date for each stakeholder group.
Audience	Frontline stakeholders, frontline mid-level managers.
Messenger	The Primary Sponsor and the QI team.
Message	**Introduction: the big picture** Share the hospital's Vision and Mission and commitment to excellent care. Share the role of the unit in facilitating the Hospital's commitment. Highlight the excellent work the unit (area, department) is doing. **The problem** What is the problem we are trying to fix (the "what" and the "why")? How does it affect our patients / customers? How big is the problem? Do we have a metric? Where is the data coming from? Do we have a story? Share examples. **The burning platform** Why are we addressing the problem now? What is wrong with what we are doing now? What are our current information gaps? What are our shared goals and desired results? What should be the expected level of performance? What will happen if a change is not made?
Channel	Staff meeting; faculty meeting.
Feedback	Evaluate the achievement of the desired goal and clarify misunderstandings.

The Communication Planner: Phase II	
The goal	What is our current performance? What are our findings? Share the magnitude of the problem; share data and the facts.
Timing	After mapping and the analysis of baseline performance.
Audience	Frontline stakeholders, frontline mid-level managers.

(Continued)

TABLE 25-2   (Continued)

The Communication Planner: Phase II	
Messenger	Primary Sponsor and the improvement team.
Message	**The reality** • What is the magnitude of the problem? • What data do we have, and how did we collect it in order to define the current performance (baseline data)? • Do we have a chart (graphic analysis)? • How are we performing compared to peer organizations? • Do we have any information gaps?
Channel	Staff meetings, email, bulletin boards.
Feedback	Evaluate the achievement of the desired goal and clarify misunderstandings.

The Communication Planner: Phase III	
The goal	Share causes; define the barriers to improvement; inform of possible solutions; explain the change.
Timing	After finding causes and possible solutions.
Audience	Frontline stakeholders, front line mid-level managers.
Messenger	Primary Sponsor & the improvement team.
Message by the Primary Sponsor	**The change** • What is the nature of the change? • How does the change align with our vision? • How will the change impact the hospital / department / unit? • What changes do we anticipate? • What will not change? • Who will be impacted the most and who will be impacted the least? • Who will make the decisions? **The timeline** • What is the time frame to implement the changes? **Define success** • How will we know the change has been successful? • What are the specific metrics we are going to measure? What are the goals? **Create hope** • Do we have previous experiences of similar changes? • Do we have a story or examples of similar change? What was the result?

(Continued)

TABLE 25-2   (Continued)

The Communication Planner: Phase III

Message by supervisors and mid-level managers	**Explain the change** • How will the change affect your day-to-day activities and the flow of work? • How will it affect you personally? If you change, what's in it for you? • What is true and not true about the change? • How will the project team help you with the change?
Channel	Staff meetings, faculty meetings.
Feedback	Evaluate the achievement of the desired goal and clarify misunderstandings.

TIPS TO ANNOUNCING A DIFFICULT CHANGE

You may need to inform your colleagues about a difficult change. The steps below describe the authors preferred approach:

- **Plan accordingly.** Make sure you have planned the meeting appropriately: invitation, agenda, venue, audiovisual aids, and equipment. Ensure all equipment, including video conferencing equipment, is fully functioning and you know how to fully utilize it. Make sure you will have enough time to make your presentation and to allow for a questions and answers session.
- **Start by describing the problem.** What are we trying to fix? How does it affect us, and who does it affect the most? Describe the magnitude of the problem. Explain how we are measuring it and where the data coming from.
- **Describe why we are addressing the problem now.** Why now? What is wrong with what we are doing now? What are our current information gaps? What would be the desired results and what performance should be expected? What will happen if a change is not made? What is the risk of doing nothing?
- **Talk about the important role of the people in the audience.** How does their work fit in the overall mission and vision of the organization? How does it fit in the mission of the department/ unit? Why is there help needed in fixing the problem?
- **Describe the change.** Highlight how the change addresses the issues. What will change and what will remain the same? Who will be impacted the most and who will be impacted the least? Who will make the decisions? How will the change affect every day work, roles, responsibilities? Will compensation change?

- **Tell them what a successful change will look like.** What should the future state look like? What are the objectives (clinical outcomes, quality, productivity, costs)? What are the specific metrics that will define success?
- **Define the strategy.** How are we going to achieve this change? What is the time frame to implement the changes?
- **Acknowledge problems.** Acknowledge the change's up-side and down-side. Acknowledge the problems and how we can address them. Acknowledge past failures and how we can avoid them.
- **Give hope.** Share success stories of other areas or departments in the hospital. Share stories of other hospitals or units. Don't oversell.
- **Listen and get feedback.** Show an interest in frontline professionals' questions and concerns. Answer the why, what, and how questions. Give a follow-up plan after the announcement.

REVIEW QUIZ

1. Communication
   A. creates awareness of the problem,
   B. creates engagement in the initiatives,
   C. allows individuals to make a personal decision as to whether they want to support the project,
   D. is a critical element of a quality improvement project, or
   E. all of the above

2. All of the following statements regarding message content are true EXCEPT
   A. Senior leadership should communicate the "why" behind the project.
   B. The message should be repeated once to enhance buy-in.
   C. Communication should be appropriate and relevant to each stakeholder group.
   D. Mid-level leaders and managers are best suited to explain "how" we are going to make a change.
   E. Senior leadership should be involved in all phases of the project communication.

3. All of the following statements regarding problems with communication are true EXCEPT
   A. Communication as a single event fails to create effective communication.
   B. Projection bias is when people in the know tend to assume others see things the same way they do and have the same information.
   C. People internalize what is said and often create their own meaning.
   D. Confirmation bias is when people confirm the facts.
   E. Cognitive dissonance is the state of anxiety created by the difference between our actions and our thoughts.

4. All of the following are reasons why we don't communicate enough during QI projects:
   A. We are too busy finding the solution.
   B. We don't want to say anything until we have a solution.
   C. We assume everybody knows (projection bias).
   D. Communication is an afterthought in the project planning.
   E. All of the above

Key: 1e; 2b; 3d; 4e

REFERENCES

1. Cooper A. (2015). Exploring the role of communications in quality improvement: A case study of the 1000 Lives Campaign in NHS Wales. *J Commun Health*; 8(1): 76–84.
2. Festinger L. (1957). *A theory of Cognitive Dissonance.* Stanford University Press.
3. Hiatt J. (2012). *Change Management: The People Side of Change,* 2nd ed. Prosci Learning Center Publications.
4. Mehrabian A. (1967). Decoding inconsistent communication. *Journal of Personality and Social Psychology* 6(1): 109–114.
5. Nolan K. (2005). Using a framework for spread: the case of patient access in the Veterans Health Administration. *Jt Comm J Qual Patient Saf* 31(6): 339–347.
6. Scarlet H. (2016). *Neuroscience for Organizational Change: An Evidence-based Practical Guide to Managing Change.* Kogan Page.
7. Van-Veen V. (2009). Neural activity predicts attitude change in cognitive dissonance. *Nat Neurosci* 12(11):1469–1474.

CHAPTER 26

How to Lead an Effective Team Meeting

Brandon, the ambulatory clinic manager, was encouraged by the director of outpatient services to pull together a team to work on reducing the clinic's no-show rate. The current no-show rate was 20%. Over the course of the next month, Brandon met with Dr. Jacobson, a newly hired clinic physician; Megan, the nursing director; and Sharon, the director for the medical technicians. While everyone on the team agreed that the clinic's no-show rate was high, they weren't able to get much done. Meetings were the problem. With a lack of a clear meeting agenda, Dr. Jacobson often derailed the planned discussion by talking about how busy he was with his patients; Megan defensively gave examples of how hard the nurses worked; and Sharon spent her time asserting that the med techs should not have to transport patients to radiology for X-rays.

Brandon was determined to get the team back on track. But at the third meeting that month, Sharon was the only one who showed up. Frustrated, Brandon complained about the meetings to the director of outpatient services who advised Brandon to put the project on hold until he could develop a strategy that would ensure progress toward the goal of reducing the clinic's no-show rate.

Why did meetings fail? What should have Brandon have differently?

The Quality Improvement Challenge: A Practical Guide for Physicians, First Edition.
Richard J. Banchs and Michael R. Pop.
© 2021 John Wiley & Sons Ltd. Published 2021 by John Wiley & Sons Ltd.
Companion website: www.wiley.com/go/banchs/quality

THE IMPORTANCE OF MEETINGS

While the project team performs the majority of the work outside of a meeting, it is during meetings that team members evaluate work, get feedback, and make key decisions that guide the progress of the project work.

> **Team meetings are an important channel for coordinating project activities when used effectively; they provide a forum for discussing the project work and the issues that arise.**

Meetings also afford the team the ability to partake in face-to-face interactions that can build trust and accountability. The team leader must use this time effectively and efficiently to support project team members' engagement, collaboration, and work completion efforts to accomplish superior results. Team meetings may feel like a burden to many staff and providers but a great meeting leaves team member feeling energized, and gives them a sense of accomplishment.

THE PROBLEM WITH MEETINGS

Studies cite unproductive meetings as one of the most underestimated problem of modern times. Yet anyone who leads and manages people understands that meetings are critical to the functioning of any organization. Meetings are the place where most major decisions are made. Now consider your own hospital and your team: What are some of the problems you have experienced with meetings? Let's face it: meetings are often a waste of time. Professionals in a hospital spend 25% to 40% of their time in meetings: team meetings, committee meetings, executive meetings, sub-specialty meetings, and the list goes on.

Studies show that on average, 33% of the time spent on meetings is unproductive and only 25% of meetings achieve their intended outcome. A recent survey revealed that 72% of hospital administrators and physician leaders spend more time in meetings now than they did five years ago, and 45% expect to spend more time in meetings four years from now. In accordance to **Parkinson's law,** "meetings expand to fill the time allotted for their completion", meaning that the more time you have, the longer meetings last and the more time is wasted. However, for such a time-consuming activity, only 33% of the surveyed leaders had formal training in how to run a meeting. While 75% said that it is "almost essential" to have an agenda, 50% admitted to using the agenda only 50% of the time.

Most healthcare professionals dread attending meetings, considering them to be a waste of their time and an interference with their work-flow. Clinicians in particular struggle to become engaged in meetings when they are focused on patient care issues.

As a result, it is imperative for project leaders to respect participants' time and competing demands by conducting meetings in an effective and efficient manner.

ANATOMY OF A GREAT MEETING

In order to make team meetings productive and an effective tool of your project strategy, consider a team meeting a process. Like any process, a team meeting should

- have a structure with phases and steps;
- be guided by rules;
- be effective, repeatable, efficient, and reproducible; and
- be continuously improved.

To make a meeting effective and efficient, give it structure and make it interesting (Lencioni 2004 & Herold 2016). To accomplish this, a team meeting should be divided in three different and very distinct phases: before the meeting, during the meeting, and after the meeting. Each phase has several steps and activities that, when followed, will lead to the meeting being productive and accomplishing its goals.

FIRST PHASE: BEFORE THE MEETING

Most of the work should be done before the meeting to decrease the work needed during the meeting and increase the likelihood of success (see Figure 26-1).

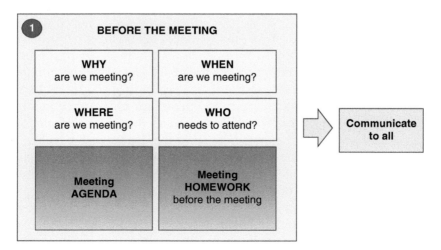

FIGURE 26-1   Anatomy of a great meeting: what to do before the meeting.

First, Ask the Question: Why Are We Meeting?

The key to a more effective meeting is first deciding if we need to meet. Differentiate between the need for one-way information dissemination and two-way information sharing. *Avoid a meeting if the same information can be conveyed in an email or brief report.*

If the purpose is to disseminate information, one can use a variety of other communication alternatives such as sending an email, posting the information on a board, or conveying the information on the hospital's intranet. If you want to be sure you have delivered the right message and people are on board, you can always schedule a meeting to simply answer questions about the information you have sent. By remembering to ask yourself, "Is a meeting the best way to handle this?", you will cut down on time wasted and convey the message that scheduled meetings are truly necessary.

Second, Ask Yourself: What Are We Trying to Accomplish?

Set objectives before the meeting. Before planning the agenda for the meeting, write down the answer to the question: "The reason we are meeting is so that at the end of the meeting we can . . ."

Depending on the focus of the meeting, how you complete the sentence may be different. It may include the need to come up with new ideas, solve a problem, or decide on an action plan. Answering the question first will help you better plan the meeting. The more concrete your meeting objectives are, the more focused your agenda will be. An additional benefit of having an objective for each meeting is to establish a concrete measure against which you can evaluate the success in meeting that objective. So according to the objective you have set, plan the agenda and decide who should attend the meeting. In general, we can identify four types of meetings: meetings to share information; meeting to discuss how to solve a problem (problem-solving meetings); meetings to create new options (creative meetings); meetings to get consensus and make decisions about issues.

Plan Where, When, and with What?

Plan for the resources you will need to run the meeting; this includes software, hardware, videoconferencing equipment, and any other item you may need. Communicate, as needed, the logistics of equipment and room arrangements. Test the technology to ensure all is functioning properly **before** the meeting. Nothing is worse than team members sitting around a table waiting for you to find the right cable or connector. This is especially true when the presenter is a Mac user and the hospital uses PCs only!

Share the Agenda

The agenda's purpose is to focus the team and improve the efficiency of the meeting. What's the most important thing you should do with your agenda? Answer: share it with the participants ahead of the meeting and then follow it closely during the meeting!

Provide the agenda beforehand to all participants. Include the time, date, and location of the meeting and any background information they may need. The agenda is the **map** that provides the leader and the team with direction. It's the leader's best weapon against the team getting off track. The agenda includes the reason for meeting, topics to be discussed, and desired outcome.

Prepare Homework

Give participants something to prepare for the meeting, and that meeting will take on a new significance.

You cannot expect a meeting to be productive if you ask for feedback on a report and you don't share it before the meeting for people to review. The same goes for resolving problems or coming up with new creative ideas. People need time before a meeting to review documents and to think about the issues before their scheduled meetings.

- For problem-solving meetings, have the team read the background information before the meeting so that they can get down to the key issues right away.
- For creative meetings, give the team member a framework for creativity; for example, ask each team member to think of one possible countermeasure to the problem to get everyone thinking about the meeting topic ahead of time.
- For consensus meetings, share with participants a summary of all the information so that they come to the meeting prepared to ask questions, and decide on the issue.

SECOND PHASE: DURING THE MEETING

This phase has several steps (see Figure 26-2).

Introductions / Break the Ice

During this step

- Introduce yourself and the participants (if it is a new team).
- Introduce the topic (for a kick-off meeting).
- Briefly go over the goals of the meeting and time allowances.
- Briefly review the ground rules (see next section).

Does Everybody Have a Role?

For any team meetings to be effective and efficient, *meeting roles need to be assigned and shared among participants.* If you can avoid it, make sure these roles are not carried out by the same team member at every meeting; roles should be rotated after several meetings.

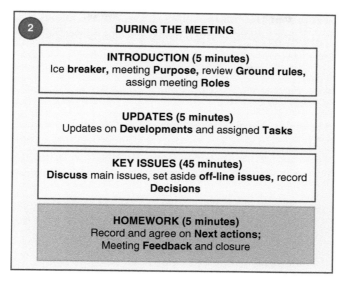

FIGURE 26-2   Anatomy of a great meeting: what to do during the meeting.

There are four main roles:

1. The **meeting leader or facilitator.** This is the person who sets the agenda, leads the meeting, and keeps the meeting on track. The meeting leader remains consistently neutral during the meeting, supporting the process, and coaching the team.
2. The **scribe.** This person captures ideas and thoughts on a white board or flip chart to stimulate the creative process, allowing the facilitator to focus on the agenda.
3. The **timekeeper.** This person keeps track of the time spent on each item on the agenda, keeps the team on task, and plays the "bad cop" by notifying the team when time is running out.
4. The **note taker.** This team member is responsible for recording both the decisions and actions moving forward. He or she should be the person responsible for distributing the follow-up assignments to the participants.

Follow the Agenda

The agenda should include

- **A quick update** (approx. 10 minutes). Allow each team member to update other participants about the most important developments as they relate to the action items from the last QI project meeting.

- **A quick review of the goals** (less than 5 minutes). Review the defining objectives of the project and note the current status and progress of each.
- **The issue section** (approx. 40 minutes). These are the key issues with an assigned order for the discussion; make sure to create a way to document overflowing topics; these topics may need to be addressed off-line or in subsequent meetings.
- **A section for decisions and actions** (approx. 5 minutes). This section helps chart all the decisions taken during the meeting and actions agreed upon. Include the time frame for the actions; discuss the team member's commitments, and get them to verbally agree to the established timeline.

Run the Meeting

- **Follow the agenda.** Complete each item before continuing on to the next. Initiate and allow open discussion for each topic. Help maintain focus and progress of the team. Make sure decisions are clarified and all members of the team understand what is going to happen and who is responsible.
- **Discuss the issues.** Run the meeting, ask questions, help clarify items, mine for productive conflict. Follow the agenda and complete each item before continuing to the next item. Maintain the focus and progress of the team and make sure everybody weighs in. . .even the quiet one in the corner! Wrap up each item after discussion in a timely manner. Summarize the issues as needed.

Remember fostering **productive conflict** is good and necessary. It is only then that all ideas and the best options arise. If you are the leader, help team members express their ideas; mine for productive conflict and wait until the end to express your own views.

Decisions, Decisions, Decisions!

Confirm that decisions are understood and recorded in the meeting minutes. Record off-topic statements and make an action item list so that you can review the issues at a later date. This will show all team members you value their input as well as their time. Discuss the potential agenda for next meeting.

What's Next?

Don't finish any meeting without deciding what to do next. During the meeting, listen for key comments that flag action items (we should. . ., why don't we. . ., it is important that we. . .) and don't let them pass by without addressing them. Make sure there is agreement on what tasks need to be done and assign them as they arise. *Finalize the meeting by summarizing all action items, identifying what needs to done, by whom, and in what time frame.*

How Did We Do?

Assign the last few minutes of every meeting to **solicit feedback** on how the meeting went and what improvements could be made. What worked well? What can we do to improve? Every participant should briefly provide a comment in the form of a suggested action. Take the opportunity to recognize good work and thank all who participated in the meeting.

THIRD PHASE: AFTER THE MEETING

Remember: "It's not over until the . . ." email reminds us of what's next!
Complete meeting notes and distribute them in a timely manner. Rather than sending a long document containing every statement made at the meeting, we prefer to send a brief document that contains only the decisions made and the action items for the next meeting (see next for template). Email the "Team Meeting Organizer" to all meeting participants and then place a copy and any other supporting document in a common drive, or web-based dropbox. Implement action items and any other assignments as needed. For those tasks that are critical to meet the team's deadlines, consider setting up reminders for the individual team members that are responsible for them.

A TEMPLATE FOR ALL YOUR MEETINGS: THE TEAM MEETING ORGANIZER

There are several templates out there to help you run productive and effective meetings. This is our preferred team meeting organizer (see Table 26-1). Our template

- follows a one-page per meeting format;
- is sent to team participants before the meeting to set the agenda and let them know what documents need to be reviewed;
- is used during the meeting as follow-up for the previous meeting's action-list, and to guide the order for discussion on the current agenda; and
- is used after the meeting as a record-keeper for: topics discussed, key decisions made, action items, and work assignments for the next meeting.

Before the meeting, the team meeting organizer is distributed among all participants with the first section completed (from "Project name" to "Agenda for this meeting"); after the meeting, the same document is sent to all participants with the second sections finalized ("Decisions made during the meeting" to "Action items"). We find the Team Meeting Organizer a very useful tool to run meetings, keep track of all decisions made and actions taken. It is an easy document to refer back to throughout the life-cycle of the QI project. We believe in the effectiveness of "one meeting, one page".

TABLE 26-1   The QI Team Meeting Organizer Template

Team Meeting Organizer	
Project name	
Meeting #	
Objective	
Why are we meeting?	
Meeting logistics	
When?	
Where?	
Who should attend?	
Documents to be reviewed before the meeting	Who will present?
Action items due from last meeting	Who is the lead?
Agenda for this meeting	
Decisions made during the meeting	

(Continued)

TABLE 26-1   (Continued)

Team Meeting Organizer		
Action items	By who?	By when?

TEAM MEETING GROUND RULES

What Are They and Why Do We Need Them?

Effective teams develop rules of conduct at the beginning of their work to help them achieve their purpose and performance goals.

If you want your team meetings to be productive, you need meeting ground rules, and you need to agree on how to use them. Having meeting ground rules can significantly improve how your team solves problems and makes decisions. Some ground rules are related to procedural issues, for example "always start on time" or "answering phones is not allowed." Others help create productive behavior. Behavioral ground rules describe specific actions that team members should take to behave in a manner that is conducive to the meeting's success. These behavioral rules need to be specific because group members may have different ideas of what "treat everyone with respect" may mean. Ground rules are crucial to maintain the self-confidence and self-esteem of the team. They ensure and maintain a constructive relationship among all participants. "Agreement on key issues help teams establish a framework upon which members can develop as a unit of effective performance" (Katzenbach 1993).

If you are going to meet more than once, it is advisable to review your ground rules at each meeting. It just makes the rules of the game clear to everyone. Late arrivals? People answering cell phones during the meeting? Notification pings on laptops and phones? Side conversations? Long speeches of unrelated topics? *The ground rules establish the guidelines for the team's dynamics and behaviors*:

- Ground rules need to be established early in the process, before conflict arises.
- They must be defined, communicated, understood and agreed upon by the entire team.
- Before each meeting, the ground rules should be reviewed.

The team makes the decisions, sets the ground rules, and enforces peer accountability. The ground rules set by the team are the tools the leader will be using to resolve issues and successfully manage productive conflict.

Steps to Developing Ground Rules

> **Meeting ground rules are the rules of engagement that help teams establish a common approach to the work that needs to be done.**

- **Agree on the need for ground rules.** Take time to discuss and develop a common understanding of what ground rules mean; this will increase the chance that the rules will be implemented consistently and effectively in different situations.
- **Develop ground rules with everybody's input.** To be effective, meeting ground rules should foster three things: strong performance, positive working relationships, and individual well-being. Ground rules are powerful tools for improving a team process.
- **Share the responsibility.** Agree that everyone is responsible for helping each other use the ground rules. Teams are too complex to expect that the formal leader alone can identify every time a team member is acting at odds with a ground rule. In effective teams, all members share this responsibility, meaning teams should agree on how individuals will intervene when they see others not following a ground rule.
- **At the end of each meeting, discuss how you can improve.** Discuss how you are using the ground rules and how to improve. Take five minutes at the end of each team meeting to discuss what you could do differently.

If the Project Charter is the leader's north star, and the agenda is the map that provides the team with direction, *the ground rules are the compass that helps the leader find his or her way when conflict arises.*

Example of Ground Rules

- **Be on time, every time.** Meetings start and finish on time; don't punish the prompt by making them wait for stragglers.
- **Stay in the meeting.** Laptops and electronic devices should be limited to making presentations, keeping notes, or looking up relevant information. Participants should not take phone calls unless there is an emergency.
- **Challenge the idea, not the individual.** Different opinions are welcomed; challenge the ideas, not the individuals. Treat others and their ideas as you want to be treated.

- **Focus on the need, not the solution.** By moving from arguing about solutions to identifying needs that must be met in order to solve a problem, you reduce unproductive conflict. State views and explain the why. Shift from monologues and arguments to a conversation in which members can understand everyone's point of view and how others reached their conclusions.
- **No sacred cows.** All ideas need to be challenged; contrary views need to be encouraged to support robust decision-making and to prevent groupthink. Every idea can be used as a building block for other ideas and workable solutions.
- **Disagree in private, unite in public.** Irrespective of how you have voted, once a decision has been made, everyone should support it and speak with one voice outside of the meeting. Be an ambassador of the project and the change initiative.
- **Silence is agreement.** It is unacceptable to remain silent during a meeting and then later say you don't agree with the group decision.
- **Everyone does real work.** No special privileges. We are united by the same goal.
- **Do what you say you will do.** Individuals are accountable for following through on agreed actions, and the group should hold each other mutually accountable.

BRUCE TUCKMAN AND THE FOUR STAGES OF TEAM DEVELOPMENT

Teams go through stages in their development. The most commonly used framework for a team's stages of development was established in the mid-1960s by Bruce W. Tuckman (Tuckman 1965). Tuckman describes four stages of team development: Forming, Storming, Norming, and Performing (see Figure 26-3). Forming a cohesive team takes time and members often go through these four recognizable stages as

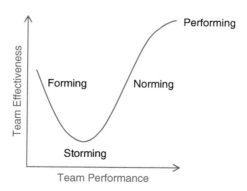

FIGURE 26-3   The four stages of team development by Bruce Tuckman.

they progressively develop maturity, establish relationships, and increase their ability to perform. Before they can work effectively, team members often struggle to find their purpose and work as a unit. In our experience, a team's stage of development is intimately connected to their ability to run effective meetings and vice-versa. Therefore, the four stages of Tuckman are a helpful framework for recognizing a team's behavioral patterns and creating a strategy for running effective and successful meetings. These stages are fluid, not linear, and should not be used as an absolute. Instead they should be used as a basis for discussion about the team's performance between the leader and team members.

> *While the maturity and ability of the team changes as it progresses through the different stages, so should the leadership style. During the four stages, the authority and freedom extended by the leader to the team increases while the control of the leader is gradually reduced. In this regard, the Tuckman model is very similar to Hersey and Blanchard's* **Situational Leadership**® **model** *described in Chapter 27 (Hersey 2012, Blanchard 2003).*

Forming Stage: The Beginning of the Team and Team Meetings

How team members feel and behave. During the first meetings, team members are polite, watchful and guarded. Communication among team members is low and the individual behavior is driven by a desire to fit in, avoid controversy or conflict. Individuals are expectant, gather information, and form impressions about each other, the team unit, the leader, and the scope of the project. Some members may be somewhat anxious. The purpose and goals of the team are unclear, and so team members feel varying degree of confusion and are unsure about their commitment. During meetings, team members tend to behave quite independently, with little interconnection, depending exclusively on the leader.

How the leader can help. At this stage, the leader plays a predominant role in the team and team meeting dynamics because team members are unclear about their place on the team and the purpose of the team. The leader should

- help the team set the ground rules that will direct team meetings,
- help clarify the goals of the project,
- clarify team member's individual roles and doubts,
- encourage discussion and exchanges,
- support the successful completion of the different assigned tasks, and
- get feedback and make sure all concerns are expressed.

The team leader should constantly refer back to the Problem Statement and Project Charter to make sure the goals and objectives of the project are clearly understood.

Storming Stage: Differences Arise

How team members feel and behave. After several meetings, team members start expressing their opinions and bid for position. Some tensions and conflict arise as member's natural different working styles collide. Work often does not progress and the team feels stuck. One of the hallmarks of this stage is for team members to be frustrated and feel overwhelmed because they don't clearly understand their role and the work strategy. They don't have a clear picture of what they should do and how work should be done. This stage can be unpleasant, especially for those who are averse to conflict. There is lower motivation to progress, and in general, team performance drops.

How the leader can help. The leader can help the team transition to the next level of performance by doing a number of things:

- Reinforce the established ground rules.
- Continuously refocus on the purpose and goals of the project.
- Emphasize tolerance of each team member and their differences with the goal to create an environment where differences of opinion are encouraged, members can express their feelings, and no judgment is passed.
- "Democratize" the team's contributions: all ideas are welcomed.
- Ask all team members to contribute and encourage productive conflict.
- Build mutual trust and commitment among team members by focusing on clarity of goals, purpose, and work strategy (see next chapter on high performing teams).
- Address and resolve conflicts as they occur.
- Remind people that productive conflict is desirable and remain positive and encourage the team to keep moving forward.

Norming Stage

How team members feel and behave. Team members start resolving their differences, accept the leader, and converge on a common purpose and common goals. The team now shares an understanding on the goals and the strategy on how to achieve them. Members are willing to give up their ideas and positions to make the team successful. Team members develop a stronger bond, are able to ask for help, and are willing to receive constructive feedback from one another. In this stage, team members feel accountable for the results. Norms and dynamics have been established.

How the leader can help. The role of the leader during this stage is to keep the team motivated and engaged during the meetings. It's about keeping the team moving forward. The leader should help team members accept the responsibility for the completion of tasks; mine for constructive conflict so that all ideas, controversial or not, are expressed; focus the team on the high leverage behaviors needed to succeed: robust discussions, mutual accountability, and follow-through (see Chapter 27).

Performing Stage

How team members feel and behave. The team functions as a unit and achieves their objectives effectively without destructive conflict or the need for external supervision. The team members are now competent, autonomous, and able to handle the decision-making process without much supervision. Different and conflicting ideas are expected and invited, and handled appropriately by the team.

How the leader can help. The leader should: delegate as much as possible and help team members achieve their goals; encourage members to challenge their own assumptions and find alternative solutions; focus on other aspects of the project such as communication with the front line and Primary Sponsor.

UNDERSTANDING DIFFERENCES IN PEOPLE'S BEHAVIOR

Differences in people are usually personality based. People very rarely set out to cause upset. People behave differently because they are different. **Personality tests** (psychometric test) can be useful to

- develop understanding of personality typology, traits, thinking styles;
- understand and improve communication among team members;
- understand the best learning style for each team member; and
- improve the knowledge, motivation, and behavior of self and others.

The most common personality tests are

- The **DISC** (Dominance, Influence, Steadiness, Conscientiousness);
- The **Myers Briggs** Type Indicator (MBTI);
- The **Thomas-Kilmann**, a conflict mode instrument; and
- The **Kolb Learning Style** Inventory.

REFERENCES

1. Blanchard K. *The One Minute Manager.* William Morrow 2003.
2. Herold C. *Meetings suck.* Lioncrest Publishing 2016
3. Hersey P. *Situational Leadership. Management of Organizational Behavior: Leading Human Resources.* Prentice Hall 2012.
4. Katzenbach JR. The Discipline of teams. *Best of Harvard Business review* 1993.
5. Lencioni P. "Death by Meeting". Wiley Editorial 2004.
6. Tuckman B. Developmental sequence in small groups. *Psychological Bulletin* 1965. 63: 384–399

CHAPTER 27

How to Help Your QI Team Become a High-Performing Team

THE USUAL REASONS WHY WE LAUNCH A QI TEAM

QI teams are usually launched in response to two situations:

1. **To address a problem of effectiveness.** An area of poor performance is affecting patients, staff, or providers. The problem must be identified and corrected so that the process delivers what the customer needs. Problems of effectiveness include safety and quality of care.

2. **To address a problem of efficiency.** A process critical to customer satisfaction is not delivering the output according to the customer's needs. Problems of efficiency include time, costs, and the resources used to deliver high-quality care.

WHAT MAKES A TEAM, A TEAM?

Professionals are grouped together in healthcare organizations to provide patient care, perform administrative functions, and complete tasks. But these associations do not constitute "teams." They are "groups" or "working groups." Professionals in these situations recognize their individual contributions to the achievements of the groups, but often their personal goals and the goals of the group do not coincide. Members of

The Quality Improvement Challenge: A Practical Guide for Physicians, First Edition.
Richard J. Banchs and Michael R. Pop.
© 2021 John Wiley & Sons Ltd. Published 2021 by John Wiley & Sons Ltd.
Companion website: www.wiley.com/go/banchs/quality

a team, on the other hand, recognize their individual contributions and understand that both personal and team goals are best accomplished with mutual support.

Working groups are groups of two or more people with potentially common interests, objectives, and a continued interaction. Teams are different. Jon Katzenbach defines a team as a **"small number of people with complementary skills who are committed to a common purpose and performance goals, and who agree on an approach for which they are mutually accountable"** (Katzenbach 1993).

Teams are not just groups of people; teams have specific characteristics that differentiate them from working groups (see Table 27-1). Without proper individual selection and careful facilitation, a group may not have the opportunity to evolve into a high-performing improvement team during a QI project.

TABLE 27-1   Characteristics of Teams versus Groups

Characteristics of Teams versus Groups		
Dimension	**Teams**	**Groups**
Goals	Teams are highly focused on achieving clearly defined, common goals.	Groups often are poorly focused or without a true common goal.
Performance	In teams, the shared individual expertise yields synergistic effects in which the sum of their combined efforts is greater than their individual contributions.	In groups, performance results from individual goal achievement.
Accountability	Teams require both individual and mutual accountability.	Groups are focused on individual accountability.
Commitment	Empathetic understanding of other members' roles, responsibilities, and workflow barriers unify their commitment to achieving a common goal.	Members of a group often avoid diving below the surface to uncover commonalities with other group members.
Trust	Team members are willing to expose their vulnerability by honestly revealing their ideas and feedback, which requires trust.	Group members may remain guarded and be unwilling to take emotional risks.
Dynamics	Team dynamics allow for breakthrough discoveries that move beyond constraints to optimal solutions and deliverables.	In groups, perceived constraints and conflicting individual objectives define the limits of the possible solutions and deliverables.
Identity	Team identity fosters motivation, higher performance, and pride in membership.	The value in group participation is not often perceived.

THE CHALLENGE FOR QI TEAMS IN HEALTHCARE

Developing effective teams is critical in quality improvement. QI projects require the coordination of defined activities that must be accomplished by specific persons based on their roles within a certain time frame. The task of building a multidisciplinary team of clinical and operational stakeholders who work together to attain the project's objectives is not easy. It requires support and structured facilitation. As we reviewed in Chapter 6, to be successful and achieve a high level of functionality, an improvement team needs to overcome three main challenges:

1. **Time.** QI teams often struggle with getting off quickly to a productive start. Finding the time to carry on their project activities is difficult. Resource constraints related to time, staffing, and scheduling requirements limit the availability of key stakeholders to participate regularly on QI project teams. Patient care is the priority of clinicians and QI activities are seen as secondary. As a result, teams are often composed in an indiscriminate way with an underrepresentation of frontline clinicians who cannot be excused from their patient care responsibilities.
2. **Silos.** Healthcare professionals often work in silos. This often creates confusion as to the true goals of the improvement efforts. Silos result in adherence to dysfunctional loyalties and competing priorities that contribute to complicate team development and performance.
3. **Pushback.** QI teams struggle with the lack of buy-in from the front lines and the successful hand-off required to get their recommendations implemented.

As a result of the functional structure that exists in many healthcare organizations, there is often a *disconnect between the clinical and the operational teams.*

- The operational teams may not understand the clinical processes sufficiently to engage in meaningful dialogue with the clinicians.
- The clinical teams may disregard or reject the input from the operational teams because they do not provide direct care for patients. It is also true that the clinical teams may not have a clear understanding of the resource limitation and constraints under which the operational teams must lead the healthcare organization.

This disconnect becomes challenging when operational teams initiate improvement projects with clinical stakeholders. Healthcare organizations, in general, present a conundrum when it comes to teamwork: healthcare professionals recognize the necessity of high-functioning teams with each patient encounter yet, the caliber of multidisciplinary team functioning within the clinical and operational areas of healthcare organizations is not always at its best.

Problems of time and silos are the most important challenges when considering how a group of professionals become a team. Without time and careful facilitation, improvement teams assembled ad-hoc may not have the opportunity to evolve into a high-performing team. Pushback is the greatest challenge to achieving the intended goals of the QI project.

FRAMEWORK FOR BUILDING A HIGH-PERFORMING TEAM

Numerous frameworks have been described:

- Allan Drexler and David Sibbet created a comprehensive model for building a high-performing team known as the **Drexler Sibbet Team Performance model.** Their model is structured around seven steps or questions that are integral to high performance and need to be resolved to allow the team to move to the next step of performance. These seven steps are: Why am I here? Who are you? What are we doing? How will we do it? Who does what, when, and where? How do we create wow? Why continue? (Drexler 2006).
- Hackman proposed the **Team Effectiveness Model** in which team composition, direction, structure, coaching, and organizational context are identified as instrumental in "providing products or services that exceed customer expectations, growing team capabilities over time, and satisfying team member needs" (Hackman 1983–2002).
- In the **Discipline of Teams**, Katzenbach and Smith's focus of four elements for high performance: Common commitment and common purpose; common performance goals; complimentary skills; and mutual accountability (Katzenbach 1993).
- **Lencioni (The 5 Dysfunctions of a Team)** proposes that teams must first develop trust in order to engage in constructive conflict. This healthy conflict supports each member's commitment to the team's work, which is required for team accountability. This shared responsibility and accountability produces the desired results (Lencioni 2000).
- **Phil Harkins** believes the four most significant behaviors consistently demonstrated by high-impact leaders driving high performance in their teams are: defining clear goals and a vision for a future; creating blueprints for action to achieve the goals; using language to build trust and create energy, what he calls "powerful conversations"; and getting the right people involved as "passionate champions" (Harkins 2006).
- **Triaxia partners** proposes a model for achieving high performance that is based on the successful achievement of six factors: A common purpose, clear

roles, accepted leadership, effective processes, solid relationships, and excellent communication (Triaxia 2015).

- Susan Annunzio from the **Center for High Performance** has focused her work on the environment in which results are achieved as the main determinant of high performance. To increase a team's performance, leaders need to focus on the single factor that is most critical to high performance – the environment of their organization and workgroups. A work environment that drives high performance is characterized by 15 attributes, organized around three drivers: valuing people, optimizing critical thinking; and seizing opportunities (Annunzio 2004).

These and other frameworks related to achieving high performance in a team share several common features of teams and their functioning that lead to exceptional outcomes. Common threads are

- The importance of leadership.
- The critical role of team selection. Without the knowledge and skills needed, a team cannot achieve its purpose and project goals.
- Need for an urgent and worthwhile pursuit.
- A collective identity that engages all team members in a shared purpose and goals (Alimo-Metcalfe 2018).
- The individual identity and the need to understand one's purpose and role in the team, membership.
- Engagement and a common work strategy to achieve the purpose and goals the team has set.
- The importance of personal achievement, self-esteem, and members contributing with their ideas and expertise.
- The key role of relationships and a climate of cooperation and communication.

The performance level of a team dictates the quality of their collective work product, which in turn, defines the degree of success they achieve with their efforts. Based on an extensive review of the literature and our own experience on the clinical front lines, we believe a team's performance is driven by four dimensions (see Figure 27-1):

1. who they are and what they know,
2. what they support and believe in,
3. how they feel, and
4. what they do.

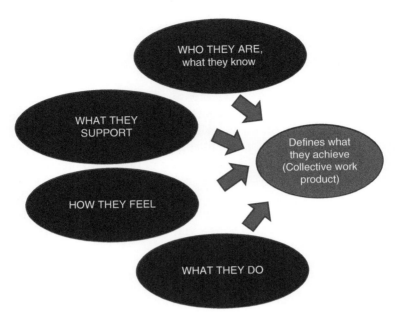

FIGURE 27-1 The four dimensions of team performance.

THE FIRST STEP TO HIGH PERFORMANCE

Having the right people is the first requirement to become a high performing team. **Who they are and what they know** is the first dimension of team performance that determines the collective work product. High-performing teams have team members with high knowledge-based proficiencies (what the team members know) and skills-based capabilities (what the team members can do), which reflect their experience and their subject-matter expertise (Lerner 2009). As we described in previous chapters, selecting the right team members becomes a critical factor in the performance of an improvement team. Members of high-performing teams are subject-matter experts and exhibit a high interactional ability to support the team dynamics necessary to reach high levels of functioning.

THE TEAM "BUILDING BLOCKS"

QI teams are established to identify and correct specific problems that affect patients, staff, or providers, and to ensure a process is functioning as efficiently as possible according to the customer's needs (problems of effectiveness and problems of efficiency). As teams work toward a **common purpose** and **goals,**

- They develop a common **commitment;** common commitment is a hallmark of high-performing teams; common commitment requires a purpose that is challenging, compelling and in which team members can believe in (Katzenbach 1993).

- They also develop commitment to a common **work strategy.**

A common purpose, a common goal, and a common work strategy is **what they support**. When team members work hard to develop a common purpose, common goals, and work strategy, they feel bound and sincerely committed to what they have developed and agreed to; this process results not only in commitment but in **trust** that all members of the team share a common view.

How team members feel towards one-another and as members of the team is of critical importance in the dynamics of high-performing teams (Katzenbach 1993). We call trust and commitment the **critical affective component** of high performing teams. The critical affective component is the third dimension of team performance or **"how they feel"** toward one another and the team. Trust and commitment develop over time and often require initial structured facilitation. Trust and commitment can overcome silo mentality and the disconnect between the clinical and operational members of the team. Open and effective communication among team members must be present to achieve this critical affective component.

Given that a central role in the performance level of teams is how team members feel, the team leader must first create the necessary conditions for trust and commitment to develop within the team. Trust and commitment develop as teams work to identify and develop their unique and common purpose and goals, even when team members initially have different views. Assuring that all members of the team share a common purpose, common goals, and a common approach or work strategy enables team members to achieve the "critical affective component." We call common purpose, common goals, and common work strategy the **team building blocks.** The team building blocks are **what the team supports and believes in,** the second dimension of team performance.

Supporting the development of trust and commitment among team members with social or work-related activities is not always feasible. This is especially true in healthcare due to the ad hoc nature of team formation and time constraints. **Clarity** around the team's purpose, goals, and work strategy is the best way to achieve the critical affective component.

Engage the Team in a Common Purpose

Define the team purpose. The team's purpose needs to be carefully considered for the QI team to achieve a high level of performance. The team's purpose needs to be **compelling** (Katzenbach 1993). That means the team's purpose

- needs to be challenging and if achieved creates a sense of accomplishment, pride, and success;
- has to have personal meaning and speak to people's beliefs and moral values;

- needs to be achievable and realistic; and
- creates a team unifying message.

Define the what's in it for me (WIIFM). The purpose of the team needs to be congruent with the individual needs of team members. People cannot connect with a purpose that is opposed to their interests and beliefs. We need to address the fact that sometimes the pursuit of a greater purpose comes at the expense of the individual needs. Assembling a QI team to improve work flow in a unit may have unintended consequences. For example, as staff finish their daily tasks earlier, they lose overtime, on which they depended to pay their bills! Teams that succeed in creating a common purpose must openly confront these issues:

- Is the WIIFM of individual members congruent and in line with the unifying purpose and goals for the team? Feedback from each team members is important to make sure everybody understands and shares in the common purpose for the team.
- Do team members believe the goals of the team can be achieved? If team members do not truly believe the goals can be achieved or have conflicting opinions about the need to launch a QI team, it will be very difficult for the project to succeed.
- Do team members have cynic views about the team charter? Decrease operating room turnover time may be a compelling purpose for the organization, but it can be easily misinterpreted as an exhortation to work harder, or a desire of the organization to improve efficiency in order to make more money. This may not be very motivating.

It is incumbent on the leader of the QI team to make sure the team agrees on a common purpose that is compelling and defines the importance of the project in the general context. Also, the individual needs (the WIIFM) are addressed. Improve clinic patient throughput may not be that appealing if the reward for efficiency is only to do more work. How can the individual beliefs, sense of accomplishment, and team spirit be addressed?

Develop a core purpose and then ask your team, "What does this mean for us as a team and as individuals?" Paint a picture of what we could achieve and what the future would look like if we could achieve it.

Connect the Team to a Common Goal

- **Set reasonable goals.** Set reasonable goals that include the performance that needs to be achieved, the time, milestones, and the objectives.
- **Create clarity around the goals.** Make sure the team's purpose is translated into goals that are clear and specific; everybody needs to understands what success looks like.

- **Define the overall strategy.** Define the overall strategy that will be used to achieve the goals; tell your team precisely what they will need to do. The more details team members get, the easier it is for them to engage; communicate the plan clearly and specifically.
- **Invite feedback.** Invite open discussion and sharing of opinions. Ask people what they think about the goals and how they think they can be achieved; giving input makes them feel empowered and it will be easier for them to commit: people support what we help create.
- **Make sure there is a level playing field.** The goals of the team need to be driven by the project and the purpose of the team, not titles, job positions, or individual agendas. This is especially important when senior physicians or hospital administrators are part of the team; the interests of a few cannot drive the goals of the project.

Define the Common Work Strategy

A common work strategy establishes a common approach or set of work processes that are going to be followed to achieve the goals. A common work strategy defines what Katzenbach calls the **social contract** (Katzenbach 1993). A common work strategy includes the specifics on schedules, meetings, roles, needed skills, decision-making processes, and how each team member contributes to the success of the team.

- **Define the rules of engagement.** Obtain consensus on the management of selected governance issues. Build a foundation upon which the team develops unity in order to achieve a higher level of performance. The "rules of engagement" defines how the team will work together.
- **Define the expectations.** Establish clear expectations on the distribution of the work; establishing clear assignment of responsibilities; make sure all the team members understand and agree on the process by which decisions are made and conflict is resolved at the initial meeting.

HIGH LEVERAGE BEHAVIORS OF HIGH-PERFORMING TEAMS

In working groups, performance is a function of how each individual performs. What matters is the individual performance, which depends on individual goals and accountability. For teams, performance is a product of both individual and collective performance, what Katzenbach calls the **collective work product** (Katzenbach 1993). The fundamental difference between teams and working groups is that teams require both individual and **mutual accountability.**

The basics of how teams are led and work together through their interactions determine the quality, quantity, and timeliness of the work that is achieved. These complex interactions are defined by the team members' **internal processes** that shape the team dynamics for all teams. Trust and commitment create the environment that allows team members to engage in robust dialogue, to demand of one another mutual accountability, and follow through with regards to the tasks they have agreed on. We have found robust dialogue, mutual accountability, and follow through to be the **high-leverage behaviors** needed for teams to become high-performing teams. High-leverage behaviors are **what they do,** the fourth dimension of team performance.

Robust Dialogue

Robust dialogue is an open, informal, and focused conversation that aims to understand the true nature of the issue and brings out reality, even when that reality is unpleasant. Robust dialogue has purpose and meaning and requires the expression of multiple viewpoints regarding the pros and cons of each available option.

Robust dialogue stimulates new ideas, generates new questions, and articulates new insights. Robust dialogue requires the team to engage in **constructive conflict**, challenging viewpoints and avoiding constrained and politicized statements, attempts to "soften reality," or maneuvers to avoid confrontation. Robust dialogue is not about wasting energy defending the old assumptions. Robust dialogue alters the psychology of a group, energizing it in the quest for new solutions. Team members strive to uncover the best answer, which means candidly sharing their ideas and acknowledging the value of the other members' contributions to the discussion. To be productive, robust dialogue must be respectful and respect personal boundaries (Bossidy 2011).

Robust dialogue can be encouraged within the project team by facilitating effective communication, conflict resolution, and decision-making practices:

- Create an environment that embraces the diversity of the team members.
- Promote the sharing of ideas.
- Coach team members on how to operationalize "robust dialogue."
- Challenge ideas but explaining that conflict must be about issues rather than people.
- Solicit feedback from team members regularly.
- Practice active listening.
- Insist on "reality" and evidence.
- Encourage team members to engage in constructive conflict to facilitate their growth, team performance, and project goal achievement.
- Use consensus decision-making processes, when appropriate.

Mutual Accountability

Approaches that support mutual accountability, or the practice in which team members hold each other responsible for the work that has been agreed-upon, include

- Require team members to adhere to the group norms that were established at the beginning of the project.
- Allow team members to set realistic deadlines for the work they are performing in accordance with the overall project work plan.
- Resolve issues with the team to ensure their input contributes to the plan.
- Empower team members to engage with each other using effective communication techniques to resolve conflicts and clarify uncertainties instead of the leader resolving the issues for them.

Follow-through

The completion of project work depends on the team's ability to follow-through on the actions and tasks that must get done. This can be facilitated by taking these steps:

- Establish a schedule with due dates for key activities and project work with the project team.
- Solicit the team members' involvement in making sure the project is on track.
- Brainstorm with the team members to generate and implement solutions to issues and action items.
- Openly discuss variances in work completion with the team.
- Develop and follow a recognition plan that acknowledges the team members' contributions and maintains their motivation for participating in the project.

When teams work diligently toward a common goal, common purpose and work strategy, trust and commitment develop. Trust and commitment allow team members to engage in robust dialogue, demand accountability of one another, and create a culture of follow-through (see Figure 27-2). Team building blocks, the Critical Affective Component, and High Leverage Behavior work as a cycle to achieve a successful work product that is engaging and energizing (see Figure 27-3).

FOCUS ON THESE SIX DRIVERS TO ACHIEVE HIGH PERFORMANCE

The specific knowledge-based proficiencies (what the team members know) and skills-based capabilities (what the team members can do) are the criteria used during the team member's selection process. The team building blocks (common purpose,

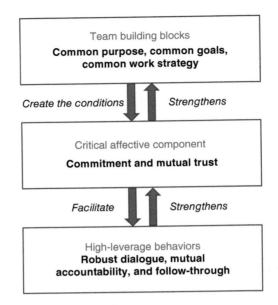

FIGURE 27-2 The six drivers of team performance.

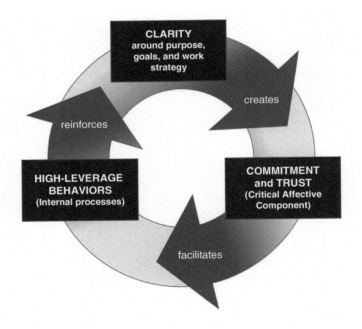

FIGURE 27-3 The team cycle drives the team to a successful work product.

common goal, and common work strategy) help develop the critical affective components (trust and commitment). As trust and commitment increase within the team, high-leverage behaviors (robust dialogue, mutual accountability, and follow-through) are enabled and become part of the fabric of the team, driving performance and goal acquisition. A common purpose, common goals, common work strategy, robust dialogue, mutual accountability, and follow-through are the essential elements of high performance leaders can incorporate into their team dynamics. They are the **six drivers of performance**. Commitment and trust are the byproducts. These six drivers must be explicitly planned, implemented, and monitored. The six drivers of high performance are the cornerstone in the team leader's strategy for leading the team and achieving the goals of the improvement initiative.

A Team's Best Practice: The Essentials

- A QI team cannot perform without securing effective organizational support: Leadership presence, appropriate resources, and time.
- A team functions at its best when it has the right people, size, mix of skills, and process knowledge.
- The ideal team leader for the QI team needs to have excellent coaching and facilitation skills.
- To achieve high performance, make sure the team shares a common purpose, common goals, and a common and clear work strategy. The team and the leaders make a commitment to following it.
- To achieve high performance, teams need to identify and agree upon a strategy to make decisions and resolve conflict.
- High-performing teams have open lines of communication and practice robust discussions, they embrace productive conflict, and insist on always addressing the reality of the situation.
- High-performing teams follow-through on their commitments and hold one another mutually accountable for the results of the team.

HOW TO IMPROVE TEAM COMMUNICATION

The quality of your team relationships has a great impact on performance. When people collaborate, they work together to understand what needs to be done and how best to go about it. As a leader, you must be able to leverage the full potential of your team so that you can tap into their diverse perspectives, skills, and experiences.

Communication is key. Communication has been defined as *a process for achieving shared understanding in which the participants exchange, acknowledge, and interpret information, ideas, and feelings.* While communication is important in every industry, the high-stakes environment, resource limitations, and time constraints inherent in healthcare organizations emphasize its criticality in this setting, not only for the provision of quality patient care but also for the successful completion of QI projects.

Communication is a vital element of the team's progressive formation and their eventual success. Communication is central to many of the team's functions and dynamics. It is important in defining the team's objectives; delineating roles and responsibilities; articulating the team's work strategy; expressing ideas and clarifying opinions; creating an environment of productive conflict, and completing the project work.

Communication failures are often implicated when the team is unable to produce the expected results. Communication is difficult, especially when communicating feelings and attitudes. The **Mehrabian formula** states that during the process of communication, only 7% of a message is in the spoken word; 38% is paralinguistic (tone, inflection, etc.), and 55% of the message is in facial expressions (Mehrabian 1971).

Expectations for team communication need to be outlined during the initial project meetings and monitored closely by the leader. Issues must be addressed promptly to restore balance to the team and resume project work. As the team matures and communication improves, so does their performance. This is because less energy is spent on internal issues and clarification of ideas and more effort is devoted to external goals and productive output.

There are several activities and practical tips to support effective communication practices:

- Clarify roles and responsibilities.
- Provide an explicit purpose and common goals.
- Create an open forum policy that welcomes all ideas.
- Standardize communication procedures for certain aspects of teamwork.
- Encourage banter and social activities among team members.
- Encourage sharing of ideas.
- Improve communication by example; practice active listening.
- Solicit feedback from team members regularly.
- Establish a mutually agreed-upon process for communication.
- Challenge the ideas, not the individual.

Developing Trust Among Team Members: the Johari Window

Effective communication requires a certain level of trust among members of a team. One way to enhance trust and team communication is by helping team members become better acquainted with one another. Initially, enhancing trust among team members may include ice-breaker-type activities at the beginning of the meetings. This helps highlight commonalities among team members and allows members to enjoy each other's company.

As the team members begin to feel more comfortable with each other, interactional exercises can promote further awareness of team member's strengths and weaknesses. An example of activities to improve communication among the members of an improvement team is the **Johari Window**. The Johari Window has been used to improve self-awareness and mutual understanding between individuals within a group.

Joseph Luft and Harry Ingham combined their first names, Joe and Harry, to name this interactional exercise the "Jo-hari" window (Luft 1955). A chosen team member is given a list of adjectives out of which they select the ones that they feel describe their personality. The other team members are also given the same list and each member picks an equal number of adjectives to describe their colleague. Examples of adjectives from the list are: Able, Accepting, Adaptable, Confident, Dependable, Friendly, Giving, Independent, Ingenious, Intelligent, Introverted, Modest, Nervous, Observant, Organized, Responsive, Searching, etc. These very adjectives are then inserted into a grid with four boxes (see Figure 27-4).

- **Quadrant 1 is called the Open Arena.** It is the part of ourselves that we see and others see. Adjectives that are selected by both the participant and his or her peers are placed into the Open Arena quadrant. This quadrant represents traits of the subjects that both they themselves and their peers perceive.

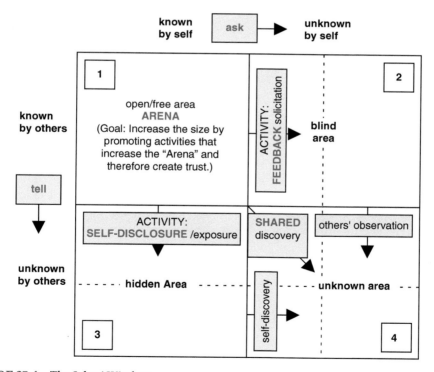

FIGURE 27-4   The Johari Window.

- **Quadrant 2 is the Blind Area.** They are the aspects that others see but we are not aware of. Adjectives that are not selected by subjects but only by their peers are placed into the Blind Area. Team members will have to decide how to inform the individual about these blind spots. Hopefully, this can be done in a respectful and safe manner.
- **Quadrant 3 is called the Hidden Area.** It is our private space, which we know but hide from others. Adjectives selected only by subjects, but not by any of their peers, represent information about oneself that peers are either unaware of or are not true but team member self-claims. It is then up to the subject to disclose this information or not.
- **Quadrant 4 is the Unknown Area.** It is the part of us that is not recognized by ourselves or others. Adjectives that are not selected by either subjects or their peers remain in the Unknown quadrant, representing the participant's behaviors or motives that were not recognized by anyone participating. This may be because they do not apply or because there is collective ignorance of the existence of these traits.

When the Johari Window exercise is completed in a respectful and constructive way, it can enhance positive team formation and communication.

WORKING WITH TEAM CONFLICT: THE KEYS TO MANAGING IT

The Role of Team Conflict

Individuals have different opinions, beliefs, or values and, under the pressure of performance, these differences can sometimes present as conflicts. *Conflict is the expression of a disagreement of points of view between two different sides.* Conflict can hinder a team's performance and must be appropriately managed. Team's conflict may be the result of: diversity of ideas; constrained resources; faulty communication and ambiguity; interdependencies of functions; incompatible work style or work habits; performance deficiencies; failure of some team members to follow team norms; differences in personal styles and personal values; and competing priorities, goals, and interests.

Many believe team conflict is the most common barrier to high performance. *Actually, experience shows that poorly written and planned charters, a lack of clear goals, inadequate ground rules, and poor facilitation skills are more likely to be the main spoilers of team progress.* As a team leader, it is very important to be able to work with conflict as the team progresses thought the phases of the project.

There are two recognizable patterns of conflict:

1. Healthy and **constructive conflict** is a component of high-functioning teams. Conflict arises from individuals' differences; the same differences that

often make diverse teams more effective than those made up of individuals with similar experiences and backgrounds. When individuals with varying perspectives, competencies, and skills are tasked with a project or challenge, their combined effort can far surpass the achievements of any group of like-minded individuals. This is because their complementary proficiencies can be utilized to challenge the status quo and generate new alternatives. The goal of the effective facilitator is not to eliminate conflict but learn to use it to the team's advantage. Conflict avoids groupthink Without conflict, team members may not be fully engaged in the activities or they may be participating in groupthink which quells innovative problem solving.

2. **Destructive conflict.** On the other hand, team members may become defensive or defiant and engage in hostile interactions. Destructive conflict is born from personal attacks that undermine the individual rather than challenge the idea. This situation stifles optimal team member participation and solution development, which negatively impacts the project's outcome.

Conflict has an ideal center point. No conflict is **artificial harmony,** which produces no engagement, groupthink and a lack of results. **Personal attacks** constitute destructive conflict. They generate withdrawal, stress, and faulty solutions (Lencioni 2000).

Conflict Models

A number of conflict style inventories have been in active use since the 1960s to understand how people deal with conflict. Most of them are based on the Managerial Grid Model developed by Robert R. Blake and Jane Mouton (Blake 1964). The **Managerial Grid Model** identified five leadership styles for managing conflict on a grid that plotted the "concerns for people" as the y-axis against the "concerns for production" on the x-axis; each axis was given values from 1 to 9.

The best known conflict style inventory is the **Thomas–Kilmann Conflict Mode Instrument (TKI)**. TKI is a conflict style inventory developed to measure an individual's response to conflict situations. It was designed by Kenneth Thomas and Ralph Kilmann to illustrate how individuals react to conflict around two dimensions. The first dimension is plotted on the y-axis and is concerned about our conflict response based on our attempts to get what we want; this is also called **assertiveness.** The other dimension plotted on the horizontal axis is concerned about our response based on helping others get what they want; this is called the **cooperativeness.** Based on these two axes, there are five basic types of responses to conflict resolution (see Figure 27-5):

1. **Avoiding.** Avoiding or withdrawing from the conflict without taking any measures to solve it. People take an unassertive and uncooperative approach to

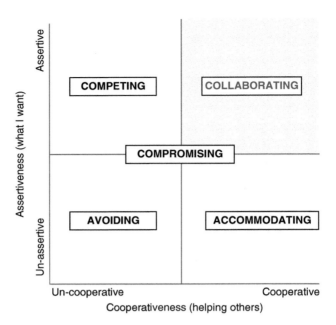

FIGURE 27-5   The Thomas-Kilmann Conflict Mode Instrument.

conflict and don't deal with it. This type is located on the bottom left of the grid. Avoidance takes the form of postponing, sidestepping, withdrawing, or ignoring the issue.

2. **Accommodating.** Accommodating or fully conceding to the other individual's position. People take an unassertive but cooperative approach. This type is at the bottom right of the grid. This takes the form of selflessness, generosity, yielding, or giving in.

3. **Competing.** Competing or forcing, or using one's power or assertiveness to coerce the other individual to accept one's solution. It's the "win–lose" method. This type is at the top left of the model. People take a wholly assertive and uncooperative approach to conflict.

4. **Compromising.** Compromising or resolving the conflict by having both individuals agree to a solution that partially meets each individual's needs but does not fully satisfy either individual's needs ("lose–lose" method). This approach is at the center of the grid. It means splitting the difference, finding middle ground, or a quick fix that partially resolves the issues; It's a quick solution but both sides give up part of what they want.

5. **Collaborating.** This option is at the top right of the grid; Collaborating, or solving the problem without requiring either side to make any concessions ("win–win"). Individuals work together to develop optimal solution. It is time-consuming and requires trust.

General Guidelines to Managing Team Conflict

Conflict will occur within the project team. It is important for the team to manage it constructively, maintaining respect for each member's differences and avoiding disruptive conflict. Certain methods of managing conflict are typically successful in resolving it while other methods tend to exacerbate the problem. Ineffective methods for attending to conflict may include ignoring the conflict, complaining about it, blaming someone for it, or hinting passively about it. *Conversely, an effective tactic for addressing the conflict involves directly clarifying what is going on and attempting to reach a resolution.* Yet, for many individuals within the team, conflict resolution is an intimidating process and makes them very uncomfortable. Often these individuals choose to do nothing about the conflict because they lack the confidence that they will handle the situation in a way that will settle it without damaging their relationships with colleagues or creating bigger issues.

There are some guidelines to manage conflict that apply to all situations as well as specific approaches to mitigate destructive conflict:

- Clarify the project's common goals, priorities, and team members' roles and responsibilities initially and during the project as needed.
- Discuss with the team members that conflict will occur during the course of the project and may be uncomfortable at times.
- Document team-selected conflict resolution techniques in the initial meetings to establish team norms for managing conflict (often part of the team's Rules of Engagement).
- Encourage team members to engage in constructive conflict to facilitate their growth, team performance, and project goal achievement.
- Model and facilitate empathy and effective communication during team interactions.
- Identify that while ineffective communication is often a cause of conflict, effective communication is usually a large part of the solution, especially when using active listening to seek common ground and clarification of the problem while soliciting frequent feedback.
- Emphasize that conflict must be about issues, rather than people, in order to foster the team's progressive development.

Specific Strategies

Specific strategies can minimize the negative effects of disruptive conflict. They include preventing it, diagnosing it, de-escalating it, and dividing it. The tactics are outlined below:

- **When possible, prevent it.** Set up conflict resolution norms in the "rules of engagement"; during discussions, ask for different points of view. Encourage the practice of active listening (paraphrasing and clarification). Encourage clarification of assumptions (ask why?). Encourage sticking to the facts of the situation, not the person. Advise the team that team issues are discussed only with the team.

- **When conflict surfaces, diagnose it.** When conflict arises, make a decision. If the conflict is not helpful, intervene to stop it. This may occur when there is a disrespectful tone or the conflict is hindering progress. If the conflict is helpful, then promote it so it yields the desired result. This may happen when the conflict is getting to a core issue and leading to a better outcome.

- **When conflict intensifies, de-escalate it.** Recognize the conflict, acknowledge its existence immediately, and discuss its impact. Then, shift the focus to securing team members' commitment to resolving the conflict. Obtain their agreement to communicate using active listening techniques. Remove ambiguity and assumptions from the conflict resolution process by listing the facts, clarifying positions and articulating team member's opinions. List the assumptions and beliefs underlying each position; document the information so that it is visible for everyone to see.

- **When conflict becomes extensive, divide it.** Form smaller teams and separate the members of the team that think alike; define and analyze the issues within the smaller groups. Use decision-making tools; reconvene the team to recap the positions, opinions, and findings of the smaller teams. Identify the next steps using techniques such as Multivoting, if necessary. At the conclusion, celebrate the team's ability to work through conflict to develop optimal solutions and complete project work.

While conflict management can be challenging for project team members, articulating team norms and ground rules in advance and monitoring specific conflict situations throughout the project can encourage the project team's engagement in constructive conflict that leads to superior results.

The project team is a highly pivotal group of individuals. *They are the cornerstone of the QI project as they collaborate to complete the work that needs to be done.* However, the team members may not have experience performing work in this manner or developing interdependencies with colleagues from other disciplines or departments. The dynamics of the team will impact the project's outcome. With proper planning and structured facilitation by the project leader and team leader, team development, communication, decision-making, and conflict resolution can be strengthened to enhance the team's performance and achieve the established project objectives.

CONFLICT RESOLUTION AND THE THOMAS KILMANN INSTRUMENT

The Thomas–Kilmann Conflict Mode Instrument is a conflict style inventory and was developed to be used to measure an individual's response to conflict situations. The Thomas–Kilmann Conflict Mode Instrument recognizes five modes of response to conflict:

1. **Avoiding.** Withdrawing from the conflict without taking any measures to solve it. We don't address the conflict. Advantage: quick solution. Disadvantage: Potential to jeopardize relationships. *This style can be used effectively when there is a time constraint – too busy with other important issues and definite advantage in waiting to resolve the situation exists.*

2. **Accommodating.** Fully conceding to the other individual's position. Advantage: quick solution to preserve the relationship. Disadvantage: Give up on one's individual solution. *This style should be used when the issue may be unimportant, other individual is the expert, other solution is superior, and preserving the relationships is important.*

3. **Competing.** Forcing or using one's power or assertiveness to coerce the other individual to accept one's solution (win–lose method). This has the potential to jeopardize relationships. *This style is often used when there is a time constraint; when able to influence the outcome based on power or position within organization and the rules and regulations must be enforced.*

4. **Compromising.** Resolving the conflict by having both individuals agree to a solution that partially meets each individual's needs but does not fully satisfy either individual's needs (lose–lose method). It's a quick solution, but both sides give up part of what they want. *It can be used when both parties are equally committed to goals that are incompatible, or when a temporary solution for a complex issue is needed.*

5. **Collaborating.** Solving the problem without requiring either side to make any concessions (win–win). Individuals work together to develop optimal solution. It is time-consuming and requires trust. *It is the preferred style to be used when issue is important or very important; preserving the relationships is important; or adequate time is available.*

REVIEW QUIZ

1. A common purpose, common goals, and common approach are called
   A. team's high performance,
   B. the needs of a team,
   C. determinants of success,
   D. a team's building blocks, or
   E. the team's abilities.

2. Successful teams develop high-leverage behaviors such as
   A. robust dialogue;
   B. mutual accountability and robust dialogue;
   C. follow through;
   D. robust dialogue, mutual accountability, and follow-through; or
   E. robust dialogue and great leadership.

3. All of the following are true of team's building blocks EXCEPT
   A. Trust and commitment among members of a team come before a common purpose, common goals and a common approach is established.
   B. A team's purpose needs to be meaningful and credible to engage its members.
   C. Individuals on a team need to understand "what's in it for me."
   D. The goals of an improvement team need to be clear.
   E. A common strategy defines the rules of engagement.

4. Of the following factors, which are the "critical affective components" of a high-performing team?
   A. Effective leadership and optimal resources
   B. Commitment and mutual trust (How the team members feel)
   C. Great level of knowledge and expertise
   D. Open communication and respect for differences in opinion
   E. Constructive conflict resolution

5. Commitment and mutual trust within the members of a QI team enables
   A. team members to know one another and understand their work needs,
   B. team members to communicate and achieve conflict resolution,
   C. achieving goals and aims of the project,
   D. quick wins, or
   E. all of the above.

6. To achieve commitment and mutual trust, a QI team needs to focus on which three team building blocks?
   A. Challenging aspirations, common goals, common results
   B. A common purpose, common goals, a common objective
   C. A common purpose, common goals, a common approach
   D. A common goal, a common approach, common results
   E. Specific performance objectives, specific work strategy, good outcomes

7. A common purpose for a high-performing team is a compelling context that drives the team to action. A common purpose can be achieved by
   A. creating a challenging aspiration for the QI team,
   B. seizing an important opportunity for action,
   C. combining elements of pride and desire to win,
   D. supplying meaning and creating emotional energy, or
   E. all of the above.

8. Common goals help teams achieve commitment and mutual trust. Which statement is NOT TRUE regarding common goals?
   A. Common goals need to be clear and specific.
   B. Common goals must be adapted to the specific titles and jobs positions of the QI team members.
   C. Specific performance objectives facilitate focus on results.
   D. Common goals help define the work product that is needed from the team.
   E. Common goals help overcome obstacles.

9. Which statement is NOT TRUE regarding a common approach?
   A. It has been called the "social contract" of team members.
   B. It defines the purpose and guides how team members work together.
   C. It defines the rules of the hospitals' approach to improvement.
   D. It defines the distribution of responsibilities and how decisions are made.
   E. It is the third building block to achieve commitment and mutual trust.

10. Regarding the work strategy of high-performing teams,
   A. The work strategy can be called the "Essential Internal Processes."
   B. It is facilitated by how team members feel about the team and each other.
   C. It leverages robust dialogue, mutual accountability, and follow-through.
   D. It allows the achievement of results and generate energizing experiences.
   E. All of the above

11. All high-performing teams agree on a common approach at the beginning of their work to help them achieve their purpose and performance goals. Critical issues teams need to agree on are
   A. attendance and rules that regulate meetings,
   B. how decisions will be made,
   C. topics of discussion and confidentiality,
   D. work distribution, or
   E. all of the above.

Key: 1d, 2d, 3a, 4b, 5e, 6c, 7e, 8b, 9c, 10e, 11e

REFERENCES

1. Alimo-Metcalfe. (2018). Five principles of high performing teams. *Personnel Today*.
2. Annunzio S. (2004). Contagious Success: Spreading High Performance Throughout Your Organization. Portfolio Hardcover.
3. Blake R. (1964). *The Managerial Grid: The Key to Leadership Excellence*. Houston: Gulf Publishing Co.
4. Bossidy L. (2011). *Execution: The Discipline of Getting Things Done*. Random House Business Books.
5. Drexler A. (2019). The Grove 2006. Accessed at www.grove.com.
6. Hackman R. (1983). *A Normative Model of Work Team Effectiveness*. Yale School of Organizational Management.
7. Harkins P. (2006). *10 Leadership Techniques for Building High-Performing Teams*. Linkage.
8. Hersey P. (2012). *Management of Organizational Behavior: Leading Human Resources*. Prentice Hall.
9. Katzenbach J. (2005). *The Discipline of Teams*. Harvard Business School Press 1993 and Best of Harvard Business Review.

10. Lencioni P. (2000). *The Five Dysfunctions of a Team*. AHA Publisher.

11. Lerner S. (2009). Teaching teamwork in medical education. *Mount Sinai Journal of Medicine*. 76: 318–329.

12. Luft J. "The Johari window, a graphic model of interpersonal awareness". Proceedings of the western training laboratory in group development. UCLA 1955.

13. Mehrabian A. Silent Messages. Wadsworth Publishing Co. 1971.

14. Parkinson N. The Pursuit of Progress. John Murray 1957. Triaxia partners at triaxiapartners.com. Site accessed September 2019.

CHAPTER 28

Steps and Strategies for Effective Decision-Making

PROBLEM-SOLVING VERSUS DECISION-MAKING

We make thousands of decisions every day. Some decisions are small and practical, and other decisions are complex, far reaching, and require analysis. **Decision-making can be defined as the selection of a course of action from a number of alternatives**. **Problem-solving** is different from **decision-making**:

- Problem-solving is a method to resolve a problem that depends on **critical** and **analytical thinking** and includes problem finding, problem shaping, and resolving.
- Decision-making is a process that is done many times during problem-solving and is the key used to reach the right conclusion.
- Decision-making
  - depends on judgment;
  - is focused on the analysis of the alternatives available;
  - considers the course of action that should be taken; and
  - looks for a final choice: the outcome being to take action or to form an opinion about a certain topic.

The Quality Improvement Challenge: A Practical Guide for Physicians, First Edition.
Richard J. Banchs and Michael R. Pop.
© 2021 John Wiley & Sons Ltd. Published 2021 by John Wiley & Sons Ltd.
Companion website: www.wiley.com/go/banchs/quality

DECISIONS: TYPES & CONDITIONS

According to the availability of information, there are two types of decisions:

- **Programmed.** Programmed decisions tend to be routine and repetitive where information is available. These decisions are made on the basis of sufficient data and usually there is a precedent that allows for the existence of a formula, structure, or algorithm; in general, programmed decisions have short-term consequences and therefore can be reversed.
- **Non-programmed.** Non-programmed decisions are new, poorly structured, and in general are made based on a limited amount or no information. Since the decision is new, there is usually no precedent to be able to make the same decision using a formula or template. These decisions tend to have long-term consequences.

In healthcare, individuals and teams are confronted with two types of decisions:

- **Clinical.** These decisions can be programmed or non-programmed and deal with the care and safety of our patients.
- **Operational.** These decisions deal with the care delivery processes. They can also be programmed or non-programmed. The general purpose is to achieve a high degree of efficiency, optimize work conditions, decrease cost, or optimize human resources.

Decisions can be made **individually** or **in groups**. In general, decisions should be made by individuals when the issues are not important and/or are routine. In healthcare, however, decisions about patient care are almost always made individually. Decisions should be made collectively when the issues are complex and require the input of multiple parties.

Decisions made by individuals or groups are made under three different conditions:

1. **Certainty.** In certainty, a decision is taken knowing all the possible alternatives, their likelihood of occurrence, and their cost and benefits. Each alternative has a definite outcome.
2. **Risk.** Under risk, all available alternatives are known, their likelihood of occurrence is also known, but the outcome is either unknown or there is doubt.
3. **Uncertainty.** In uncertainty, the available alternatives, likelihood of occurrence, and outcomes are not known. These are the most difficult decisions to make because there is a lack of knowledge and a high level of ambiguity (see Table 28-1).

TABLE 28-1   Conditions under which We Make Decisions.

Conditions under which We Make Decisions				
Condition	Available alternatives	Likelihood of occurrence	Outcome	Likelihood of failure
Certainty	known	known	known	minimal
Risk	known	known	doubt	average
Uncertainty	unknown	unknown	unknown	high

Most decisions in a QI project are **non-programmed, made in groups, under conditions of risk or uncertainty,** and generate a certain amount of **conflict.** Conflict appears because the team struggles with several options, there is uncertainty about the results, or because there are different points of view and interests among the different constituencies or key stakeholders. For these and other reasons, the decision-making process in quality improvement efforts are complex and often difficult.

SOURCES OF ERRORS AND BIASES IN PEOPLE'S DECISION-MAKING PROCESS

Faulty inputs

Decision-making is not always easy; it requires the proper input and a solid process to maximize success. Common challenges when making decisions are:

- A lack of information: We make decisions without having the facts.
- A lack of data or unreliable data: We make decisions based on no or faulty data.
- We use conflicting opinions and points of view as a basis for our decisions.
- We make decisions without considering the available alternatives and the level of risk.

The Influence of "Decision Framing" or Option Presentation

Decisions are influenced by the way we frame our choices. Framing depends on **wording** and **situations.** Frames impacts choices, especially when people are presented only with one or two frames. This tends to bias their decision process. The framing effect is one of the strongest influencers in decision-making.

Framing often comes in the form of gains or losses, as described by Kahneman and Tversky in their **Prospect theory** (Kahneman 1979). Prospect theory states that a loss is more significant and has a greater influence on the decision-making process than a gain.

> **Prospect theory shows that gains are preferred over probable gains; a probable loss is preferred over a sure loss; but when it comes to losses, a loss is perceived as much more significant than an equivalent gain.**

This means that our decisions are heavily influenced by the fear, real or imagined, of a loss. Decisions can be influenced by framing them in a positive or negative light:

- When an issue is presented in a positive light (positive frame), people tend to make the decision that is best in avoiding risk.
- When an issue is presented in a negative light (negative frame), people tend to opt for the risky alternative to avoid loss at all cost (Tversky 1981).

Heuristics

Heuristics are rules, strategies, or mental shortcuts used by our brain to resolve a problem or confront a situation. Some people call them the "mini-maps."

> **Heuristics are fast mental shortcuts we use when we need to make fast and automatic decisions.**

They play an important role in both problem-solving and decision-making. Heuristics

- rely on forming templates and mini-maps in our brain that depend heavily on previous experiences and emotional states,
- help us make quick decisions by scrutinizing a limited amount of information, and
- streamline the decision-making process and diminish the work of retrieving information from memory.

Because they do not engage the areas of our brain responsible for complex thinking (the prefrontal cortex, for example), heuristics avoid considering the long-term consequences of our decisions.

Heuristics can be positive or negative and affect our perception of things. However, while heuristics can speed up our problem-solving and decision-making process, they can introduce errors and biases in our judgments (Dale 2015).

Common examples of heuristics are

- **Availability heuristic.** The tendency to judge the frequency or likelihood of an event by the ease with which it comes to mind. This heuristic operates on the assumption that if something can be recalled easily, it must be more important than the alternative solution. As a result, people tend to weigh their judgments toward more recent information, making old information less relevant.

When we are asked to think about the likelihood of a problem, we ignore the statistical probabilities and rely on how easily we can think of an example.

- **Anchoring heuristics.** The tendency to rely too heavily on the first piece of information or experience to make a decision. Once an anchor is in place, judgments are made on the basis of comparison to the anchor. We judge the likelihood of the event by using an anchor and then making adjustments up or down.

- **Representativeness heuristic.** The tendency to make a decision by comparing information to our mental "map" or stereotypes. We judge the likelihood of an event by comparing it to the typical case, ignoring rules of chance, independence, and norms.

Biases

A bias or cognitive bias is a systematic error in thinking that affects our decision. Biases can result from the use of heuristics. Heuristics play a major role as sources of error in our decision-making process. However, not all biases come from heuristics. Some biases come from errors in the way we process information, process memory, focus our attention, or from the tendency to make attributions. Common examples of biases are

- **Confirmation bias.** People favor information that conforms to existing beliefs while discounting or ignoring the evidence that supports a different conclusion.
- **Attentional bias.** The tendency to pay attention to some information or things, while simultaneously ignoring others.
- **Overconfidence bias.** The tendency to overestimate the reliability of one's judgment, ability, performance, or level of control.
- **Actor-observer bias.** The tendency to attribute one's actions to external causes (decrease culpability), while attributing other people's behavior to internal causes (increase culpability).
- **False consensus effect.** The tendency to overestimate how many people agree with one's point of view.

The Effects of Time

Time pressure has a negative effect on the decision-making process:

- It reduces our ability to review data and to seek alternative options.
- It reduces our creativity.
- It reduces the ability to properly evaluate and predict potential outcomes.

Time pressure, however, may have a beneficial effect by allowing us to raise the most practical or simple option to the top.

Making decisions with time improves creativity. It allows for the review of additional data, allows us to consider alternative options and choose the best ones, and allows for evolution in our decision-making process. Individual's preferences can evolve over time until a decision is reached (Bursemeyer 1993).

Excessive time may have a negative impact on decision-making because it may allow for the appearance of additional biases. Too much time and we may succumb to **decision paralysis.**

THE DECISION-MAKING PROCESS

People make better decisions when they follow a sequential and structured approach. Most of the existing models consider the decision-making process as a six-step approach: identify and diagnose the problem; identify alternative options; evaluate alternative options; select the best option; implement the decision; evaluate and learn (see Figure 28-1).

1. **Identify and diagnose the problem.** The first step is to recognize that there is a problem. This requires us to identify the problem in precise terms, review the existing data to confirm the existence of the problem, diagnose the true cause, and agree to take actions.
2. **Identify alternative options.** The second step is to identify the range of alternatives available. We can choose from an existing range or design situation-specific approaches.

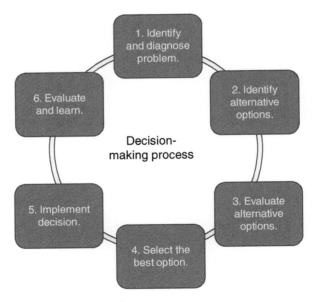

FIGURE 28-1　The six-step decision-making process.

3. **Evaluate alternative options.** We must then evaluate each alternative in order to choose the best one. For each alternative, consider the advantages and disadvantages, time that it will take, cost-versus-benefit ratio, and the possible results after the decision is made. Consider that each possible alternative may have a range of outcomes depending on the different scenarios under which it may be implemented.

4. **Select the best option.** Alternative options may be suitable or not suitable. If the alternative options are not suitable, the process must start again. If the alternatives seem suitable, these may be clearly different or have a great number of common features – in which case, judgment should prevail. Each option may have specific requirements, trade-offs, and require different resources. Each option may be different in terms of ease of implementation.

5. **Implement the decision.** Once the decision has been made, it is time to implement it. Implementation is the key to the decision-making process. Effective implementation depends on making sure people responsible for the implementation understand why it is implemented, how the choice was made, and are fully committed to making it work.

6. **Evaluate and learn.** After the decision has been made, evaluate the results. Make sure the most appropriate decisions were made. Follow-up enables the identification of errors and learning from the decision-making process.

FOUR WAYS QI TEAMS CAN MAKE DECISIONS

There is considerable evidence that teams are more effective in making decisions than individuals. In general, teams benefit from more knowledge and expertise, the ability to generate more options, greater depth in the analysis of alternatives, and a greater commitment and buy-in toward the implementation of the solution. Decision-making in teams, however, may be negatively affected by peer pressure, status and influence, and time delays. Teams must also overcome **groupthink** and **escalation of commitment**, a pattern in which an individual or group facing a negative outcome continues on the same path instead of analyzing the options and altering the course.

There are four common ways for a team to make a decision: direction, consulting, consensus, and voting.

- In **direction**, the decision is made by the leader or the person assigned to make the decisions.
- In **consulting**, the leader consults the QI team, but makes the final decision.
- In **consensus**, the leader and the team participate in the decision-making process; once the decision is made, all members of the team support the decision both publicly and privately.
- In **voting**, decisions are made unanimously or approved by the majority vote when all team members have a significant stake in the outcome and the cost

of making a bad decision is extremely high in terms of safety, jobs, financial considerations, etc.

Team decisions using **consensus** require several conditions:

- All team members must have presented their perspectives and preferences regarding the decision to be made.
- There has been sufficient time for discussion and feedback.
- All team members agree with the decision or have a clear understanding of why the final decision /conclusion is different from the one they chose.
- There is a statement that summarizes the decision in writing and is shared with all the members of the team to make sure there is agreement. This statement should be reviewed and each team member should commit to the final decision, fully supporting the team both publicly and privately.

Consensus by its nature is slow and there is always the risk of missing an opportunity. Teams should opt for consensus when the potential harm of a bad decision is much greater than the cost of missed opportunities. In general for less risky decisions, teams should try and strive for direction or consulting.

IMPROVING THE EFFECTIVENESS OF A TEAM'S DECISION-MAKING PROCESS

As the QI project progresses, team members will need to make many decisions. Teams often struggle with making decisions as a group, for any of several possible reasons:

- They are not accustomed to working together.
- The process of how to make a decision is not clear.
- Hierarchy is ambiguous.
- Simply because empowerment to make decisions is new for some of the front line team members accustomed to only following protocols and practice guidelines.

Unclear roles, missing information, and a general lack of team consensus about the issues can make the decision-making process even more difficult. To improve the decision-making process, teams and their leaders should

Bring the right people to the table. Bring the people with the expertise and the right mix of skills to the table. Make sure there is diversity in the opinion pool and that everybody that needs to be included is included. Share the information needed ahead of the meeting: people need time to review the information so that they can come prepared.

Establish the level of autonomy given to the team. Occasionally, decisions are made by a team only to be reversed by the Primary Sponsor. This creates frustration and feelings of futility among team members. Instead, set the level of autonomy for the team; be explicit and clear. What can the team decide on and what needs the leadership's input? Establish the decision-making authority in advance of team meetings:

- The **Project Charter** should clearly specify the team's level of authority and the limitations for developing and implementing solutions.
- If it's not clear, the team leader should clarify the team's decision-making authority directly with the **Primary Sponsor** ahead of the meeting. The team leader may choose to invite the Primary Sponsor to attend the meetings, in which case, key decisions requiring the Sponsor's approval will need to be made at the meeting before the team's work can proceed.

Define the ground rules. Meeting ground rules can help the team with the decision-making process. Make sure everybody knows them. A structured environment is key so people can share ideas and opinions freely. This is especially important when leaders are present. If this is the case, senior members should speak last to avoid influencing the team or dominating the discussion.

Establish the process by which the team is going to make decisions. When the process by which decisions are made is not clear, a number of things can happen:

- The team struggles to make decisions.
- Team members forget how decisions were made and don't support them.
- There are lingering disagreements, so decisions are not unanimously supported by all members of the team.

Before making a decision, a team should decide on the process by which the decision will be made to ensure: the decision-making process matches the issue at hand; there is an opportunity for every team member to weigh-in; there is clarity among all team members; and there will be buy-in on the final decision. Agreement of the decision-making process should include

- the objective,
- the available time,
- the need for technical expertise, and
- the degree of acceptance required.

When the rules are set at the beginning of the meeting, team members are clear on the expectations and methods for making decisions. As with all processes, decision-making should be effective, efficient, repeatable, and reproducible.

Establish a time frame for making decisions. Decisions need to be subjected to a time constraint. Nevertheless, for some, the decision-making process will take too long, resulting in "analysis paralysis," whereas for others, the decision will feel "rushed."

Concentrate on the issues, not the solutions. At the beginning of the meeting, define the problem, not the solution. When we define the problem by the solution, we create a narrow-minded focus that, at best, restricts creativity and, at worse, sets in motion a process that may end up in a bad decision. As you progress through the decision-making process, consider all the alternatives so that the team is not steered toward any preconceived opinions. Be mindful of the flaws of group decision-making:

- Ask probing questions and challenge all the options.
- Encourage the team members to disagree with one another.
- Mine for productive conflict.

Focus on the big picture, don't sweat the details. Parkinson's law of triviality argues that members of a group often give a disproportionate weight and spend much more time on trivial issues than on the important issues. It is not a bad idea at the onset of the meeting to let people know what will be deliberated and decided by the team, and what can be and will be decided by the leader. The team should focus on what is important. This will save time and energy.

Use tools to enhance your decision-making process. Several tools are available to make better decisions. Examples are

- **Ladder of Inference:** a tool to overcome biases and assumptions. The ladder of inference exposes the chain of reasoning and path to decision-making so that we are better able to find the best options among multiple possibilities.
- **Marginal analysis:** an analysis of options is based on benefits versus costs.
- **SWOT diagram:** an acronym that stand for Strengths, Weaknesses, Opportunities, Threats.
- **Pareto analysis.**
- **Bowtie diagram.**

REFERENCES

1. Bursemeyer J. (1993). Decision Field Theory: A Dynamic-Cognitive Approach to Decision Making under an Uncertain Environment. *Psychological Review* 100 (3): 432–459.
2. Dale S. (2015). Heuristics and biases: The science of decision-making. *Business Information Review* 32 (2): 93–99.
3. Kahneman D. (1979). Prospect theory: An analysis of decision under risk. *Econometrica.* 47: 263–291.
4. Tversky A. (1981). The framing of decisions and the psychology of choice. *Science 30*; 211 (4481): 453–458.

CHAPTER 29

What Neurosciences Can Teach Us to Motivate People to Change

STORIES FROM THE FRONT LINES OF HEALTHCARE: "MAKE IT HAPPEN"

It was clear! The hospital was spending too much money purchasing different types of intravenous tubing. Time had come to take advantage of economies of scale and stick to one single vendor. Tom Briezniak, the CFO (chief financial officer), asked Edward, the director of Materials Management and Wendy, the CNO (chief nursing officer) to "make it happen."

A select committee of leaders were brought in to study the issue. After several weeks of analysis and interviews, a single vendor was chosen to supply the entire hospital with all its intravenous tubing needs. Five months later, Tom Briezniak realized the total expenditure for intravenous tubing had gone up despite a lower per-unit purchasing price! To make matters worse, there had not been any significant increase in hospital census since the changes in i.v. tubing has taken effect that could account for the increased cost. Surprised and annoyed, the CEO called Wendy. As he learned, there had been a lot of push-back from providers in the OR and ICUs. Providers felt they had not been consulted and their needs had not been considered. As it turns out, the new tubing did not have a proximal port and made administering drugs more difficult. Upon patient arrival to the OR and ICUs, the intravenous tubing used on the inpatient units was being thrown out and replaced with the old i.v. tubing that was still being purchased.

What was the problem? How did hospital administration make the choice for the new IV tubing? What was the result?

The Quality Improvement Challenge: A Practical Guide for Physicians, First Edition.
Richard J. Banchs and Michael R. Pop.
© 2021 John Wiley & Sons Ltd. Published 2021 by John Wiley & Sons Ltd.
Companion website: www.wiley.com/go/banchs/quality

THERE IS NO IMPROVEMENT WITHOUT CHANGE

Albert Einstein is quoted as having said that "the definition of insanity is doing the same thing over and over again and expecting different results." This quote first appeared in 1981 in a document published by Narcotics Anonymous, a guidebook for addicts trying to overcome their condition. The authors were trying to convince its members that continuing to use narcotic drugs and expecting that something would change on its own was a "folly."

Whether this quote has been correctly attributed to Einstein or not, the message is clear: We cannot keep doing the same thing and expect different results. To improve means to change, and every change requires healthcare professionals to do something differently. Doing something differently requires a change in behavior, and as we all well know, trying to make people change their behavior is generally met with varying degrees of pushback and resistance.

As a member of a QI team, you can always expect some measure of pushback with every new idea you try to roll out. This is an inevitable reaction to change in human beings. This is especially noticeable in a change-averse culture like healthcare. People's reaction to change is different. For some, change triggers some pushback while for others, any change triggers a strong opposition. Some in the healthcare environment prefer a "wait-it-out" approach to improvement, hoping to revert to their former approaches when the change pressure subsides. It's surprising how professionals often adopt a conservative approach to patient care for fear of change even when this practice is incongruent with their results and evidence-based recommendations.

The role of the improvement team is to understand the fears, expectations, and desires of the frontline professionals who will be impacted by the proposed change while, at the same time, focus their efforts on identifying and implementing the optimal solutions to the problem.

> *Quotable quotes: "Successful change is about making smaller changes, measuring the ripples on the pond, and deciding when the next stone should go and how big it should be." Ian Coyne,* **Make Change Happen**

WE THINK OF CHANGE IN TERMS OF OUR OWN INTEREST

We do not naturally push back on every single change that comes our way. We accept change if we believe it will help us and it is in our best interest. We push back, however, when we believe change is not in our best interest **whether this is true or imagined.**

Our task as leaders of an improvement effort is to do three things:

1. Understand the issues that will affect the front line when we roll-out a change; how will the change affect staff and providers? What are the challenges? What are the advantages and disadvantages?

2. Understand the points of view, concerns, perspectives, and beliefs the front line espouses towards the change.

3. Design a change strategy that addresses both challenges and perceptions.

Understanding the **reality** and the **perceived reality** should guide our efforts when trying to change resistance to engagement and support.

> **Quotable quote: "Change is like heaven, everybody wants to do it (go there), but not right now." Chinese quote**

THE TRADITIONAL APPROACH TO MAKING CHANGE HAPPEN

The traditional approach to rolling-out change in many healthcare organizations is ineffective. It often relies on a document, a single meeting, or a bolt-on last-minute effort shortly before full-scale roll-out. Common approaches are

- **A well-crafted document.** Buy-in and acceptance of a change cannot rely only on a well-written document or email. A document can fulfill a critical human need for information and establish the framework upon which individuals can make a personal choice to change. But a single document does not generally result in the motivation to change.

- **A change management meeting.** Verbal persuasion, logic, and data cannot alone create the willingness of the front line to change. These are not by themselves strategies; they are elements of a bigger construct. Verbal persuasion and logic must be incorporated into a broader approach to change. Even the best PowerPoint presentation cannot by itself change minds.

- **By decree.** This is the top-down implementation. Leaders and the improvement team come up with several ideas and change is implemented top-down. With this type of strategy, people don't understand the need for change, don't feel motivated, and push back against what is perceived as an imposition. Staff and physicians are the key stakeholders in any change initiative. Change cannot be driven from the top down with the steps and the actions required already prescribed. When change is implemented this way, the result is usually resentment, cynicism, and widespread resistance at the front line. Remember, people support only *what they help to build*. Force alone is a bad strategy to achieve change. Force may temporarily achieve the desired goal, but it will also result in resentment and lost relationships. Pushing people to change may be an occasional measure needed to achieve a critical goal, but it is not the best approach. Leaders can create a burning platform to encourages change, but evidence shows that pushing too hard and forcing change will not yield the results we expect. Force causes people to feel stressed and anxious and people eventually disengage.

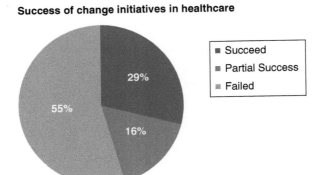

Success of change initiatives in healthcare

FIGURE 29-1   Success of change initiatives in healthcare.

Organizations often search for the **magic bullet** that will achieve the change they seek. Change is a complex, dynamic process that requires a multi-pronged approach. We should not assume people's behavior and motivation are influenced by a single factor. We should avoid trying to achieve change with a single approach. Even if the proposed solution can potentially address all the problems, it does not guarantee the frontline professionals will see the need to change. Buy-in and adoption of a solution does not stem from the characteristics or appropriateness of the solution, but from the successful transition of people through their own change line.

Using this traditional approach, the success of change initiatives in healthcare, defined as achieving all the objectives within the time frame and budget alloted, has been modest at best (see Figure 29-1).

TO UNDERSTAND CHANGE, WE NEED TO UNDERSTAND THE DRIVERS OF HUMAN BEHAVIOR

The Central Organizing Principle

During the last decades, scientists have gained a better understanding of human behavior by integrating psychology and neurosciences. Research using imaging technologies such as functional MRI, positron emission tomography (PET) scanning, and quantitative electroencephalography (QEEG) have allowed researchers to pinpoint the areas of the brain responsible for a good number of brain functions. Combined with psychology, these advances have helped us map the brain and understand why people behave the way they do.

Our relation with the environment is governed by an overarching principle of the brain called the **Central Organizing Principle** (Gordon 2000). The Central Organizing Principle aims to **minimize threats** and **maximize rewards**. That is, our brain is constantly assessing the environment to detect threats and avoid them and seeking opportunities for reward (Scarlet 2016). At the core, the Central Organizing Principle aims to assure our survival.

To maximize rewards, the brain uses a **reward system.** This is a dopaminergic network of neurons that links the prefrontal cortex (PFC) to the hippocampus, hypothalamus, thalamus, amygdala, ventral tegmental area, nucleus accumbens, caudate nucleus, putamen, and substantia nigra, among others. Activation of this dopaminergic network also enhances the formation of memories in the hippocampus and positive emotions in the amygdala.

To detect and avoid threats, the brain uses the threat **response system.** This is a fast-reacting serotoninergic system of interconnected neurons that links the PFC to the limbic system among others. The limbic system includes the orbitofrontal cortex (OFC), hippocampus, hypothalamus, thalamus, basal ganglia, cingulate gyrus, and the amygdala. When we perceive a threat in the environment, our brain initiates a cascade of events known as the **fight-or-flight** response. The amygdala has a leading role in the threat response, and the activation of the fight-or-flight response is often known as the **amygdala hijack.** One of the hallmarks of a fight-or-flight response is the diversion of blood flow away from the PFC, the part of the brain where we do the planning and analytical thinking, to the areas of the brain that enable us to defend ourselves or run (see Figure 29-2).

A threat response (fight-or-flight) increases adrenaline and **cortisol** productions, decreases dopamine production, and diverts blood flow from the central core to the muscles. A threat response also **diverts blood** from the PFC, the area for higher executive functions, to limbic system. Preferential blood flow to the limbic system, particularly the amygdala, results in a generalized state of anxiety and defensiveness; it impairs analytical thinking, creative insight, and problem solving.

The Brain's Mini-Guides

Our brain stores information in the form of templates, blueprints, or mini-guides called **schemas.** These schemas are beneficial because they allow for the organization of information and the ability to quickly recall it and infer reality based on small pieces of information. Schemas allow us to *selectively focus on a single piece of information, draw a conclusion about the meaning of the information, and execute an appropriate response.* Schemas are, in essence, shortcuts to interpreting available information.

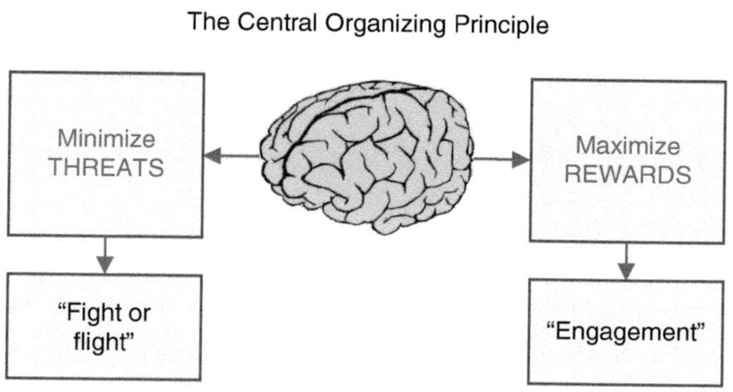

FIGURE 29-2   The brain's Central Organizing Principle.

Schemas are formed using our knowledge and experiences. They influence how we perceive and respond to stimulus and information from the environment based on the information stored from similar objects, people, and events. Schemas are also susceptible to our own biases and the way we organize information.

We are constantly scanning the environment looking for threats and when a stimulus arrives, we use schemas to give it a meaning and take action. Stimuli are first sent to the basal ganglia and the amygdala for quick processing because these structures are faster and more efficient than processing the information at the level of the PFC. This serves the purpose of detecting threats and quickly reacting. Information arriving at the basal ganglia and amygdala is quickly compared to existing information stored in the memory banks, searching for commonalities and patterns relating to previous experiences.

- If memory banks (schemas) exist, and the experience is seen as positive and nonthreatening, an appropriate response is then generated by the PFC and the motor cortex.
- If memory banks (schemas) exist, and the experience is seen as negative and threatening, a "fight-or-flight" response is initiated.
- When there are no patterns in the memory banks (schemas), an error signal is generated by the basal ganglia. The information void is usually filled by a new schema created from similar memory banks. This new schema, however, is substantially edited and reshaped with our unique perceptions, beliefs, and emotions, and often results in significant distortion and misleading interpretation of the environmental cues.

In general, we are more attuned to threats than to rewards. The brain has five times the number of neural networks assigned to the threat response than to the reward response. The natural reaction of people to environmental cues is to perceive them as threatening rather than a reward. Gordon uses the term **negativity bias** to describe the phenomenon by which "humans pay more attention and give more weight to negative rather than positive experience or other kinds of information" (Gordon 2000). The tendency to process ambiguous information as negative and threatening has an important evolutionary role that has assured our survival. Our brain prefers to err on the side of caution making sure we do not misinterpret critical information that threatens our survival. The threat response creates far more arousal in the limbic system, more quickly, and with longer-lasting effects than a reward response (Baumeister 2001).

How the Central Organizing Principle affects our interpretation of change

The Central Organizing Principle aims to **minimize threats** and **maximize rewards**. To avoid threats, we need to **predict** what is going to happen. But with change, we can't predict (Scarlett 2016). Change begins with **uncertainty** about the future. There are no templates or blueprints in our brains that help us know what to expect. We do not know exactly what will happen; we can only try to imagine it. If we can't predict, we become anxious because our brain feels it may not be able to avoid a threat. When it comes to change, we tend to assume the worst. Because the perception – real or imagined – is threatening, our brain's Central Organizing Principle directs us to **avoid it. When confronted with change and the inability to predict how it is going to affect us, we become anxious.** We increase adrenaline and cortisol productions and divert blood from the PFC to the limbic system. Amygdala activation impairs our analytical thinking and creative insight. We become **defensive** and **push back.**

TO UNDERSTAND CHANGE WE NEED TO UNDERSTAND THE DRIVERS OF SOCIAL BEHAVIOR

Social Needs

The behavior of humans in social groups is driven by the need to minimize the loss and maximize the gains in relation to a number of needs. When our needs are met, there is a favorable response. We feel at ease, engaged, and part of the group. When our needs are not met, we feel anxious and threatened and do everything we can to have our social needs fulfilled. The brain's neural pathways that drive social behavior are the same as the brain pathways used by the Central Organizing Principle. Therefore as with our environment humans imbedded in social groups are constantly seeking rewards (social gains) and avoiding threats (social loss) (Lieberman 2009).

> *Hilary Scarlet uses the acronym* **SPACES** *to describe the six needs or drivers of social behavior: Self-esteem, Purpose, Autonomy, Certainty, Equity, and Social Connection (Scarlett 2016). David Rock uses the acronym* **SCARF**. *The SCARF model involves five domains of human social experience: Status, Certainty, Autonomy, Relatedness, Fairness. These domains activate either the primary reward circuitry – is there a gain? – or the primary threat circuitry – is there a loss? (Rock 2008). Daniel Pink considers purpose, autonomy, and mastery as the main drivers of social interaction (Pink 2011). Now consider together the Central Organizing Principle and the drivers of social behavior. Change may be seen as a threat because it brings* **uncertainty;** *so is the strategy used to roll out change if it results in a loss of* **status**, **identity**, **purpose**, **autonomy**, **connectedness**, *and* **fairness** *(see Figure 29-3).*

How We Roll-out Change Impacts our Social Needs

The strategy we use to roll out change may negatively impact our social needs. *A change that is perceived as a loss of one or more of these needs is seen as a threat; a change that is perceived as a gain of social needs is seen as a reward* (see Figure 29-4). Understanding the drivers of social behavior can be very valuable in designing an effective strategy for change:

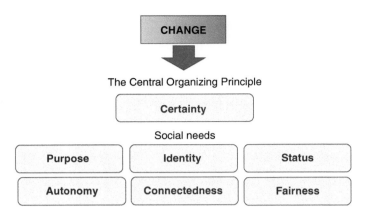

FIGURE 29-3   Change affects our behavior through the Central Organizing Principle and our social needs.

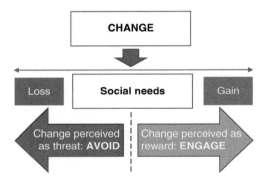

FIGURE 29-4   The effects of change on our social needs.

- **Certainty.** We need to be able to predict and know what is going to happen. We seek what is familiar. We need clarity about our responsibilities so that we can achieve our goals. Certainty is rewarding and increases the dopamine levels in the brain circuits. Change is uncertainty and the unknown. With change, we can't predict. We perceive change in a better light when we understand what is asked of us, where we stand, and what is going to happen. We need to remove uncertainty to create safety. We perceive change as a loss of certainty and therefore something unpleasant or threatening we want to avoid when we do not know how change will affect us and what will happen to us.
- **Purpose.** Purpose gives us meaning and direction; purpose energizes and motivates us. We want to know that we matter and that our purpose is worthwhile. Change threatens our sense of purpose. We may see change more positively when we understand why change is needed and we believe in the

change. Change feels like a threat when we don't understand why we are asked to change, or we don't believe in the reasons for change.

- **Identity.** The way we do things – our habits – provide us with a sense of comfort, stability, and confidence in our abilities. The way we see things is grounded in our values, beliefs, and attitudes. The way we do things and the way we see things is our identity. We feel attached to the ideas we hold sacred and feel a sense of loyalty to the people and organizations that helped us see things the way we see them. Change requires us to find new ways of performing our work and thinking about things. It requires a change in our habits, beliefs and attitudes. Change challenges our sense of competency and forces us to question and redefine aspects of our identity (Linsky 2002).

- **Status and self-esteem.** Status refers to the feeling of importance relative to others, the sense of achievement and value. We need to feel valued, to be recognized by our colleagues and leaders, and receive positive feedback. Change often threatens our self-esteem. Change can affect our area of responsibility, our budget, our title, or influence. Change may mean we lose status because we are not part of the QI team, entrusted with finding the source of the problem and creating new solutions. When this happens we feel our opinion does not matter.

- **Autonomy.** The ability to self-determine without constraints is what we call autonomy. Autonomy is the sensation of control over events and the environment that surrounds us. When we have autonomy, we have a choice. Even when we only have limited autonomy, we feel positive: we can influence the circumstances around us. When we are part of co-creating solutions, we gain autonomy and with it a sense of control. We see change in a more favorable light when we have some measure of choice. Change can feel constraining, especially when it is imposed. Change can feel like a threat; it takes away our autonomy and our ability to self-determine. We feel we have no choices and no say over the outcome.

- **Connectedness.** We are social beings. We have a need to be connected to other people, to feel we are accepted and part of the "in-group" (Scarlett 2016). Connectedness makes us feel safe and enhances our sense of purpose. By belonging to a group, we feel as if we are a part of something bigger and more important than ourselves. The need to belong involves gaining acceptance, attention, and support from other members of the group. The brain associates social inclusion with something positive: a reward. When we feel socially connected, our brains respond by increasing the levels of dopamine. Change may threaten connectedness. We feel we are not with the group in charge of making decisions; we feel our opinions are not considered.

- **Fairness.** We want to know we are being treated fairly compared to others and relative to our expectations. We want and need transparency. When we feel change will affect us more than others, we perceive it as a threat.

CHANGE IS PSYCHOLOGICALLY PAINFUL

The working memory – required for perception and creation of thoughts and ideas – resides in the PFC. The working memory requires high levels of energy; it is a complex structure but fatigues easily and can only hold a limited amount of information. The brain is 2% of the body's weight but consumes 20% of the energy (Raichle 2002). To save energy, the brain shifts routine activities from the PFC to the basal ganglia. Basal ganglia requires much less energy than the working memory does, in part because the basal ganglia does not need to process information in the same way the PFC does. The basal ganglia instead uses mini-guides, or schemas, and templates shaped by experience and training to perform certain activities. Any activity done repetitively forms a habit and is then stored in the basal ganglia. This frees up the processing resources of the PFC for other tasks. For example, we can drive and talk at the same time. Driving is done automatically; talking requires a higher brain-processing center.

With a change, we can't predict. This means that we cannot use the information stored in the basal ganglia, and have to constantly engage the PFC to process and interpret information. Change requires something "new" that draws on working memory from the elegant but easily fatigued PFC. Work that has been hardwired in the basal ganglia is all of a sudden pushed to the top of the consciousness. The PFC is more energy intensive and when engaged, requires an effort that is often experienced as uncomfortable and "painful". Change is experienced as psychological pain – even when the change appears to be in an individual's best interests – because it requires the brain to switch to a different, more energy intensive, processing circuit.

Quotable quote: "Not until the pain of the same is greater than the pain of change does one embrace change." Dave Ramsey

BASIC PRINCIPLES FOR LEADING A SUCCESSFUL CHANGE INITIATIVE

Start with the leader. As we discussed in Chapter 5, the leader has a crucial role in the QI team's ability to manage change. The leader is the project facilitator and needs to become the **change leader.** Heifetz defines the change leader as "the person that provides the technical solution while preparing people for the adaptive change by understanding their loss, providing hope, and explaining the process" (Heifetz 2002).

Be the facilitator, not the architect. The role of the improvement team is not to find solutions and implement change management plans. The role of the QI team is to create the conditions that engage the front line. Frontline providers and staff need to be engaged in understanding the problem and co-creating solutions. The improvement team is there to provide the front line with information, data, support, and the tools they need to create a change.

Change needs a comprehensive strategy. Change does not happen as a result of a "magic bullet." Human behavior is influenced by multiple factors, and a strategy for change must identify and address the effects of change on these factors. Change is not a single event but a process.

Culture "eats" strategy. Individuals, groups, and units have idiosyncratic cultures that differentiates them from the rest of the organization. Each area has its unique culture, which influences the success of QI projects. A change strategy must address the unique needs of each area. Understanding the culture of each area is a necessary first step of a successful change strategy. **Edgar Schein** defines culture as a "pattern of shared basic assumptions learned by a group as it solves its problems of external adaptation and internal integration, which has worked well enough to be considered valid and, therefore, to be taught to new members as the correct way to perceive, think, and feel in relation to those problems" (Schein 2010). **Gareth Morgan** defines organizational culture as the "set of beliefs, values and norms, together with symbols like dramatized events and personalities, that represents the unique character of an organization and provides the context for action in it and by it"(Morgan 2006).

Buy-in depends on how people experience the process of change. Change is less likely to succeed when it is rolled top-down and is imposed. Change should be a shared experience that harnesses the position of senior leadership and the hands-on experience of the front line professionals. Successful adoption of a change comes from the personal experience of being engaged in co-designing the change. Successful change must be "socially constructed where everybody discusses the causes, diagnoses barriers, and generates possible solutions" (Hammel 2014). The need to find solutions and the responsibility to implement a change needs to be shared with those that are affected by the problem. Change cannot be sustained without the engagement and commitment of the front line. "Change comes naturally when individuals have a platform that allows them to identify shared interests and to brainstorm solutions" (Hammel 2014).

Be patient: Change does not happen all at once. Change is not homogenous; individuals and groups have their individual pace of change. Change happens at different rates. Change efforts need to be adapted to an individual's specific change needs and stages. Change is driven by the organization but happens at the individual level (Hyatt 2012). "Change management is only effective when the processes and tools for changing the organization are combined with the processes and tools for changing" the frontline healthcare clinician (Hyatt 2012).

Quotable quote: "You cannot change your destination overnight, but you can change your direction." Jim Rohn

THE WINNING CHANGE STRATEGY

The change-resistant culture characteristic of healthcare organizations necessitates incorporation of a change strategy. QI projects and their change initiatives stand the best chance of success when they focus on making the change feel **safe**, create the **right conditions**, and leverage leaders, peers, and the environment to influence

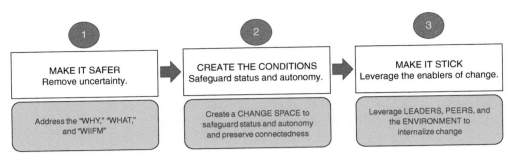

FIGURE 29-5　The Change Strategy.

behaviors. People will be more likely to engage in change if they understand "why" change is needed, "what" is asked of them, and believe change is worth it ("WIIFM", or what's in it for me). (**See Figure 29-5**).

FIRST, MAKE IT SAFE: REMOVE UNCERTAINTY

Uncertainty creates psychological discomfort. A winning strategy starts with making change feel safer by removing uncertainty about "why" change is needed, "what" is the change we are proposing, and "how" will it affect me. People prefer to know rather than not know, even if change will affect them negatively.

Help People Understand "Why" Change Is Needed

The problem. To know the "why" is a human need. People want to know, "Why do I need to change?", "What is wrong with what I am doing now?", "Why change now, and what will happen if we don't change?" People often don't want to be part of a change because they don't know why change is needed. When the purpose of change is not clear, people push back. The lack of awareness of why the change is needed is the most common cause of initial resistance (Hiatt 2012). A lack of awareness of why change is needed is often the result of poor communication, either because the message did not reach the people it was intended for, or because it was misinterpreted. Change often fails because it is implemented without defining the "why", without leadership support or credible data.

　　The solution. Start a change initiative by removing uncertainty. Define "why" we need to change and "what" is going to change. Create a compelling purpose that can bring the front line together. The reasons for change must be clearly understood, even when change may negatively affect some aspects of our daily work.

- The **Primary Sponsor** or senior leader should be the first one to address the coming change: It will legitimize the change effort. The Primary Sponsors should explain the "why" and the "what" of change; leaders need to create clarity around the purpose.

- It may help to develop a **change story** or consistent messaging for all stakeholders to understand where the organization is headed, why it is changing, and why this change is important. Change stories not only help get the message out but are also powerful change tools.

- Address the **challenges** of the change, and at the same time, provide **hope** that the challenges can be overcome and change will be successful.

- Make sure every informative session has an allotted time for questions and answers; **feedback** is an important component of any change strategy so that you can understand what issues trouble the front line and assess how the "change story" is being received.

- Start early in the project life cycle; a proactive approach is better than a reactive approach.

- **The change story.** The change story should answer most of the questions the front line may have. Here are some suggestions: What's the background? What's the problem? Who does it affect? What is the patient's perspective? What metrics are we currently using to measure the problem? Where is data coming from? What is the current performance? What is the key output metric that needs to be improved? Why are we addressing the problem now? What would be the ideal performance? What is the gap between our current state and the ideal state? What needs to happen? What benefits can we expect for our patients, staff, physicians, and the healthcare organization? How does this project support /relate to the overall strategic goals of our organization?

Help People Understand What the Change Entails

The problem. People often don't want to change because they are confused about what exactly is asked of them. They need to know what needs to change, what they need to do, and what should stay the same. Sometimes, despite our best efforts, there is a lack of clarity about what we are asking people to do. Leaders frequently overestimate the extent to which the front line understands the problems and shares in their beliefs and opinions – a tendency known as the **false-consensus effect**. The front line is often confused and unsure about the expectations regarding a change.

The solution. Be clear around the expectations. Define what change is needed; explain how to achieve the desired behavior; set clear standards; define the goals we are looking for; show people what success looks like.

Help People See Change Is in Their Best Interest: Explain the "WIIFM"

The problem. People may understand the reasons for change and what the change entails but may not want to change because they do not think the change is in their best interest. They don't see the benefit or WIIFM (what's in it for me). If there is nothing to be gained, there must be a lot to lose! If there is no extrinsic or intrinsic motivation to change, there is no need to go through the pain of change.

The solution. People need to see a reward in order to engage in change. Without this reward, there may be no motivation to support the change. The reward can be extrinsic. However, extrinsic rewards produce short-lived and unintended results. Intrinsic rewards, however, are very powerful motivators of human behavior. There are different ways to create intrinsic rewards:

- Engage people in co-creating the change; make people feel they are part of a unified team.
- Give people autonomy and the responsibility to make change.
- Change the perception of change to something that has personal meaning, moral value, or the greater good (Patterson 2008).
- Appeal to people's vocation and their drive to want to help.
- Make it a game or a competition.

Staff and physicians are the key stakeholders in any change initiative. The reasons for change must be clearly understood and the perception that the change may negatively affects roles and responsibilities addressed. Communicate constantly. Frequent and open communication about the problem, the project, the need for change, the type of change, and the consequences of not changing are the key. Remove uncertainty, preserving purpose and identity.

SECOND, CREATE THE RIGHT CONDITIONS TO SAFEGUARD STATUS AND AUTONOMY

Create a Change Space

The problem. Sometimes people find it difficult to support a change because leaders come up with solutions and then implement them top-down without any say from the front line. There is no awareness of why the change is needed and people feel their opinion is not valued.

The solution. Change should be "socially engineered" (Hammel 2014). Co-creating change preserves frontline professionals' sense of status and autonomy. Efforts of senior leaders and the QI team should be directed toward creating a **change space,** where frontline professionals can come to their own insights about the problems, barriers to improvement, and the possible options to solving them (Hammel 2014). A change space has multiple advantages:

- Being part of the improvement process preserves status and connectedness: We feel we are part of a team and part of something that matters. Having information removes uncertainty and reduces anxiety.
- If we are part of the team, we have insight and a better understanding of the issues. Insight feels rewarding to the brain (Scarlett 2016). It is a gain in status and self-esteem.

- Identifying problems and barriers to improvement builds engagement and commitment to change.
- Allowing people to find solutions and reach their own conclusions about what needs to change creates a sense of accomplishment and feels rewarding (Scarlett 2016).
- Participating in the design of the solution preserves our sense of autonomy and helps us focus on what we can control.

Engaging the front line in co-creating change may seem difficult at first, but the efforts to create a change space has a great return on investment. Healthcare professionals see and understand the challenges our patients face. Their understanding of the process and proximity to the patients makes them uniquely suited to identify and deliver potential solutions that can improve care and the healthcare experience. Staff and physicians have a pivotal role and are the linchpin that drives the success of the improvement efforts.

. . .and Then Provide Them with the Knowledge and Tools They Need to Succeed

The problem. Even when people want to adopt a new behavior, they don't embrace the change because they don't know how. They don't have the knowledge and tools they need. Leaders sometimes take for granted that people at the front line have the skills they need. They find it difficult to imagine that others don't know something that they themselves do know; it's the **"curse of knowledge."** All attention is focused elsewhere, taking for granted that people can do the tasks we ask them to do. There is no attention to personal ability; there are no training programs and leaders don't see the need to coach and support frontline professionals.

The solution. Preserving people's status and self-esteem includes making sure they have the ability to perform the new tasks change requires. Status and self-esteem should be safeguarded:

- setting clear standards and defining mini goals,
- providing training and coaching, and
- giving frequent feedback and positive encouragement.

THIRD, MAKE IT STICK AND INTERNALIZE THE CHANGE

Leverage the Influence of the Leader

The problem. Change is more difficult or fails when leaders are not present or not involved. When leaders are not involved it sends a clear signal change is not important. Change efforts can also fail when the behavior of the leader is incongruent with the change that is being proposed or when the leader is not able to resolve the cross-functional issues that arise. An ineffective change sponsorship is one of the most important reasons for change to fail (Hiatt 2012). The role of the **opinion leaders** (we call them the Local Sponsors) is also critical; change fails when the opinion leaders at the front line do not support change.

The solution. Leverage the influence of the leader. The leader must demonstrate the values and behaviors that drive the change and show improvement efforts are not just a sidebar activity. Leaders must behave in a manner that is congruent with the change they are asking the front line to do. They must be visible and active facilitators. Leaders should:

- use their influence and networking capacity to engage people to talk about change;
- use public forums to legitimize change;
- provide resources, training, support, and coaching;
- show an active involvement and be present during critical phases of the project; and
- show a "personal cost" and share in the drawbacks of the change (Patterson 2008).

The behavior of leaders during change and towards the change is the most important determinant of the behavior of the front line professionals during the change. The **local leaders (mid-level leaders and managers)** also play a crucial role as change partners. They are the **Local Sponsors.** The Local Sponsors are in the best position to operationalize the required change. They support change activities, communication, training and coaching.

Leverage the Influence of Peers

The problem. Humans need to be socially connected with their group. When humans are part of a group, they feel fulfilled. When they are rejected, they feel psychological pain. Matthew Lieberman showed that the brain processes physical and emotional pain using the same areas (Lieberman 2009). When a significant number of members of a group discourage change, other members of the same group may push back against change even if they want to change for fear of being rejected by the group. Change is more difficult for people when other members of the same group act in a manner that is incongruent with what they believe. Solomon Asch conducted an experiment to investigate the extent to which social pressure from a majority group could affect a person to conform to giving the wrong answer in a test, even when the correct answer was clear. Asch found that participants conformed to a majority view, even when the majority was clearly wrong, in about 30% of the time.

The solution.

- **Leverage peer pressure** by creating a sense of belonging where everybody is part of a team struggling to make the change work. Identify opinion leaders and ask them to support the changes. Make sure everybody has the needed resources (information, equipment . . .). Foster an environment where people encourage one another and openly discuss the right and wrong way of doing things.

- **Demonstrate fairness** and make sure there are no "special privileges" where one group of people can continue with the old way of doing things.
- Make sure **the system of rewards and accountability** is congruent with the desired changes. In this system, the right behavior is rewarded, the wrong behavior has consequences, and the system must apply to all.

Leverage the Influence of the Environment

The problem. People sometimes have a hard time with change because the system is a barrier to making the change. System design such as leadership structure, policies and procedures, processes, and the layout of the work environment may be impediments to the successful implementation of a change.

The solution. If the system is a barrier, it needs to be redesigned to support change. Policies and procedures must be reviewed; front lines must have the tools and resources they need; and the work layout must help with the desired behavior (change).

REFERENCES

1. Baumeister S. (2001). Bad is stronger than good. *Review of General Psychology.* December 1.
2. Coyne, Ian. (2014). *Make Change Happen: Get to Grips with Managing Change in Business.* Pearson Education.
3. Gordon E. (2000). *Integrative Neuroscience: Bringing Together Biological, Psychological and Clinical Models of the Human Brain.* CRC Press.
4. Hammel G. (2014). *Build a Change Platform Not a Change Program.* McKinsey Company.
5. Heifetz R. (2002). *Leadership on the Line.* Harvard Business Review Press.
6. Hiatt J. (2012). *Change Management. The People's Side of Change.* Prosci Learning Center Publications.
7. Higgs M. (2010). Building change leadership capability: "the quest for change competence." *Journal of Change Management.* 1(2) 116–1340.
8. Lieberman M. (2009). The pains and pleasures of social life: a social cognitive neuroscience approach. *Science.* 323 (5916): 890–891.
9. Morgan G. (2006). *Images of Organization.* SAGE publications.
10. Patterson K. (2008). *Influencer. The Power to Change Anything.* Vital Smarts.
11. Pink D. Drive. (2011). *The Surprising Truth about What Motivates Us.* Riverhead Books.
12. Raichle ME. (2008). Appraising the brains energy budget. *PNAS 2002.* 99 (16): 10237–10239.

13. Rock D. (2008). SCARF: A brain-based model for collaborating with and influencing others. *Neuroleadership Journal*, June 15.

14. Scarlett H. (2016). *Neurosciences for Organizational Change. An Evidence-Based Practical Guide to Managing Change*. Kogan Page.

15. Schein E. (2010). *Organizational Culture and Leadership*, 4th Edition, Jossey Bass.

CHAPTER 30

How Does it All Fit Together? The MRI Suite at St. Mary's Hospital

SIMULATION BACKGROUND

St. Mary's Hospital is a 285-bed medium-size community hospital located in the Willamette Valley. It provides a wide spectrum of services including primary care, maternity, inpatient care, surgery, and on-site laboratory and diagnostic imaging services.

Dr. Amanda Alluck is the current chief medical officer (CMO). She has been increasingly concerned about the number of complaints she has received from the Medical and Surgical Services regarding a long wait list to schedule routine and nonemergent inpatient MRI (Magnetic Resonance Imaging) studies. An initial assessment done by her office staff confirmed a significant backlog of patients, and revealed an apparent low patient throughput in the outpatient MRI suite when compared to other hospitals of similar size, acuity, and patient volume.

The MRI suite is located in the outpatient building and is equipped with two 1.5 and one 3.0 Tesla scanners. Currently, the MRI technicians perform an average of 24 scans per day shift (7:00 a.m. to 7:00 p.m.). Day shifts are staffed with a front-desk clerk, three MRI technicians, a day shift Supervisor, and a Registered Nurse (RN). Outpatient and nonemergent inpatient MRIs are scheduled from Monday to Friday. Weekends, after hours, and emergent MRIs are performed in the in-patient MRI scanner located on the third floor of the main hospital.

Concerned about the current situation, Dr. Alluck spoke with Mr. John McLain, the director of Imaging Services, and asked him to "assess the problem and find me a

The Quality Improvement Challenge: A Practical Guide for Physicians, First Edition.
Richard J. Banchs and Michael R. Pop.
© 2021 John Wiley & Sons Ltd. Published 2021 by John Wiley & Sons Ltd.
Companion website: www.wiley.com/go/banchs/quality

solution." Overwhelmed with the responsibility, McLain walked to Dr. Robert Dow's office to ask for his help. Dr. Dow was the associate head for Outpatient Services, an experienced project manager, and a well-regarded leader in the organization. After a brief conversation, Dow and McLain agreed to work on the problem. They would assemble a team and launch a QI project. Dr. Dow offered to lead the team.

THE FIRST "R": THE RIGHT PROJECT

Dow knew the first order of business was to properly frame the project. This is a critical step to the success of any improvement initiative. After a couple of phone calls and a thorough review of the CMO's staff report, he sat at the computer to write a first draft of a Problem Statement. The Problem statement is a clear, concise, and specific explanation of the problem that does not include any causes of the problem. As the report stated, the average number of work days per month (without weekends and the 10 US holidays a year) is 20.9 days. The outpatient MRI suite currently performs an average of 24 scans a day or 502 scans a month. To address the current patient backlog, the MRI suite would need to perform an additional 125 cases a month for an average of 30 scans per day.

Problem Statement

"Ideally, patient throughput in the outpatient MRI suite would meet the hospital's Medical and Surgical needs. It has been estimated an average 30 scans per 12-hour shift are needed to satisfy current demand. Data provided by the CMO's office on the current performance shows the MRI suite performs an average of 24 scans per 12-hour shift, which is allowing for a significant backlog of patients to develop. It should be noted that current throughput is considered well below the performance level of other outpatient MRI suites in hospitals of similar size, acuity, and patient volume. This leaves a gap of 6 scans per 12-hour shift between demand and current capacity.

Project Charter

The next step would be to write a Project Charter to gain agreement among all parties as to the nature, scope, goals, and timeline of the project. Dr. Dow knew it was important to get everybody on the "same page" The Project Charter would serve as an informal "contract" between all key stakeholders and the QI team. Dow sat at the computer and wrote his first draft:

PROJECT CHARTER
Title: *Improving patient throughput in the outpatient MRI suite*
Start date: *January 6, 2020, and Completion **date**: July 10, 2020*

Primary Sponsor: *Mr. John McLain*
Team Leader: *Robert Dow, MD*

Reasons for action/Background

Scheduling outpatient and non-emergent inpatient MRI studies is made difficult by a significant patient backlog, the result of a low MRI patient throughput. Data provided by the CMO's office shows the MRI suite performs an average of 24 scans in a 12-h day shift (7:00 a.m. to 7:00 p.m.), which is insufficient to meet the needs of the Medical and Surgical Services. The current performance is considered below the performance level of other hospitals of similar size and patient volume. The inability to schedule elective MRI studies impacts the ability of physicians to make accurate diagnoses, initiate treatments, and admit or discharge patients from the hospital. It may also result in delayed diagnoses, increased complications, and an overall low quality of care. The current causes for a low MRI patient throughput are not known.

Project Scope and Boundaries

<u>In scope</u>: *Improve patient throughput in the outpatient MRI suite for elective outpatient and non-emergent inpatient studies.*

<u>Out of scope:</u> *Patient throughput in the inpatient MRI scanner (weekends, after hours and emergent MRIs).*

Key Metric (Primary Project Metric)

*"Wait time from provider request to MRI results" seemed an optimal metric. But it was unclear if targeting this metric for improvement should be done now. Factors that influenced "wait time from provider request to MRI results" were numerous, and included the diagnostic assessment and reporting by the radiologists. Dr. Dow struggled with the idea and realized the organization did not have the resources to commit to such an ambitious endeavor at this time. Instead, he decided on improving the **"Average daily patient throughput in the outpatient MRI suite."** This was selected as the key metric for this project. Average daily patient throughput was defined as the **"average number of MRI studies performed on a 12-hour day shift using three scanners."***

Project Goals

After a discussion with McLain and several other senior members of the C-suite, Dr. Dow set a goal to improve the average patient throughput by 25% in order to meet current demand. Patient throughput would have to increase from 24 to 30 per 12-hour shift. This was an aggressive but achievable goal (SMART goal). As it was customary, this goal would need to be discussed with members of the QI team and key stakeholders in the MRI suite to get their support and buy-in.

Timeline

- *Project "go-live": January 6, 2020*
- *Project boundaries, VOC, VOS, CTQs, and Process Map by January 17*

- *Data collection planning, baseline data, and baseline process performance by February 21*
- *Identify and confirm the most likely causes by March 31*
- *Ideas, pilots, and full-scale roll-out by May 29*
- *Monitoring, summary findings, control plans, and project closure by July 10*

Electronic Signatures

The Project Charter would be signed by the QI project Leader (Dr. Dow), and the Primary Sponsor (McLain) when completing the final draft.

THE SECOND "R": THE RIGHT PEOPLE

Organize a QI Team

It was time to organize the team. Dow knew for this project it would be important to assemble a team of people that actually did the work. Without firsthand knowledge of the process, improvement ideas could risk being counterproductive and not applicable to the situation at St. Mary's. Technical expertise and process knowledge of the intimate details of how scanning was done would be invaluable.

Later that day, Dow met with Kiara Smith, the outpatient MRI day-shift supervisor. After a friendly banter, Dow explained the problem and told her about the QI project and the need for her to be part of the team. Sensing Mrs. Smith's initial apprehension, Dow reassured her that this was going to be a partnership and nothing would be done without her knowledge and support. Dow proceeded then to explain how the project would unfold and told Mrs. Smith he would need her help and advice to assemble the QI team. After a brief discussion, Dow and Smith agreed on the team roster. The team would include two MRI technicians, Dr. Dow and her. Mrs. Smith also proposed to speak to Dr. Bretislava, one of the attending radiologists, to ask her to be part of the QI team. Dr. Bretislava would bring additional process knowledge and her well-known ability to organize people and get things done.

The next morning Dr. Dow called the outpatient vascular clinic and enrolled Dr. John Cusamano, one of the attending vascular surgeons, who agreed to speak for the "customer" on the team and, as he put it, be the "voice of dissent." The QI team roster was now completed and the team was ready for the project kick-off and first team meeting (see team roster in Table 30-1).

A week later, the QI team met for their first meeting. Dr. Dow introduced himself to all participants and gave each team member the opportunity to do the same. He then introduced the topic, briefly describing the problem and how it affected the organization. He explained the purpose and goals of the QI project and set the timeline for each project phase. A schedule of team meetings was drafted, and the team members then agreed on a common set of team meeting ground rules. The Problem Statement and Project Charter were reviewed, eliciting a lively debate and numerous

TABLE 30-1   The QI Team Roster at St. Mary's Hospital

TEAM ROSTER: Who Is on the Team?	
Primary Sponsor: John McLain, Director of Imaging Services	
Team Leader: Robert Dow, MD, Associate Head for Outpatient Services	
Team members	Unit / Department; role.
Kiara Smith	MRI day shift supervisor
Helen Cheung	MRI technician
Petra Johnson	MRI technician
Irene Bretislava	Attending physician, Department of Radiology
John Cusamano	Attending surgeon, Division of Vascular Surgery

changes to the original draft. However, all members of the team agreed on the metric and the project goals. The meeting ended with a summary of action items, identifying what needed to be done, and the assignment of tasks to each member of the QI team.

The First Tollgate Review

Several days later, Dr. Dow and the rest of the QI team briefly met with the Primary Sponsor, John McLain, for their first tollgate review. They discussed the planned project activities, reviewed the Problem Statement, and discussed at length the Project Charter. All parties agreed on the project scope, metric, goals, and timeline and agreed to proceed to the next phase.

THE THIRD "R": THE RIGHT PROBLEM

After several rounds of emails, the team agreed to divide the project tasks. Mrs. Smith and the two MRI technicians agreed to create their first SIPOC diagram and to get the Voice of the Stakeholders (VOS); Drs. Dow, Bretislava, and Cusamano would work on validating the Voice of the Customer (VOC) with patients and providers.

The Project Scope and Boundaries: the SIPOC Diagram

With the help from one of the project managers in the hospital's QI department, Kiara Smith, Helen, and Petra created their first high-process map or SIPOC diagram. The SIPOC diagram was an important tool to provide all interested parties clarity on the scope and boundaries of the project, and specifically the beginning and the end of the process targeted for improvement. The process boundaries would help define the project scope, keep the team on the same page, and serve as an effective way for making decisions about project activities. Using their process knowledge, Kiara, Helen, and Petra identified the customers and then proceeded to create a list of suppliers, inputs, and outputs. Using small Post-it self-sticking notes on a wall, they identified and recorded six high-level steps making sure to clearly mark the beginning and end of the process. With this information in hand, Mrs. Smith returned to her office. Using Microsoft Visio®, she created a digital copy of her first SIPOC diagram (see Figure 30-1). As she would later explain, the process targeted for improvement starts at "Patient arrival to MRI suite" and ends at "Patient discharged".

The Voice of the Customer

Dr. Dow knew the first step in finding the "Right Problem" was to identify the customer and understand the problem from the perspective of the customer. In this project, customers were patients (external customers) and their referring physicians (internal customers). The VOC (Voice of the Customer) would help the team understand the main drivers of quality and customer satisfaction, focus improvement efforts, and set the priorities, scope, and goals for the project. Dr. Dow spoke with several colleagues, surgeons, and other providers and recorded some of their statements:

- *"I need to be able to schedule an elective outpatient MRI in less than two weeks."*
- *"The only way I can get my patients in the OR is if the MRI is done."*
- *"We need to do a better job: after a patient comes to my clinic, I need the MRI in a matter of weeks."*
- *"...the MRI is usually the limiting factor: I should be able to make a diagnosis for my cancer patients without having to wait for weeks."*

It was clear: Patients wanted to get their scans in a timely manner and physicians needed to be able to make accurate diagnoses, initiate treatments, and admit or discharge patients without having to wait to get their patient's MRI study scheduled.

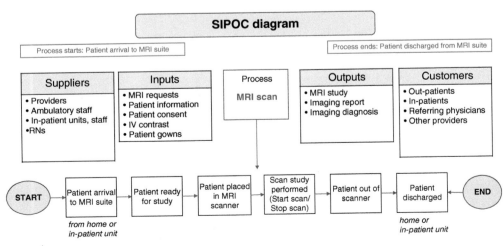

FIGURE 30-1   The project scope and boundaries: the SIPOC diagram.

The Voice of the Stakeholder

The perspectives of the frontline stakeholders is always important in any QI project. Their issues and challenges need to be considered to get a clear understanding of the problem and develop optimal solutions. Kiara Smith quickly understood the MRI staff could not fully address the needs of patients and their referring providers without getting help addressing the challenges they were experiencing. The perspective of the front line is critical to understand the nature of the problem, the drivers of stakeholder's performance and motivation, and ultimately to gain stakeholder's project buy-in. Stakeholders, needs and the ability for the stakeholders to fulfill customer requirements are intimately interrelated.

At an MRI staff meeting the next day, Kiara spoke to the rest of her staff. She informed them of the project and asked them for their help. She assured them the goal of the project was not to evaluate their performance, make them work harder, or blame them for the unit's performance. The goal was to find the best way to increase their ability to provide quality care while decreasing their work burden. With a smile, knowing her staff was probably sckeptical, Kiara said: "Let's try and find a way to work smarter, not harder." Kiara sat down with each member of her staff for a brief conversation and recorded their statements:

- *"Kiara, the problem is that there are numerous delays with patient arrivals."*
- *"I know it is not my place to make a judgement, but I can tell you: often the MRI study is not indicated; this takes valuable resources from doing MRI of patients that really need it."*
- *"Not all information needed for the MRI study is in the chart; we often have to call providers to clarify information or get the additional information we need. We have to page them, and as you can imagine, they're busy and take a long time to return the page. You cannot expect patients to know if their implants are MRI compatible or not!"*
- *"I am often waiting in-between patients; not that I complain, because this gives me time for myself, but to be honest...I'd rather get the work done quickly."*
- *"Even when we are ready, in-patients are not ready...the nurse, transport, who knows?...there is always something."*
- *"In-patients needing IV contrast come down without an IV. Then I have to spend the next 15 minutes trying to find one. This is especially frustrating in patients with difficult IV access."*

Based on their discussions with the entire staff and their own experience, Karen, Helen, and Petra developed the Voice of the Stakeholder (VOS) and created a Critical needs tree (see Figure 30-2).

The Second Tollgate Review

Several weeks later, Dr. Dow called the administrative assistant for Mr. McLain to schedule their second tollgate review. Dr. Dow and the other team members briefly met before meeting with McLain to make sure they were ready and on the same page.

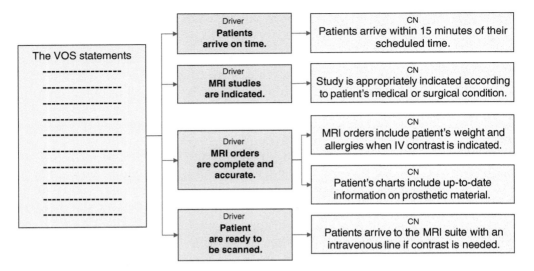

FIGURE 30-2   The Critical Needs tree for the MRI staff.

They reviewed information, discussed deliverables, and each team-member agreed to be responsible to present their part of the project work. The team concluded their meeting by briefly going over the second tollgate review checklist. Data and deliverables were then emailed to Mr. McLain for his review ahead of the meeting.

The next day, armed with their newly developed knowledge, the team briefly met with McLain. They discussed the ongoing project activities, reviewed deliverables, and talked about the importance of the project. Mr. McLain asked some questions and team members responded confidently. It was clear the project was on track and all parties agreed they should proceed to the next phase.

THE FOURTH "R": THE RIGHT CAUSE

Visit to the Gemba and Process Map

It was time to go to the gemba to directly observe the process and uncover undisclosed information and conditions that may be impacting work flow efficiency and effectiveness. Kiara, Helen, and Petra would also be joining the rest of the team. All members of the team knew perfectly well every search for the cause of a problem must start with a visit to the gemba, the place where value is created. Without a clear understanding of how work is being done, a team risks missing valuable insight and clues. Dr. Dow set a time and date that would be convenient for all. The team set several goals:

- directly observe the work being done;
- understand the sequence and order of the steps, actions, and decisions of the processes;
- elicit the input and perspective of the stakeholders; and

- collect any additional information that would enable them to draw a Basic Process Flow map.

At the agreed time, Drs. Dow, Bretislava, and Cusamano arrived at the MRI suite. There they were met by Kiara, Helen, and Petra. After communicating the purpose of the visit to the MRI technicians on-duty, the entire team walked the process from beginning to end. They took notes, asked questions, and in turn elicited feedback form the MRI staff. The team was able to observe staff perform the process at different times and got a clear picture of the most common way of performing the process. Kiara and Petra took the opportunity to explain to their physician team colleagues the MRI zones, the scanning process, and the scanning protocols.

The next day, the entire team met in the Hospital's conference room to review their findings and complete a process map. Using a large Post-it 25 × 30 paper stuck to the wall, the team was able to recreate the entire process sequence. Each step was written on a sticky note and was placed on the Post-it paper in the order it was observed; actions and decisions were recorded and additional notes added on the margin. Steps were then connected with arrows and any pertinent notes or information about the step was added under the step. Each step was numbered. The team then briefly discussed and highlighted the steps where most issues occurred and documented this on the map. Using Microsoft Visio, Dr. Bretislava created a digital copy and posted it on the team's common drive for all to share (see Figure 30-3).

During their visit, the team also identified and recorded several examples of waste: Transport, Inventory, Motion, Waiting, Overproduction, Overprocessing, and Defects (TIM WOOD). Findings were discussed with key stakeholders and ideas for their elimination noted for future action (See Table 30-2).

Metric Selection and Collection of Baseline Data

Based on the information gathered by the team (Problem Statement, Project Charter, VOC, VOS, and Basic Process Flow map), a number of additional measurements (secondary metrics) were selected (see Table 30-3).

The team agreed to meet the following week to plan data collection. A Data Collection Planner and data collection sheets were created to make the data collection process effective, repeatable, efficient, and reproducible. The team agreed that

- Data collection would follow an Operational definition; use the Principle of Stratification; and data would be collected in a time-ordered sequence (the three rules of data collection).
- Data would be collected over the next month, at predetermined intervals, and would include a total of 90 randomly selected patients.
- Data collection would be stratified by date, time, patient type (ambulatory vs. in-patient unit), patient race, insurance type, diagnosis, ICD-10 classification, type of study, ordering physician, MRI technician, level of the MRI technician's experience, and MRI supervisor.

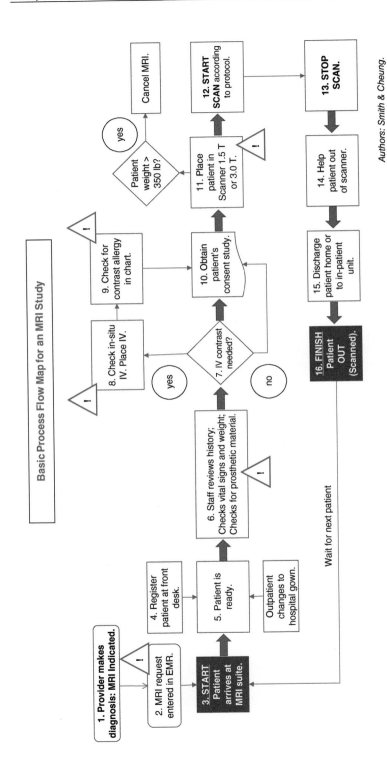

FIGURE 30-3   A Basic Process Flow map for an MRI study.

TABLE 30-2   Quick Wins: Waste Identification

Waste Identification

Transportation (Relocation of patients, materials, supplies to complete a task; traveling)

Staff going to distant storage areas to get needed supplies, forms, blankets

Inventory (More material, patients, items at hand than are required to do the work)

Excessive storage of supplies, forms, and linen noted in storage areas, drawers, control desk

Motion (Wasted movement of people, equipment that does not add value; problems with layout)

Excessive motion of patients and patient stretchers noted

Staff seen walking around suite looking for charts, forms, and information

Waiting (Idle time created when people, information, equipment or materials are not at hand)

Staff noted waiting for patients to arrive from home

Staff waiting for return phone calls from in-patient units, physicians, and nursing staff

Staff noted waiting for transport to arrive from in-patient units

Overproduction (Making something in excess that was is needed; tests and activities "just-in-case"

Nursing staff preparing multiple IV sets at the beginning of the shift that would not be needed

Referring physicians scheduling MRIs that were not indicated

Referring physicians scheduling follow-up MRIs that where not needed

Overprocessing (Using complex equipment for simple tasks; duplications of work)

Staff checking multiple times the same chart looking for the same information

Multiple forms containing the same information

Defects (Work that contains errors or lacks something of value)

MRI orders requesting the wrong study

In-patient charts missing current patient weights and other information

No documentation on patients with pacemakers, or history of aneurysmal brain clipping

Patient charts missing information on prosthetic material and contrast allergies

TABLE 30-3   The QI Project Metrics

Project Metrics		
Type	Metric	Definition
Primary Metric	Average daily patient throughput	Average number of MRI studies performed per day shift (12 hrs., 7:00 a.m. to 7:00 p.m.) using three scanners.
Metrics of efficiency	Lead time	Time from patient entering the MRI suite (patient-in, step 3) to patient exiting the MRI suite (patient-out, step 16).
	Wait time	Time from patient arrival to MRI suite (patient-in, step 3) to START scan (step 12).
	Scan time	Time to complete a study protocol from START SCAN (step 12) to STOP SCAN (step 13).
	Scanner idle time (Scanner TOT)	Time from STOP SCAN (step 13) for previous patient to START SCAN of next patient, also called Scanner Turn-over-time.
Metrics of effectiveness	% monthly MRI studies not indicated	MRI studies that do not follow existing evidence, current guidelines, or best-practice indications, and are deemed unnecessary by a panel of experts.
	% Charts defective	A defective chart is an incomplete chart: it does not include the patient's weight, allergy to i.v. contrast, or information regarding prosthetic material or pacemaker MRI compatibility.

- The Data Collection Planner would need to include the rationale for data collection; the metrics and their operational definitions; the stratification factors; and a checklist of steps to ensure data collection would proceed as planned.

Calibration of the instruments (measurement system accuracy or bias) and a Measurement System Analysis (MSA) would not be needed since time could be determined using any of the standard tools. Dr. Dow explained to the team that the MSA is a study of how much variation in the measurement is assigned to the measurement tool, measurement method, and the data collector. A standard stopwatch would be used to assess the time for each step and the time in between steps.

Armed with their stopwatch, Data Collection Planner, and data collection sheets, members of the QI team returned to the MRI suite for data collection. They arrived early and briefly discussed with the MRI staff the purpose of their visit, reassuring them once more the objective was not to blame them or assess individual performance but to better understand the process. Again the team was able to observe the process in full, at different times, and performed by different staff members. Steps were timed at repeated intervals and data was manually entered in the data collection sheets. Averages were calculated and entered at the bottom of the columns. Additional

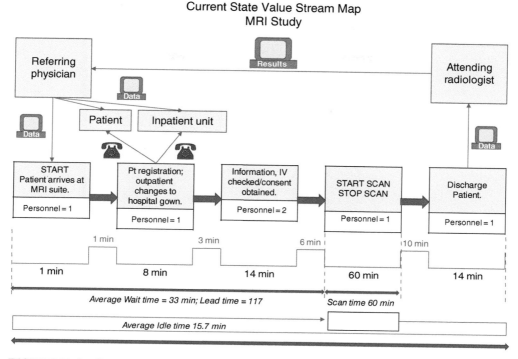

FIGURE 30-4 Current state Value Stream map for an MRI study.

observations were also noted on the margins. After all the information was reviewed, the team met briefly to create a current state Value Stream Map (see Figure 30-4).

Data Analysis and Baseline Process Performance

Data analysis was performed using a standard software package. Summary statistics were obtained, graphs created, and the variation in the data was characterized using the appropriate tools. A baseline process performance was obtained. After the analysis, Dr. Dow and the team met for an in-depth discussion of their findings. Several things were worth highlighting:

- No statistical significant difference was found in the percentage of patients undergoing an MRI study that were inpatient (48%) versus outpatient (52%). As the team had originally thought, the lower patient throughput could not be assigned to a higher number of sicker and more complex inpatient MRI studies (see Figure 30-5).
- No differences could be found in patient demographics, insurance type, diagnosis, ICD-10 classification, ordering physician, MRI technician, or MRI supervisor.
- The most commonly selected scan protocol was 60 minutes. Note: MRI scan protocols are a combination of various MRI sequences designed to optimally

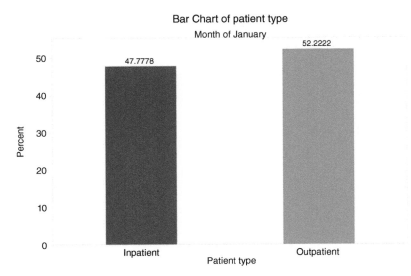

FIGURE 30-5 Bar chart comparing the percentage of inpatients to outpatients.

assess a particular anatomic region according to the pathologic process under study. Each anatomic area has a specific protocol design. Scan times are therefore based on standard protocols according to the types of MRI study requested. These protocols are stored as menus from which technicians select the sequence that best fits their patient's needs. While scan duration is measured in time (continuous data), protocols are independent units that can be sorted in distinct, separate, and nonoverlapping categories and therefore can be graphed using tools for discrete data. Taken as continuous data, the average duration of an MRI scan was 60 minutes (see Figures 30-6 and 30-7).

- Scanner idle time (turnover time between the last patient and the next patient or TOT) was found to be surprisingly high, averaging 15.7 minutes with a SD of 3.5 minutes. Data was normally distributed (the Anderson-Darling normality test showed a p value = 0.229). Scanner idle time was on average one quarter of the average scan time; based on the average scanner idle time, in a 12h day shift, the scanner was idle for 2½ hours! (see Figure 30-8).

- Variation in "Scanner idle time" was assessed to look for nonrandom patterns in the data indicative of Special Cause Variation. A process showing Special Cause Variation would be under the influence of factors outside of the design of the process that could explain the inflated "Scanner idle time" average.

  o A Run chart or time-series plot of "Scanner idle time" showed no violation of rules 1, 2, 3, 4. There were no shifts, trends, extreme points, or an unusual number of runs. Data was homogeneous and variation was characterized as random (noise) or Common Cause Variation. Given these findings, we can conclude there were no external factors influencing the results, the process was stable, and would continue to produce the same results (predictable) if nothing was changed (see Figure 30-9)

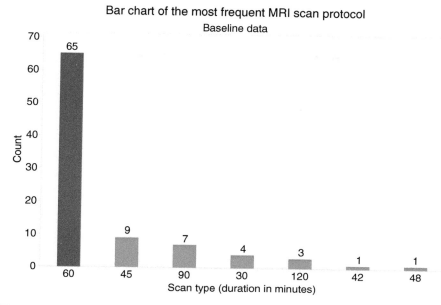

FIGURE 30-6   Bar chart showing the most common MRI scan protocol used.

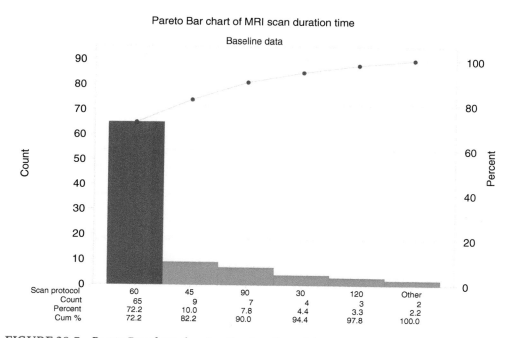

FIGURE 30-7   Pareto Bar chart showing the duration of the most common scan. Chart created with Minitab® Software package. Printed with permission of Minitab, LLC. All rights reserved.

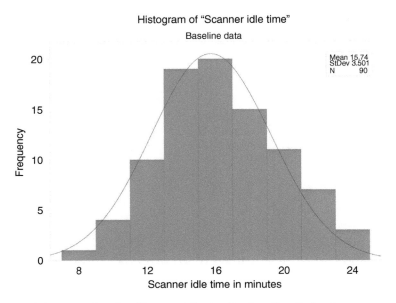

FIGURE 30-8   Histogram showing "Scanner idle time" at baseline (before improvement).

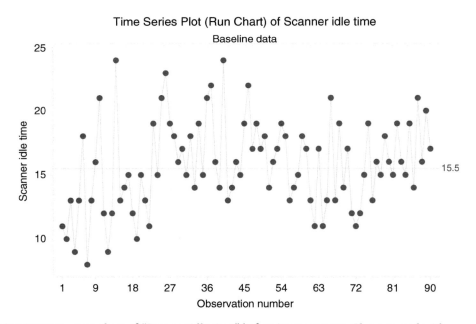

FIGURE 30-9   Run chart of "Scanner idle time" before improvement. Chart created with Minitab® Software package. Printed with permission of Minitab, LLC. All rights reserved.

o An Individuals and Moving Range (I-mR) chart of "Scanner idle time" also showed a stable process, with an average Scanner idle time of 15.74 minutes, and an upper control limit (UCL) as high as 25.73 minutes. The I-mR chart also shows significant variability, with a range as high as 12.26 minutes. (see Figure 30-10).

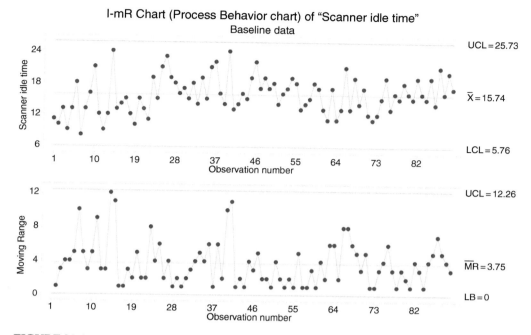

FIGURE 30-10 I-mR chart of "Scanner idle time" before improvement. Chart created with Minitab® Software package. Printed with permission of Minitab, LLC. All rights reserved.

- A Capability Analysis of "Scanner idle time" was performed to compare the Voice of the Customer VOC (what the customer wants or the performace the hospital needs) to the Voice of the Process (what the Scanner idle time really is and the process delivers) to quantify how the process is actually performing. The Capability Analysis showed that during the study period, scanners were idle more than 10 minutes (the USL or Upper Specification Limit) in more than 90% of the turn-over time between patients (see Figures 30-11 and 30-12). Note: In discussions with the Primary Sponsor and key stakeholders in the MRI suite, the QI team set a limit of 10 minutes for the turn-over time, or time the scanner should be idle. During the visit to the Gemba, the QI team realized most of the steps during "Wait time" (Steps 3 to 12) in preparation of a patient to be scanned were being done while the previous patient was still in the scanner (in parallel). The main determinants of patient throughput were therefore "scanning time" and "Wait for next patient". Keeping the scanning interval between patients (Scanning idle time) to less than 10 minutes would address the current patient throughput needs in the MRI suite.
- The team was informed by a panel of experts convened at the request of the Primary Sponsor that 22% of the MRI studies submitted for evaluation were not indicated.

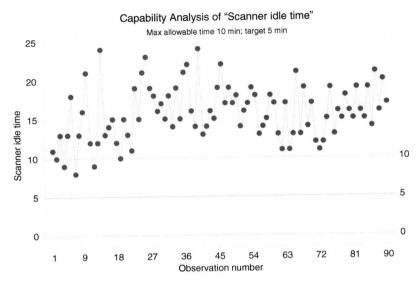

FIGURE 30-11   A Time Series plot (Run chart) of "Scanner idle time" shows the performance of the process (Voice of the Process) to the requirements set by the customer (Voice of the Customer). Chart created with Minitab® Software package. Printed with permission of Minitab, LLC. All rights reserved.

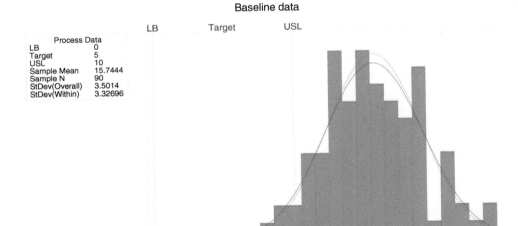

FIGURE 30-12   Capability analysis of "Scanner idle time" shows a 50% defect rate (amount of data above the Upper Specification Limit (USL) set at 10 minutes). Chart created with Minitab® Software package. Printed with permission of Minitab, LLC. All rights reserved.

- On a thorough review, the team also found that 24.4% of charts had one or more defects: did not include the patient's weight, information on the patient's allergy to IV contrast, prosthetic material, or pacemaker MRI compatibility.

Identify and Confirm the Most Likely Cause

Members of the QI team returned to the outpatient MRI suite to collect data on an additional 95 cases in order to better understand and document the causes of prolonged turnover time (defined as a turnover time or scanner idle time of more than 10 minutes). A total of 45 cases (47%) of turnover time greater than 10 minutes were identified. After identifying the specific cause(s) for each, a Pareto Bar chart was created. It showed the following (see Figure 30-13):

- Waiting for the next patient (71.1%) was the most common cause for delay
- Waiting for the referring physician to return call (11.1%)
- Difficulty with IV placement (8.9%)
- Difficulty with positioning the patient in scanner (4.4%)
- Other causes (4.4%)

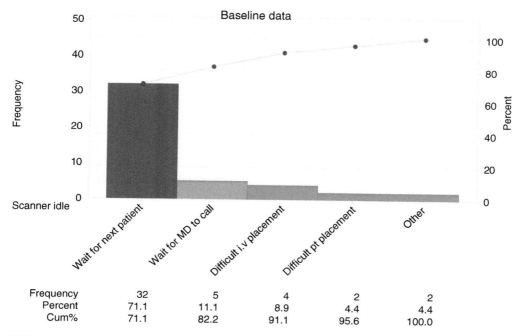

FIGURE 30-13   Pareto Bar chart showing the most common causes of turn-over time (scanner idle time) greater than 10 minutes. Chart created with Minitab® Software package. Printed with permission of Minitab, LLC. All rights reserved.

Given the Pareto Bar chart in Figure 30-13 follows the Pareto Principle, the team decided to focus on "Waiting for the next patient" as the target of their improvement efforts. This was the most common cause (71%). Early morning the next day, the team met to brainstorm ideas and generate a list of possible causes for "Waiting for the next patient". All members of the team contributed freely to generate ideas and all ideas were recorded before passing any discussion or judgment as to the merits of each. After the brainstorming session, a fishbone diagram was created to provide the structure and template on which to arrange and organize all the ideas generated To create the fishbone diagram, the team facilitator wrote the problem or effect ("Waiting for next patient") at the head of the fishbone skeleton; using a large sheet of paper on the conference's room wall, they then labeled the main branches and wrote down the major categories for the arrows entering the "spine"; the team organized the ideas from the brainstorming session according to the main categories created (see Figure 30-14).

A week later, the team met again. Using the fishbone diagram from the previous session, the team Multivoted to filter and prioritize the most likely causes of "Waiting for the next patient." Given the inherent difficulties in obtaining data specific to each cause identified during the brainstorming session (causes entering the main branches of the Fishbone diagram), the team decided to narrow it down and collect data on the main categories displayed by the fishbone diagram. Over the ensuing weeks, 31 cases of "Waiting for next patient" were analyzed and a Pareto Bar chart created (see Figure 30-15). Findings revealed:

- 12 cases of "waiting for an ambulatory patient" (38.7%)
- 7 cases of "waiting for inpatient transport" (22.6%)
- 6 cases of "waiting for the unit RN" (19.4%)
- 6 cases of "patient issues" (12.9 %)
- 2 cases of "other" (6.5%)

Given the limited number of cases and the fact that the resulting Pareto Bar chart did not fulfill the conditions for the Pareto principle (The first bar is not 2 to 3 times larger than the rest of the bars; 70-80% of the total is achieved by the third bar, which represents almost all the causes), the team decided to move forward and consider all causes of "Waiting for the next patient" as targets for improvement.

The Third Tollgate Review

One week after, the QI team met with their Primary Sponsor. John McLain was surprised to hear how the team had found that "waiting for the next patient" was the most common cause of a prolonged turnover time (Scanner idle time). He reviewed the Pareto Bar chart of "waiting for the next patient" and agreed with the team they should include all causes as targets for improvement. After a brief discussion, all team meeting participants agreed the project was on track and decided to proceed to the next phase. The meeting adjourned as McLain repeated his commitment to help the team with the final stages of the project.

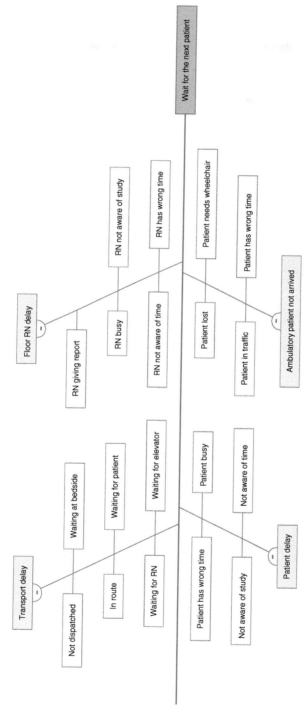

FIGURE 30-14 Fishbone diagram of possible causes of "Waiting for the next patient." Chart created with Companion by Minitab® Software package. Printed with permission of Minitab, LLC. All rights reserved.

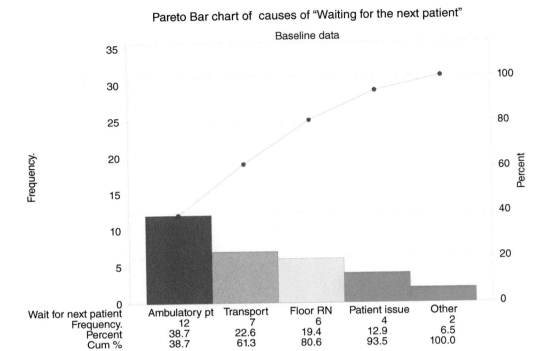

	Ambulatory pt	Transport	Floor RN	Patient issue	Other
Wait for next patient Frequency.	12	7	6	4	2
Percent	38.7	22.6	19.4	12.9	6.5
Cum %	38.7	61.3	80.6	93.5	100.0

FIGURE 30-15　Pareto Bar chart showing the most common cause of "Waiting for the next patient." Chart created with Minitab® Software package. Printed with permission of Minitab, LLC. All rights reserved.

THE FIFTH "R": THE RIGHT SOLUTION

Develop and Prioritize Improvement Ideas, and Run Pilots

Dr. Dow found and distributed articles, literature reviews, and best-practice recommendations ahead of their next team meeting. Finding and distributing material before a team meeting may facilitate creative thinking and may make the improvement team more open to finding evidence-based solutions to address the causes of the problem they discovered in the previous phase. A site visit was attempted but Dr. Dow was unable to confirm the visit to a nearby hospital's MRI suite. On the day of the scheduled meeting, the entire team met to conduct a free brainstorming session. Dr. Dow placed a flipchart on a tripod for everyone to see and proceeded to record every idea the team members came up with. At the end of the session, all contributions were categorized into groups, and the team voted to select the best ideas (Multivoting). An Impact/Effort matrix was then created to prioritize the list of possible solutions according to their impact on the problem and the amount of effort required for implementation.

A number of ideas were selected for testing and implementation (see Table 30-4). These ideas were presented by the team to Mr. McLain, the Primary Sponsor, and

TABLE 30-4   List of Ideas for Improvement

Ideas for improvement	
Causes & problems	**Improvement idea**
Waiting for an ambulatory patient (38.7%)	• MRI technician will call all patients to confirm appointments 3 days before. • All outpatients will receive an automated reminder call the day before the scheduled MRI study. • All patients are given contact numbers and are encouraged to call to report changes.
Waiting for inpatient transport (22.6%)	• Elective MRI studies will be included in the SurgiNET Cerner® OR Schedule; a copy of the schedule is to be shared the day before with the Patient Transport Services (PTS) office. • MRI technician will confirm the MRI schedule in a.m. with the Patient Transport Services office to assure timely transfers.
Waiting for unit RN (19.4%)	• Elective MRI studies will be included in SurgiNET Cerner® OR Schedule and is to be distributed the day before to all inpatient units. • The MRI Supervisor on-duty will call the inpatient unit Supervisor the night before to confirm the MRI schedule and assure patients are ready when transport arrives. • MRI Supervisors will confirm first-case of the day in am.
MRI study not indicated (22%)	• All completed MRI studies will be reviewed monthly by an expert panel of MDs: 1 Radiologist, 1 Internist, and 1 Surgeon. • A monthly report with the total number of studies, types of studies, and ratio of studies that do not meet criteria will be sent to all department heads. Department heads should discuss performance with individual providers.
Chart incomplete or defective (24.4%)	• Scheduling an MRI study will require completing three mandatory fields in the EMR: patient weight, i.v. contrast allergy, history of prosthetic material.

Dr. Amanda Alluck, the CMO, to assure their buy-in, the availability of resources, administrative assistance, and IT support. A commitment was made by senior leadership to support the team and to provide the needed resources for training, coaching, and a full-scale roll-out.

Roll Out Full-Scale Change and Project Summary

Over the next weeks, changes were implemented. Members of the team helped with training and coaching activities. Proposed changes were presented at the monthly Executive Committee meeting for their approval. Chris Wang, the head of IT, assigned one of his team members to create the needed EMR mandatory fields for the MRI orders.

After several weeks, the team collected additional data on 90 cases. The analysis showed the following results:

- There were no significant changes in the percentage of inpatient (52%) versus outpatient (47%) MRI studies. The most commonly selected scan protocol continued to be 60 minutes (68.9%).
- The average Scanner idle time after rolling out the proposed improvements was reduced to 6 minutes (SD 2.5). Data was normally distributed (Anderson-Darling normality test showed a p value = 0.059) (see Figure 30-16). The comparison of the before and after histograms side by side shows a clear improvement (see Figure 30-17).
- An Individuals and Moving Range (I-mR) chart of "Scanner idle time" or turnover time showed a stable process, Common Cause Variation, an average TOT of 6 minutes, and an upper control limit of 14.28 minutes (see Figure 30-18). The before-and-after QI project Individuals chart clearly shows the difference in process behavior (performance) between the two periods. The mean was significantly lowered from 15.74 to 6.07 (p=0.001). The Standard deviation was reduced by 18.9% (p=0.001) (see Figure 30-19).
- A Process Capability report for "Scanner idle time" after improvements showed a defect rate that had been significantly improved and lowered from 94.44% to 5.56 (observed), or in other words, 94% of turn-over time between patients is less than 10 minutes. The process mean changed significantly and is now closer to the target (p<0.01), and the process Standard deviation has been significantly reduced. (see Figures 30-20 and 30-21).

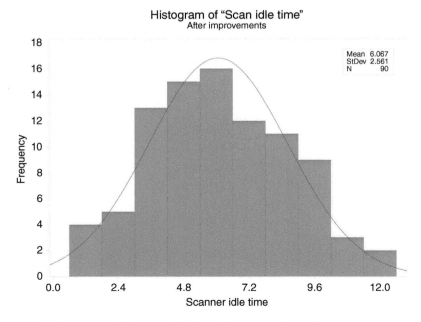

FIGURE 30-16   Histogram of "Scanner idle time" (turn-over time) after improvements.

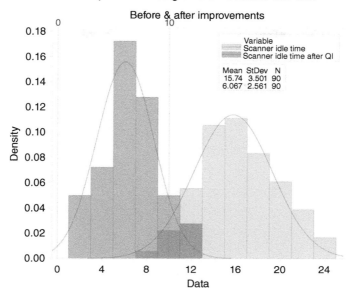

FIGURE 30-17 Histograms comparing "Scanner idle time" before and after improvements. Chart created with Minitab® Software package. Printed with permission of Minitab, LLC. All rights reserved.

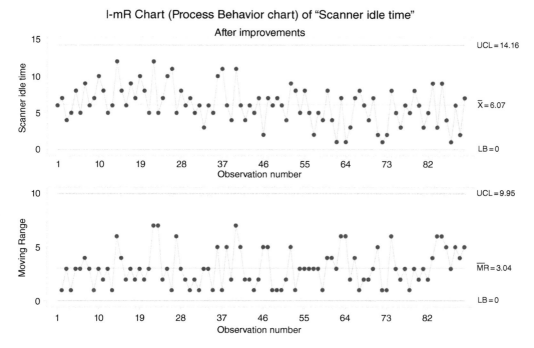

FIGURE 30-18 An I-mR chart of "Scanner idle time" after improvement shows Common Cause Variation. Chart created with Minitab® Software package. Printed with permission of Minitab, LLC. All rights reserved.

Individuals Chart of "Scanner idle time" before & after improvements

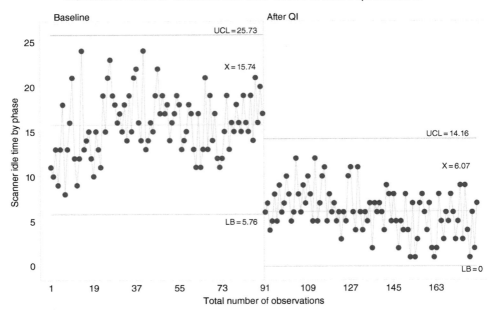

FIGURE 30-19   Before and after Individuals chart of "Scanner idle time." Chart created with Minitab® Software package. Printed with permission of Minitab, LLC. All rights reserved.

Process Capability Report for "Scanner idle time"

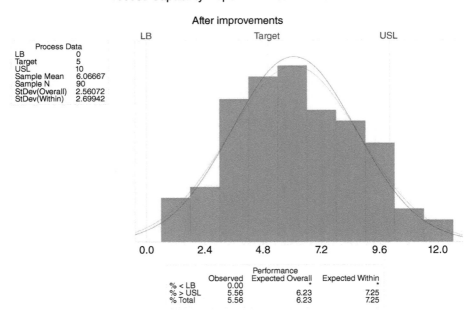

FIGURE 30-20   A Process Capability report of "Scanner idle time" after improvements shows a defect rate of 5.56 %. Chart created with Minitab® Software package. Printed with permission of Minitab, LLC. All rights reserved.

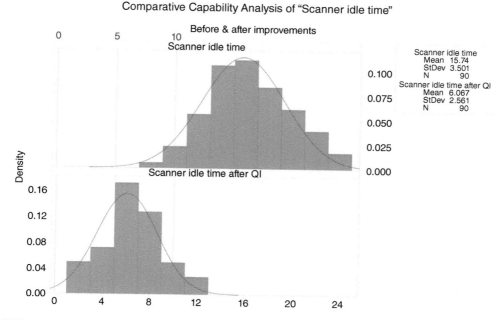

FIGURE 30-21 Capability Analysis of "Scanner idle time" before and after improvement. Chart created with Minitab® Software package. Printed with permission of Minitab, LLC. All rights reserved.

- After monthly reports for MRI studies were shared with department heads, only 8.8% of MRI studies were found not to be indicated. Changes in the way an MRI was scheduled in the EMR achieved a significant reduction in the defect rate: Only 3.3% of charts were incomplete.

Summary findings were presented at a subsequent meeting between the QI team, Primary Sponsor, and senior leadership. The average scanner idle time was reduced from 15.7 minutes to 6 minutes (62%), resulting in an increase of the average daily patient throughput from 24 to 30 scans per 12-hour shift. There are 720 minutes of available scanning time per scan and day shift (12h). Staff breaks are covered by other staff. Given the most common MRI scan protocol is 60 minutes (72%) and 94% of the "Scanner idle time" is below 10 minutes (70 minutes), current MRI scan capacity was increased from an average 8 scans to 10 scans per scanner per day (720/70), or 30 scans per 12 h day shift. The target (primary metric and goal) of the QI project was achieved. Likewise, the percentages of monthly MRI studies not indicated and the percentage charts defective were decreased. Lead time and wait time decreased without a significant change in the scan time (see Table 30-5).

The Fourth Tollgate Review

Dr. Dow and the team met with the Primary Sponsor to review the results of the QI project. The team agreed on a monitoring plan and set the appropriate metrics for

TABLE 30-5   Summary of QI Project Results

Summary Findings			
Metric	**Before**	**After**	**Change**
Average daily patient throughput (Primary metric)	24 scans per 12 h shift	30 scans per 12 h shift	**25%**
Lead time	117 minutes	94 minutes	**20%**
Wait time	33 minutes	16 minutes	**51%**
Scan time	60 minutes (72%);	60 minutes (68.9%) Average 60 min	No significant change
Scanner idle time (Scanner TOT)	Average 15.7 min (SD 3.5)	Average 6 min (SD 2.5)	**62% (p < 0.001)**
% monthly MRI studies not indicated	22.2% (n=22)	8.8% (n=8)	**60% (p < 0.009)**
% Charts defective	24.4 % (n=22)	3.3% (n=3)	**86% (p < 0.001)**

tracking current performance and monitoring future performance. All project documentation was updated and the process was completely transferred to the process owners. Several Power Point presentations were made at the C-suite. A small celebration was scheduled to properly recognize and reward the QI team.

APPENDIX

Appendix I: Common Improvement Tools and Techniques

5S. 5S is an acronym that stands for Sort, Set in Order, Shine, Standardize, and Sustain. 5S is a systematic way to organize a workspace to allow work to flow in a safe, efficient, intuitive, and sustainable manner. Key points: 5S allows the frontline professional to quickly confirm the availability of needed equipment and supplies, increase efficiency, safety, and the reliability of the process.

5 "Whys" diagram. A quick, basic, and focused technique used to explore potential causes of a problem by asking "why" five times to drill down to the root level of the causes. The answer from the preceding question serves as the basis for the following question.

Assumption busting. Assumption busting is a brainstorming technique that generates a list of potential ideas by doing two things: Identifying and challenging conventional assumptions, and eliminating them if they are obstacles to optimal solutions.

Bar charts. A graph that displays data counts within each category in bar format and allows comparisons between categories.

Basic Process Flow map. A graphic depiction of an entire process that outlines the sequence of the individual steps, actions, and decision used to provide a service or patient care. Key points: to create a Basic Process Flow map, "walk" the process; "see it" for yourself; make sure you record the beginning and the end of the process; schedule multiple observations, as not all work is done in the same manner every time; engage key stakeholders to validate the map's accuracy.

Box plot. A box plot or box-and-whiskers plot (or diagram) is a method for graphically depicting groups of numerical data through their quartiles.

Brainstorming. A basic analytical or creative technique where members of a QI team contribute spontaneously to generate a large list of ideas. Key points: leverage your team and generate a large quantity of ideas; welcome all ideas; withhold criticism until the end; modify, extend, or add to existing ideas; combine and improve ideas to generate additional ideas.

The Quality Improvement Challenge: A Practical Guide for Physicians, First Edition.
Richard J. Banchs and Michael R. Pop.
© 2021 John Wiley & Sons Ltd. Published 2021 by John Wiley & Sons Ltd.
Companion website: www.wiley.com/go/banchs/quality

Capability Analysis.   A tool that compares the Voice of the Customer (what the customer wants, or VOC) to the Voice of the Process (what the process delivers, or VOP) to quantify the percentage of time the specifications (customer attributes and requirements) are met.

Cause and Effect Matrix.   A tool used to quantitatively evaluate a set of inputs versus a set of outputs to determine the likely relationship between inputs and outputs in a process.

Communication plan.   A plan that details the audience, message, channels, speakers, date, and strategies when communicating with key sponsors and stakeholders; communication is the key to establishing a collaborative platform that will achieve buy-in from the front lines.

Control chart.   A Control chart or Process Behavior chart is a graphical display of time-ordered data used to detect signals or nonrandom patterns of variation that are indicative of the presence of Special Cause Variation.

Correlation coefficient.   The correlation coefficient is a measure that determines the degree to which two variables are associated.

Critical Needs.   A tool to translate the Voice of the Stakeholder into critical requirements of frontline performance. Key points: by clearly identifying the stakeholders' needs, you gain a better understanding of the problem, the drivers of stakeholder's performance, and the barriers to providing customer satisfaction.

Critical to Quality.   The CTQs are used to translate the broad customer needs (VOC) into specific, actionable, and measurable performance requirements that provide direction for the project's activities. Key points: The CTQs focus the problem by understanding what drives satisfaction from the "customer's" perspective; project metrics often derive from the CTQs.

Data Collection Planner.   Tool used to plan data collection, making data reliable and relevant to the key questions the project is trying to address. The Data Collection Planner makes data collection effective, efficient, repeatable, and reproducible. The Data Collection Planner records the rationale for data collection; the metrics; the operational definitions; the stratification factors; and the steps and activities for data collection (checklist).

Fishbone diagram.   A basic analytical tool that provides the structure and template on which to arrange and organize all the ideas generated during a brainstorming session; the fishbone diagram is a useful tool for identifying the potential causes of a problem.

FMEA.   Failure Mode and Effects Analysis (FMEA) is a highly structured, systematic techniques for failure analysis. It is used to proactively evaluate a process to identify where and how it might fail, the possible causes of failure, their relative impact, the steps or parts of the process involved, and the strategies to mitigate or eliminate that risk.

Gemba.   The place where people "do the work" and generate "value" for the customer.

Graphic Summary.   A summary display of data using graphs, charts, tables, or diagrams. For continuous data, a Graphic Summary may include a histogram, box plot, or Individual Value plot. For count or attribute data, a Graphic Summary may include a Bar chart, Pie chart, or Pareto chart.

Histogram.   A histogram, also called a frequency plot, is the preferred tool to graph continuous data when we have at least 50 points in the data set. A histogram displays bars representing the count within different ranges or intervals.

How-Now-Wow matrix.   The How-Now-Wow matrix is an idea selection tool that forces people to categorize ideas based on their originality and the ease of implementation counteracting the tendency to select only ideas that are the most familiar.

Hypothesis testing.   Hypothesis testing is used to make comparisons between two or more groups of data to determine if their differences are due to random variation, or if they come from different populations and are actually different.

Impact/Effort Matrix.   The Impact/Effort matrix provides a quick way to prioritize possible solutions according to their impact on the problem and the amount of effort required for implementation.

Individual Value plot.   The Individual Value plot is a graph that shows a dot for the actual value of each observation in a group.

Mistake Proofing.   The use of a device or method that either makes it impossible for an error to occur, or makes the error immediately obvious once it has occurred.

Multivoting.   A technique designed to facilitate a collaborative decision-making process. Participants cast multiple votes to identify their priorities and narrow down possible options from a list of ideas generated during a brainstorming session. Each team member can cast multiple votes equal to one-third to one-quarter of the number of items. Each team member can cast more than one vote per item or choose to place all votes on one item.

Negative brainstorming.   Negative brainstorming is an idea-generation method that, unlike the conventional brainstorming session, focuses on how not to solve the problem.

Opportunity flowchart.   A basic process mapping technique that stratifies process steps into value-added (VA) steps, non-value-added (NVA) steps, and business value-added (BVA) steps in order to allow for the elimination of steps that do not add value.

Pairwise Comparison.   The Pairwise Comparison or Paired Comparison Analysis is a selection technique for weighting potential ideas against each other.

Pareto Bar chart.   A specialized bar chart used with count and attribute data that presents a graphical visualization of the frequency of the individual causes displayed in decreasing order using cumulative percentages. Key point: The Pareto Bar chart follows the Pareto principle. The Pareto principle states that, for many events, roughly 80% of the effects come from 20% of the causes.

PDSA cycle.   A PDSA cycle is a localized controlled trial of a possible solution in a small scale in order to test its effectiveness and understand its limitations before full implementation; PDSA is an acronym at it stands for Plan-Do-Study-Act.

Pearson correlation coefficient.   The Pearson coefficient (r) is a type of correlation coefficient that represents the relationship between two variables that are measured on the same interval or ratio scale. The Pearson coefficient represents the strength and the direction of the relationship.

Pie charts.   A graph that presents data in a circle divided into a number of sections, each of which designate a proportion of the data collected.

Pilots.   A pilot study is a localized controlled trial of a possible solution in a small scale in order to test its effectiveness and understand its limitations before full implementation.

Positive deviants.   Positive deviants are people within a certain area or department whose uncommon but successful behaviors or strategy enables them to find better solutions to a problem than their peers, despite facing similar challenges and having no extra resources.

Problem Statement.   A clear, concise, and specific explanation of the problem; the Problem Statement should not include the potential causes of the problem or the possible solutions to resolve it. By properly defining the problem, you will find better solutions. Key points: A problem statement should answer questions about the nature of the problem, the magnitude of the problem, the gap between the current state and the ideal state, and why we should address the problem now. When writing a Problem Statement, try to understand the problem from the perspective of the people affected by the problem.

Project Charter.   The Project Charter is a document that establishes an agreement between the primary sponsor and the project team on the criteria for the successful completion of the project. It concisely delineates the high-level who, what, when, where, how, and why of the project; the Project Charter is a "live" document that should be updated as more information becomes available. Key points: the Project Charter helps focus the activities of the QI Team regarding the nature, scope, goals, and timeline of the project.

Project Selection matrix.   This matrix is a tool that combines project selection criteria with weighted scores used to prioritize the most relevant projects.

Pugh matrix.   A Pugh matrix is an idea selection technique that can be used to develop and refine potential ideas by comparing a set of criteria for each idea against a standard idea.

Regression analysis.   Regression analysis is a tool that uses data on relevant variables to develop a prediction equation model.

Risk Priority Number (RPN).   The RPN is a numerical ranking of the risk of each potential failure and its cause, calculated from the arithmetic product of the Severity Index, Occurrence Index, and Detection Index.

Run chart.   A Run chart, or time-series plot, is a graphical display of time-ordered data used to detect signals or nonrandom patterns of variation that are indicative of the presence of Special Cause Variation.

SCAMPER.   An acronym for an idea-generating method that is based on the notion that everything new is a modification of something that already exists.

Scatter Plot.   A scatter plot or Scatterplot is a graph consisting of a set of data points plotted on a horizontal and vertical axis used to see patterns that allow us to establish a relation or correlation between two variables.

SIPOC diagram.   A high-level map of the process showing Suppliers, Inputs, Process, Outputs, and Customers that defines the scope and boundaries of the project. Key point: a SIPOC diagram helps clarify the beginning and end of the process targeted for improvement, and helps to get everyone on the "same page."

Solution Desirability Matrix.   A solution desirability matrix is a team-based decision tool for evaluating various improvement proposals against weighted criteria established by either the organization or the team according to the goals of the project.

Spaghetti diagram.   The Spaghetti diagram, also called the transportation or work-flow diagram, is used to show movement and physical flow of people, staff, providers, work, and materials in a process. Data regarding the distance traveled, the amount of time expended during the movement, and the number of trips required to perform the steps of the process can be added to the diagram. The Spaghetti diagram is used to identify and eliminate waste, and to improve the physical layout of a space.

Sponsor Analysis.   The Sponsor Analysis is a structured approach for identifying and assessing the sponsors and their willingness to advocate for and positively impact the outcome of the project. The Sponsors have the greatest role in promoting the acceptance of the change and the success of the QI project.

Sponsor Strategy.   The Sponsor Strategy uses the information gathered in the Sponsor Analysis to create a plan for engaging the sponsors and opinion leaders in supporting the QI project.

Stakeholder Analysis.   Stakeholder Analysis is the systematic collection and analysis of data to determine the stakeholders' interests that should be considered when developing and/or implementing a policy, process, program, or project.

Stand in the Circle.   Stand in the circle is a tool used to identify the seven types of waste. The goal is not the circle but, using your eyes and ears, to "see" and understand the process in order to unroot the waste. Key points: There are seven types of waste that form the acronym TIM WOOD: Transport, Inventory, Motion, Waiting, Overproduction, Overprocessing, and Defects.

Swim Lane chart.   The Swim Lane chart is a basic flowchart used to see the sequential steps of the work flow as well as who is involved with each step. This chart is the preferred mapping tool to identify work-loads and hand-off points.

Team Roster.   A team roster is a list of the improvement team members, position, and their role in the organization. Key point: Cultivate the diversity in your team members' skills and expertise to achieve your objectives; team members should be selected from upstream and downstream the process that needs to be improved; ensure that your team is comprised primarily of frontline stakeholders; the preferred sequence for team members is front line > supervisors > mid-level leaders.

Value Stream map.   The Value Stream is the specific sequence of steps required to provide service or care to the customer. The Value Stream map is a high-level view process map that shows the individual operational steps of a process, along with the flow of people, equipment, and information used to achieve the desired outcome. The Value Stream map is one of the preferred mapping techniques to eliminate waste.

Visual Management.   Visual Management is a way to create a visual workplace or work environment that is self-explanatory and makes "doing the right thing" easier. With Visual Management the workplace environment "talks" through visual cues, so that instructions, workflow, steps, and limits are easily understood, and the correct work is performed. Visual Management creates a work environment where the outliers are immediately obvious, and health professionals can easily correct them, making work safer.

Voice of the Customer (VOC).   The VOC is the expression of the collective needs, wants, preferences, and expectations of the customers (patients, staff, and providers). Key points: the VOC helps us understand the main drivers of quality and customer satisfaction, and set the priorities, scope, and goals for the project.

Voice of the Stakeholder (VOS).   The VOS is the expression of the needs and requirements of the front line professionals (staff and providers). Key points: the VOS uncovers the barriers faced by front line professionals when they try to do their job.

Waste Rounds.   Waste is anything other than the minimum amount of equipment, material, technology, space, staff, and time that are essential to add value. Waste rounds or waste walk is a tool to identify the seven types of waste.

Appendix II: Glossary of Improvement Terms

Change Management. Cyclic process of steps and activities that a QI team must carry out throughout the life cycle of the project to get buy-in, manage resistance, and successfully implement a change.

Common Cause Variation. Variation that is due to the random effects of factors that are always present, and are an intrinsic component of the design of a process.

Convergent thinking. Once divergent thinking is complete, information and ideas are structured and organized using convergent thinking. In the convergent thinking phase, a team works towards organizing, prioritizing, and selecting the most likely cause or the best solution. Convergent thinking involves refining and narrowing down the best ideas, bringing together different ideas from different sources or fields, and prioritizing the best ideas.

Critical-to-Quality (CTQs). The CTQs translate general and difficult-to-measure customer needs or desires into very *specific* and *measurable* attributes and requirements of customer satisfaction. The CTQs are the quantifiable expectations of the customer.

Critical Needs. The Critical Needs (CNs) translate very general and difficult-to-measure requirements of stakeholders (VOS) into very specific and measurable needs and requirements of the front line's ability to deliver quality care.

Critical-to-Quality tree. The CTQ tree is a diagram-based tool used to organize identified specifications of an outcome's attributes and requirements the customer expects.

Customer. The person who receives the work product of the process that is the target for improvement; the end user of the product, service, or care.

Defect rate. A defect rate is a metric of effectiveness that represents the percent of outcomes that fail to meet the customer's specifications for quality.

Defect. A failure to meet customer expectations for quality, defined by the attributes and requirements of the product, service, or care.

The Quality Improvement Challenge: A Practical Guide for Physicians, First Edition.
Richard J. Banchs and Michael R. Pop.
© 2021 John Wiley & Sons Ltd. Published 2021 by John Wiley & Sons Ltd.
Companion website: www.wiley.com/go/banchs/quality

Divergent thinking.   During the divergent thinking phase, a team works to generate as many ideas as possible. In this phase any filtering or selectivity is minimized, and the objective is to come up with a great number of possible ideas. Divergent thinking calls for generating ideas, making combinations, changing forms, and identifying connections among different possibilities.

Flow.   How work progresses through a process. When a process is working well, steps and actions are executed in synchrony and the people, information, services, equipment, supplies, and patients in that process move through it steadily and predictably.

FMEA.   Failure Mode and Effects Analysis (FMEA) is a highly structured, systematic techniques for failure analysis. It is used to proactively evaluate a process to identify where and how it might fail, the possible causes of failure, their relative impact, the steps or parts of the process involved, and the strategies to mitigate or eliminate that risk.

Gemba.   The place where work is being done and value is created.

Ground Rules.   A team's rules established at the beginning of a QI project to help create a productive environment for team meetings.

Homogeneity.   The homogeneity question of data analysis tests the assumption all data comes from a single process (universe).

Map.   A graphical depiction of the sequence of the process steps, actions, and decisions.

Measurement.   A measurement takes a concept and describes it in terms of a number, usually referred to as data.

Metric.   A numeric value that represents the measurement of the relationship of one or more dimensions of a process used to define the current state and goals of a project. A metric is used to understand, compare, or track performance.

Operational definition.   An operational definition is a concise statement that clearly defines the data collection criteria, gives a communicable meaning to the metric, and makes the data collection process both repeatable and reproducible.

Primary Sponsor.   The senior leader who has access to the necessary resources and the authority to ensure the success of the improvement project or change initiative.

Problem Statement.   A clear, concise, and specific explanation of the problem that does not include any causes of the problem.

Process.   A series of steps, actions, and decisions that are used to transform inputs into outputs.

Project Charter.   A document that serves to gain agreement between the Primary Sponsor and the QI team as to the nature, scope, goals, and timeline of the project. The Project Charter concisely delineates the who, what, when, where, how, and why of the project.

Quality.   The Institute of Medicine defines quality along six dimensions: effective, efficient, timely, safe, patient-centered, and equitable.

Risk Priority Number (RPN).   A numerical ranking of the risk of each potential failure and its cause, calculated from the arithmetic product of the Severity Index, Occurrence Index, and Detection Index.

Special Cause Variation.   Variation arising from factors that are not always present in a process and have a dominant effect; Special Cause Variation signals a process has changed or is operating under different conditions.

Stakeholders.   The people that "do the work" and will be directly affected by the improvement project; the frontline healthcare professionals with the subject-matter expertise.

Standard Work.   An agreed-upon set of work practices that establishes the best and most reliable method and sequence of tasks for each clinician and support staff member to follow.

Stratification.   Stratification refers to collecting and organizing data according to specific subcategories in order to identify patterns and trends that will allow us to observe the independent variables affecting the outcome we want to improve.

System.   A planned, organized, and purposeful structure with interrelated and interdependent elements that follow a set of detailed methods, procedures and routines to create and deliver a product, provide care, or achieve a goal.

Systems thinking.   Systems thinking is a way to view a problem from a broad perspective that includes seeing the system and its overall elements, structures, cycles, feedback mechanisms and handoffs as contributors to the problem or undesirable outcome.

TIM WOOD.   TIM WOOD is an acronym for the seven types of waste: transport, inventory, motion, waiting, overproduction, overprocessing, and defects.

Tollgate review.   The analysis and review conducted by the QI team with the Primary Sponsor on the project status to date.

Value.   The outcomes achieved (therapeutic intervention + patient experience) divided by resources used in achieving the outcomes. Value is also any item or step that is done right the first time; changes information, product, or improves the course of a disease; the customer or end user is willing to pay for.

Variation.   The differences that occur in the outcome of a process that are due to the influence of factors that are intrinsic or extrinsic to the design of the process.

Voice of the Customer (VOC).   The expression of the needs and requirements of the people that receive the work product of the process we are trying to improve.

Voice of the Process (VOP).   The VOP is how the process communicates performance against customer needs and expectations, and this communication is done through process measures and in the form of data.

Voice of the Stakeholder (VOS).   Expression of the needs and requirements of the people who actually do the work.

Waste.   Anything other than the minimum amount of equipment, material, technology, space, staff, and time essential to add value.

Additional Resources

BOOKS

1. Arthur J. (2011). *Lean Six Sigma for Hospitals*. McGraw Hill.
2. Black J. (2008). *The Toyota Way to Healthcare Excellence*. American College of Healthcare Executives.
3. Bossidy L. (2002). *Execution. The Discipline of Getting Things Done*. Crown Business.
4. DeCarlo N. (2007). *The Complete Idiot's Guide to Lean Six Sigma*. Breakthrough Management Group.
5. Brook Q. (2010). *Lean Six Sigma & Minitab. The Complete Toolbox Guide for all Lean Six Sigma Practitioners*. Opex Resources.
6. Carey R. (2003). *Improving Healthcare with Control Charts. Basic and Advanced SPC Methods and Case Studies*. ASQ Quality Press.
7. Furterer S. (2014). *Lean Six Sigma Case Studies in the Healthcare Enterprise*. Springer.
8. George M. (2005). *Lean Six Sigma Pocket Toolbox*. McGraw Hill.
9. Graban M. (2012). *Healthcare Kaizen. Engaging Front-Line Staff in Sustainable Continuous Improvement*. CRC Press
10. Graban M. (2009). *Lean Hospitals*. CRC Press.
11. Hiatt J. (2012). *Change Management. The People Side of Change*. Prosci Learning Center.
12. Hiatt J. (2006). *The Prosci® ADKAR® Model. A Model for Change in Business, Government and Our Community*. Prosci Research.
13. Institute of Medicine. (2001). *Crossing the Quality Chasm: A New Health System for the 21st Century*. National Academies Press.
14. Institute of Medicine. (1999). *To Err is Human: Building a Safer Health System*. National Academies Press.
15. Jimmerson C. (2010). *Value Stream Mapping for Healthcare Made Easy*. CRC Press.
16. Kornacki MJ. (2012). *Leading Physicians through Change*. ACPE.
17. Kotter J. (1996). *Leading Change*. Harvard Business School Press.

18. Langley G. (2009). *The Improvement Guide*. Jossey Bass.

19. Linsky M. (2002). *Leadership on the Line*. HBR Press.

20. Orin G. (2012). *Fundamentals of Health Care Improvement*. IHI.

21. Plsek P. (2014). *Accelerating Health Care Transformation with Lean and Innovation*. CRC Press.

22. Provost LL. (2011). *The Health Care Data Guide. Learning from data for Improvement*. Jossey Bass.

23. Jackson T. (2013). *Rona Consulting Group. Kaizen Workshops for Lean Healthcare*. CRC Press.

24. Jackson T. (2013). *Rona Consulting Group. Mapping Clinical Value Streams*. CRC Press.

25. Jackson T. (2012). *Rona Consulting Group. Standard Work for Lean Healthcare*. CRC Press.

26. Carlson S. (2016). *Rona Consulting Group. Mistake Proofing for Lean Healthcare*. CRC Press.

27. Jackson T. (2009). *Rona Consulting Group. 5S for Healthcare*. CRC Press.

28. Scarlet H. (2016). *Neurosciences for Organizational Change*. Kogan Page.

29. Wheeler D. (2000). *Normality and the Process Behavior Chart*. SPC Press.

30. Wheeler D. (2000). *Understanding Variation. The Key to Managing Chaos*. SPC Press.

31. Zidel T. (2006). *A Lean Guide to transforming Healthcare*. ASQ Quality Press.

ARTICLES

32. Benn J. (2012). Using Quality Indicators in Anaesthesia: feeding back data to improve care. *BJA*.

33. GE CAP Model. (1990). The Change Acceleration Process Equation. Jack Welsh.

34. Gisvold S. (2011). How do we know we are doing a good job. Can we measure the quality of our work? *Best Practice & Research in Clinical Anaesthesiology* 25.

35. Hamel G. (2016). Build a change platform, not a change program. *McKinsey & Company*.

36. Katzenbach J. (1993). The Discipline of Teams. *Harvard Business Review*.

37. Kotter J. (1995). Leading Change: Why Transformation Efforts Fail. *Harvard Business Review*.

38. Lleape L. (2009). Transforming Healthcare: a safety imperative. *Quality & Safety Health Care* 18: 424.

39. National Academies Press (2002). Health Professions Education: A Bridge to Quality.

40. Nicholay CR. (2012). Systematic review of the application of quality improvement methodologies from the manufacturing industry to surgical healthcare. *British Journal Surgery* 99: 324–335.

41. Norman D. (2013). Find the right problem, find the right solution. *Design of everyday thinking. UX Magazine* 1168.

42. Prosci. (2014). Best Practices in Change Management. Prosci Benchmarking Report.

43. Rever H. (2016). Five Elements to Process Improvement Project Success. Paper presented at PMI® Global Congress 2008—North America, Denver, CO. Newtown Square, PA: Project Management Institute.

44. Shojania K. (2005). Evidence-Based Quality Improvement: The State of the Science. *Health Affairs.* 24 (1): 138–150.

45. Varughese A. (2010). Improving Quality in Pediatric Anesthesia. *Pediatric Anesthesia* 20: 684.

46. Vonderheide-Liem D. (2004). *Applying Quality Methodologies to Improve Healthcare. HC Pro.*

WEBSITES

The Lean Enterprise Institute at www.Lean.org

The American Society of Quality at www.asq.org

International Project Leadership Academy. Why do projects fail? http://calleam. com/WTPF/.

The Institute for Healthcare Improvement at www.IHI.org

Index

The Quality Improvement Challenge: A Practical Guide for Physicians, First Edition.
Richard J. Banchs and Michael R. Pop.
© 2021 John Wiley & Sons Ltd. Published 2021 by John Wiley & Sons Ltd.
Companion website: www.wiley.com/go/banchs/quality